DrExam™ Part B MRCS OSCE Revision Guide: Book 1

Applied Surgical Science & Critical Care, Anatomy & Surgical Pathology, Surgical Skills & Patient Safety

Editors:

B.H. Miranda
K. Asaad
Prof. S. P. Kay

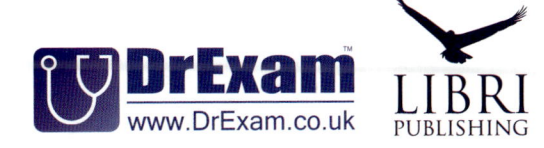

Second edition first published in 2017 by Libri Publishing

Copyright © DrExam

ISBN 978-1-911450-06-1

All rights reserved. No part of this publication may be reproduced, stored in any retrieval system or transmitted in any form or by any means, electronic, mechanical, photocopying, recording or otherwise, without the prior written permission of the copyright holder for which application should be addressed in the first instance to the publishers. No liability shall be attached to the author, the copyright holder or the publishers for loss or damage of any nature suffered as a result of reliance on the reproduction of any of the contents of this publication or any errors or omissions in its contents.

A CIP catalogue record for this book is available from The British Library

Design by Carnegie Publishing Ltd
Diagrams by BH Miranda

First edition published in 2010 by Libri Publishing

Printed in the UK by Hobbs the Printers

Libri Publishing
Brunel House
Volunteer Way
Faringdon
Oxfordshire
SN7 7YR

Tel: +44 (0)845 873 3837

www.libripublishing.co.uk

CONTENTS

About the Editors..xi
Authors & Contributors..xiii
Acknowledgements...xvi
Preface..xvii
Dedication..xviii
Introduction (Important – Read Me!)..xix
- How to Use this Book xx
- Introduction to the MRCS OSCE xx
- Approaching the OSCE Stations..xxiv

SECTION A: APPLIED SURGICAL SCIENCE & CRITICAL CARE 1

Chapter 1: **Radiology**..3
A Hameeduddin, BH Miranda, A Malhotra

Radiography 4
- Systematic Interpretation of the Chest Radiograph 5
- Chest Radiograph OSCE Cases 7
- Systematic Interpretation of the Abdominal Radiograph 15
- Abdominal Radiograph OSCE Cases 21

Computed Tomography 29
- Systematic Interpretation of Computed Tomography Scans 31
- Computed Tomography OSCE Cases 33

Magnetic Resonance Imaging 41
- T1 & T2 Weighted Sequences 42
- Systematic Interpretation of Magnetic Resonance Imaging Scans 42
- Magnetic Resonance Imaging OSCE Cases 44

Chapter 2: **Critical Care**..51
BH Miranda, N Sivasathan, BS Ghoorun

Anaesthetics 52
Arterial Blood Gases 55
Burns 58
Pulmonary Artery Catheters 61
Cardiopulmonary Bypass 63
Head Injury & Cerebral Autoregulation 64

Nutrition 68
Renal Failure 70
Renal Replacement Therapy 74
Fluids 75
Respiratory Failure 78
ALI & ARDS 79
Oxygen Therapy & Mechanical Ventilation 81
Pancreatitis 82
SIRS, SEPSIS & MODS 84
ICU Admission 87
Brainstem Death 88

Chapter 3:   Physiology **89**
            BH Miranda, BS Ghoorun
Calcium Homeostasis 90
Peripheral Nerves 92
Nerve Action Potential 93
Neuromuscular Junction & Muscle Relaxants 94
Blood Pressure Regulation 96
Arterial Waveform & Cardiac Cycle 98
Cardiac Action Potentials 100
Cardiac Output 102
Shock 104
Lung Function 108
Oxygen Transport 110
Thermoregulation 112
Renal Function 115

SECTION B: ANATOMY & SURGICAL PATHOLOGY 117

Chapter 4:   Anatomy **119**
            BH Miranda, K Asaad, L Clarke, W Birch
Head & Neck 120
- Atlanto-Axial Joint & Vertebrae 120
- Mandible & Temperomandibular Joint 122
- Tongue 123
- Parotid Gland & Facial Nerve 124
- Thyroid Gland 127
- Triangles of the Neck 128

Trunk & Thorax 130
- 1st Rib 130
- Mediastinum 132
- Heart 134
- Lungs 136
- Diaphragm 138
- Liver 140
- Abdominal Aorta & Related Structures 142
- Penis & Scrotum 144

Limbs, Spine & Vascular 146
- Upper Limb Vessels 146
- Rotator Cuff 148
- Antecubital Fossa 150
- Carpal Tunnel 151
- Dorsum of the Hand 153
- Femur & Hip Joint 154
- Lower Limb Vessels 157
- Femoral Triangle 158
- Femoral Sheath 160
- Inguinal Canal 161
- Adductor Canal 162
- Knee Joint 163
- Popliteal Fossa 165
- Lower Leg Compartments 166
- Ankle & Foot 168

Neurosciences 170
- Skull 170
- Lateral Cerebral Hemisphere 172
- Medial Cerebral Hemisphere 173
- Cerebrospinal Fluid 174
- Cranial Nerves 175
- Ascending & Descending Spinal Pathways 176
- Brachial Plexus 177
- Carotid Sheath 178
- Circle of Willis 179

Chapter 5: **Surgical Pathology** 181
BH Miranda, K Asaad, DJ Tobin

Biochemistry 183
- Plasma Proteins 183
- Calcium 183
- Hyperuricaemia 184
- Hepatic Function & Jaundice 185

Growth, Differentiation & Morphogenesis Disorders 187
- Atrophy, Hyperplasia & Other Common Phenomena 187
- Urinary Calculi 188
- Gallstone Disease 190
- Amyloid 191

Haematology 192
- Anaemias Including Fe^{2+}, B12 & Folate Deficiency 192
- Sickle Cell Anaemia 194
- Thalassaemia 196
- Polycythaemia 198
- Haemostasis, Platelets & Clotting Cascade 199
- Disseminated Intravascular Coagulation 201
- Blood Groups Including ABO & Rhesus Systems 202
- Blood Transfusion & Blood Products 203
- Blood Transfusion Reactions & Substitute Blood Products 206
- Oedema & Lymphoedema 207

Immunology 210
- Hypersensitivity, Cytokines & Mediators 210
- Complement Cascade 212
- Immunity & Immunoglobulins 214
- Transplantation 216

Inflammation 218
- Acute Inflammation 218
- Chronic Inflammation 219
- Cyst, Abscess, Pus & Other Common Phenomena 220
- Wound Healing 222

Microbiology 223
- Surgical Site & Wound Infections 223
- Pneumonia 224
- Urinary Tract Infection 226
- Endotoxin & Exotoxin 228
- Commensal Bacteria 230
- Nosocomial Infection 230
- Immunisation & Vaccination 231

Neoplasia 232
- Cell Cycle 232
- Tumour Markers 233
- Carcinogenesis 234
- Malignancy 236
- Paraneoplastic Syndromes 238

Vascular 240
- Clot, Thrombus, Embolus & Virchow's Triad 240
- Atheroma 241
- Infarction & Ischaemia 241
- Aneurysm 242

SECTION C: SURGICAL SKILLS 245

Chapter 6: Operative Surgery & Procedures 247
W Bhat, S Fraser, Q Bismil, BH Miranda, K Asaad

Head & Neck 249
- Thyroidectomy 249
- Parotidectomy 251
- Central Venous Access & Central Venous Pressure (CVP) Lines 252
- Surgical Airways 254

Trunk & Thorax 258
- Mastectomy 258
- Cardiac Pericardiocentesis 262
- Chest Drains 264
- Laparotomy 266
- Principles of Bowel Anastomoses 267
- Hartmann's Procedure 268
- Right Hemicolectomy 269
- Anterior & Abdominoperineal Resection of the Rectum 270
- Cholecystectomy 273
- Splenectomy 276
- Appendicectomy 280
- Inguinal Hernia Repair 283
- Femoral Hernia Repair 284
- Haemorrhoidectomy 285
- Suprapubic Catheterisation 288
- Renal Trauma & Nephrectomy 289
- Testicular Torsion 292
- Orchidectomy 294

- Circumcision 295
- Vasectomy 297
- Hydrocoele Repair 299

Limbs, Spine & Vascular 300
- Carpal Tunnel Decompression 300
- Approaches to Hip Joint 301
- Zadek's Procedure & Ingrown Toenail 303
- Fasciotomy & Compartment Syndrome 305
- Tendon Repair 307
- Amputations 309
- Femoral Embolectomy 312
- Varicose Vein Surgery 313
- Abdominal Aortic Aneurysm Repair 315

Neurosciences 319
- Burr Hole & Craniotomy 319
- Intracranial Pressure (ICP) Monitor Insertion 321
- Lumbar Puncture 322

SECTION D: PRINCIPLES OF SURGERY & PATIENT SAFETY 325

Chapter 7: Bones & Soft Tissues 327
K Asaad, BH Miranda, SP Kay

Bones 328
- Bone Structure 328
- Fractures 328
- Osteomyelitis 333
- Septic Arthritis 336

Soft Tissues 338
- The Reconstructive Ladder 338
- Scars 339
- Muscle 341
- Cartilage 343

Chapter 8: Endocrinology 345
K Asaad, BH Miranda, SP Kay

Multiple Endocrine Neoplasia (MEN) 346
Gynaecomastia 346
Hyperparathyroidism 348
Cushing's Disease / Syndrome 349
Carcinoid Syndrome 351
Hypo / Hyperthyroidism 353

Chapter 9: **Oncology** **355**
K Asaad, BH Miranda, SP Kay

Oncological Principles 356
- Screening 356
- Staging & Grading 358

Skin Cancer 359
- Basal Cell Carcinoma (BCC) 359
- Squamous Cell Carcinoma (SCC) 361
- Malignant Melanoma 363

Thyroid 367
Salivary Glands 368
Breast 370
Liver 372
Pancreas 374
Renal Tract 376
- Renal Cell Carcinoma (RCC) 377
- Transitional Cell Carcinoma (TCC) 378
- Wilms' Tumour 379

Intestinal Polyps & Colorectal Carcinoma 380

Chapter 10: **Perioperative Care & Surgical Technology** **385**
K Asaad, BH Miranda, SP Kay

Perioperative Care 386
- Clinical Trials 386
- Thromboprophylaxis 388
- Patient Positioning 389
- Patient Safety for Theatre 391

Surgical Technology 392
- Theatre Design 392
- Disinfection & Sterilisation 393
- LASER 394
- Tourniquets 395
- Diathermy 397
- Suture Materials 400
- Drains 402
- Dressings 403

SECTION E: ADDITIONAL OSCE PRACTICE 407

Chapter 11: Additional OSCE Questions 409
E Ewart, BH Miranda

Burns Assessment: 410
- Case 1: Lund & Browder Chart 410

General Surgery: 412
- Case 2: Epigastric Pain & Vomiting 412
- Case 3: Painful Groin Lump 414
- Case 4: Duodenal Ulcer Perforation 416
- Case 5: Necrotising Fasciitis 417
- Case 6: Dysphagia 419
- Case 7: Referral to Coroner 421

Trauma & Orthopaedics: 422
- Case 8: Acute Gout 422
- Case 9: Scaphoid Fracture 424
- Case 10: Fractured Neck of Femur 425
- Case 11: Osteoarthritis 429
- Case 12: Fractured Tibia 430

Urology: 432
- Case 13: Acute Testicular Pain 432
- Case 14: Haematuria 433
- Case 15: Renal Trauma 435
- Case 16: Intravenous Urography (IVU) 436

Cardiorespiratory: 437
- Case 17: Preoperative Assessment 437
- Case 18: Post-Operative Chest Pain 438
- Case 19: Pneumothorax 440
- Case 20: Mediastinal Mass 441

Index **449**

ABOUT THE EDITORS

Ben Miranda ALCM, BSc, MBBS (Lond), MRCS (Eng), PhD

Ben is a Specialty Trainee (ST) Registrar on the London Deanery Plastic Surgery & Burns Training Rotation. He was previously a Research Registrar at the Plastic Surgery & Burns Research Unit, University of Bradford. His research interest in hair follicle biology & growth control led him to complete a PhD within three years. Having graduated from the Royal Free & University College Hospital School of Medicine (London) in 2004, he has now won 14 academic prizes & awards, primarily at postgraduate level. He has 35 published / accepted journal papers, features & books, including a front cover publication in the *British Journal of Dermatology* on part of his PhD research & 50 international / national presentations at high-end conferences. Ben has had training exposure to a wide variety of surgical specialities, including A&E, Burns, ENT, Gastrointestinal, Neurosurgery, Plastic Surgery, Urology & Vascular Surgery.

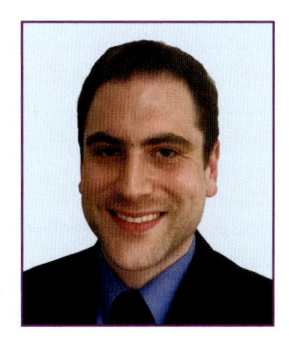

Ben's passion for education developed since 1998, when he began teaching Mathematics to GCSE & A-Level students. He continued this throughout medical school & in 2006 was drafted to teach Royal Free & University College Hospital School of Medicine MBBS finalists. In 2007 he helped to establish DrExam as a leading provider of postgraduate surgical education, in association with & in support of the Plastic Surgery & Burns Research Unit. His dedication to surgical education & the future progress of surgery has been proven by his many extracurricular activities. These include integral participation in the well-publicised £100,000 fundraising appeal for the Research Unit's 25th anniversary in 2010.

Kamil Asaad BSc (Lond), MB ChB, MRCS (Eng), MPhil

Kamil is a Specialty Trainee (ST) Registrar on the Oxford Deanery Plastic Surgery & Burns Training Rotation. He graduated from Leeds University Medical School in 1999 & undertook an intercalated BSc at Imperial College School of Medicine (London) in 1997. During this time he researched antigen-presenting cells in inflammatory bowel disease at the internationally renowned St Mark's Hospital. He has previously been a Research Registrar, completing his MPhil placement in 2007 at the Plastic Surgery & Burns Research Unit, University of Bradford. His research interest here was the structural variability of skin at different sites of the body, relating this to scarring potential & he developed a new histological stain. He has 11 academic prizes & awards,15 publications & 30 international / national presentations.

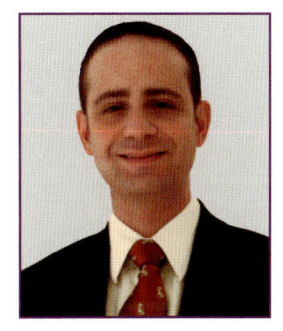

Kamil has maintained an active interest in teaching since qualifying. He has regularly taught on DrExam MRCS revision courses since 2007, having helped design & establish the OSCE course in response to the changes in the MRCS examination. Kamil has had training exposure to a wide variety of surgical specialities & several years experience in Plastic Surgery & Burns. He has been key in fundraising for the Plastic Surgery & Burns Research Unit in Bradford during its 20th & 21st anniversaries. He has worked as an expert reviewer for the London Student Journal of Medicine as well as a Medical Consultant for several film & television projects.

Professor Simon P Kay FRCS, FRCS (Plas), FRCS Ed (Hon)

Professor Kay is a fellow of the Royal College of Surgeons of England & Edinburgh, Consultant Plastic & Hand Surgeon, Leeds General Infirmary & Professor of Hand Surgery, University of Leeds. He is an Honorary Visiting Professor in Plastic & Hand Surgery, Faculty of Medicine, Umea University, Sweden. He is a member of the British Association of Aesthetic Plastic Surgeons. He is a past President of the British Association of Plastic Aesthetic & Reconstructive Surgeons & of the British Society for Surgery of the Hand.

Professor Kay has developed a multidisciplinary hand surgery service & a children's hand surgery service that is now one of the largest such clinics in the UK. His research experience includes children's hand reconstruction, brachial plexus surgery & nerve repair in collaboration with the Department of Hand Surgery in Umea. He has published extensively in the fields of children's hand surgery, brachial plexus surgery & plastic surgery. He has edited the world's major textbook in children's hand surgery, has received numerous awards & was recently the Editor of The Journal of Plastic Reconstructive & Aesthetic Surgery.

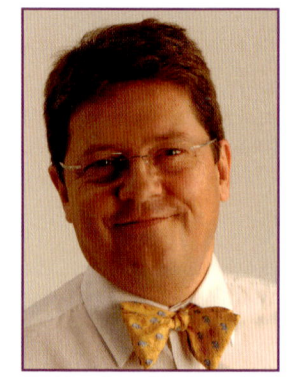

AUTHORS & CONTRIBUTORS

Mr Sharif Kaf Al-Ghazal MS, MD, FRCS
Consultant Plastic Surgeon
Bradford Teaching Hospitals
Honorary Senior Lecturer
School of Medicine, University of Leeds

Dr John Annaradnam MB BS, MRCGP
General Practitioner
The Southgate Surgery, London

Mr Kamil Asaad BSc, MB ChB, MRCS, MPhil
Plastic Surgery Registrar
St Thomas' Hospital London

Mr Omar Baldo MBBS, MRCS
Specialty Registrar Urology
Yorkshire Deanery

Dr M Bauer
Consultant Dermatologist
Bradford Teaching Hospitals NHS Foundation Trust

Carly Betton MA, BA (Hons), MIMI, RMIP
Senior Clinical Photographer
University Hospitals Birmingham NHS Foundation Trust

Mr Waseem Bhat MuDr, MA, MRCS
Clinical Fellow Plastic Surgery
Castle Hill Hospital, Cottingham

Wendy Birch BSc (Hons), MSc, MBIE, LIAS
Anatomist & Dissection Room Manager
Research Department of Cell and Developmental Biology
University College London Medical School

Mr Quamar MK Bismil MB ChB (Hons), MRCS, Dip SEM, MFSEM, FRCS (Tr & Orth)
Specialty Registrar Trauma & Orthopaedics
London Deanery

Professor Peter EM Butler MD, FRCSI, FRCS, FRCS (Plast)
Professor of Plastic Surgery & Honorary Senior Lecturer
Royal Free & University College Hospitals London

Laurence Clarke MBIE, LIAS, FAAPT
Senior Anatomy Technician
Research Department of Cell and Developmental Biology
University College London Medical School

Paul Creasey BSc MIMI, RMIP
Senior Clinical Photographer
Bradford Teaching Hospitals NHS Trust

Antony Dook BSc, MIMI, RMIP
Chief Clinical Photographer
Bradford Teaching Hospitals NHS Trust

Mr AD Ebinesan MB ChB, MRCS (Eng)
Specialist Registrar in Trauma & Orthopaedics
North Western Rotation

Dr Marc Epstein BSc, MBBS, MRCGP, MRCP
General Practitioner

Ms Edwina Ewart BSc (Hons), MBChB, MRCS (Ed)
MD Research Registar
Northern Lincolnshire & Goole Hospitals NHS Trust

Carol Fleming BSc, FIMI, RMIP
Principal Clinical Photographer & Medical Illustration Manager
Bradford Teaching Hospitals NHS Foundation Trust

Mr Ivan Foo FRCS Eng (Plast), FRCS Ed
Consultant Plastic & Reconstructive Surgeon
Bradford Teaching Hospitals NHS Foundation Trust

Miss Sheila Fraser MB ChB MRCS
Specialty Registrar General Surgery
Yorkshire Deanery

Dr Brian Geffin MB BCh, MRCGP
General Practitioner
The Southgate Surgery, London

Dr Brijanand Sharma Ghoorun MD, FRCA
Consultant ICU & Trauma Anaesthetist
Huddersfield Royal Infirmary

Katherine Grice BA, MIMI, RMIP
Senior Clinical Photographer
Bradford Teaching Hospitals NHS Trust

Dr Ayshea Hameeduddin MBBS, BA (Hons) Med Journalism, FRCR
Specialist Trainee in Radiology
Royal Free Hospital, London

Dr Brian Holloway MRCS, FRCR
Consultant Radiologist
Royal Free Hospital, London

Mr Jonathan A Joseph BSc, MBBS, MRCS, DOHNS
Specialist Registrar in ENT
Oxford Deanery

Mr Vishal Kakar BSc, MBBS (Lond), MRCS (Eng)
Specialty Registrar Neurosurgery
Northern Ireland Deanery

Mr Senthil Kamalasekaran MB ChB, MS (Orth), MRCS
Trauma & Orthopaedics Registrar
Barnet & Chase Farm Hospitals NHS Trust

Professor Simon P Kay FRCS, FRCS (Plast), FRCS Ed (Hon)
Professor of Plastic & Reconstructive Surgery & Surgery of the Hand
Leeds Teaching Hospitals NHS Trust

Mr Malcolm Keene MBBS, FRCS
Consultant ENT Surgeon
Barts and the London NHS Trust

Mr R Linforth MD, FRCS Ed, FRCS (Gen Surg)
Consultant Breast & Oncoplastic Surgeon
Bradford Teaching Hospitals NHS Foundation Trust

Dr KM London
Consultant Dermatologist
Bradford Teaching Hospitals NHS Foundation Trust

Ms Joanna Lorains BSc, MB ChB, MRCS
Specialty Registrar General Surgery
North Western Deanery

Dr Anmol Malhotra BSc (Hons), MRCP, FRCR
Consultant Radiologist
Royal Free Hospital, London

Mr JC May MB, BCh, FRCS Ed (Gen)
Consultant General Surgeon
Bradford Teaching Hospitals NHS Foundation Trust

Ms Laura K McMurray BSc, PGCMCH, PGCCBT, PGDipCBT
Psychological Therapist
Isllington Psychological Assessment & Treatment Service, London

Mr Benjamin H Miranda ALCM, BSc, MBBS (Lond), MRCS (Eng)
Plastic Surgery & Burns Research Registrar
Plastic Surgery & Burns Research Unit
University of Bradford

Mr Jabir Nagaria MBBS, FRCS (Surgical Neurology)
Consultant Neurosurgeon
Royal Victoria Hospital
Belfast

Mr Marios Nicolaou BMedSci, BMBS, MRCS, PhD
Specialty Registrar in Plastic Surgery & Burns
Oxford Deanery

Dr Selva Nithiyananthan MB BS, MRCP, DipMedRehab, MRCGP
General Practitioner
The Southgate Surgery, London

Dr Stephen Oakey MBBS, FRCA
Consultant in Anaesthesia & Burns Critical Care
St Andrew's Centre for Plastic Surgery & Burns
Broomfield Hospital, Chelmsford

Mr Kanak K Patel FDS, RCPS, FRCS (OMFS)
Consultant Oral & Maxillofacial Surgeon
Bradford Teaching Hospitals NHS Foundation Trust

Mr Mark James Portou MB ChB (Hons), MRCS
Specialty Registrar in General Surgery
London Deanery

Mr N Rhodes FFDRCS, FRCS (Plast)
Consultant Plastic & Reconstructive Surgeon
Bradford Teaching Hospitals NHS Foundation Trust

Mr J Saksena BMSc (Hons), MB ChB, MRCS, FRCS (Tr&Orth)
Consultant Orthopaedic & Trauma Surgeon
The Whittington Hospital London

Professor DJA Scott MD, MB ChB, FRCS, FEBVS
Professor of Vascular Surgery
Division of Cardiovascular and Diabetes Research
Leeds Institute of Genetics, Health and Therapeutics

Professor David T Sharpe OBE, MA, Bchir, FRCS
Professor of Plastic & Reconstructive Surgery
Plastic Surgery & Burns Research Unit Director
University of Bradford

Mr Masha Singh MBBS, BSc, MRCS
Department of General Surgery
Bradford Royal Infirmary

Mr Niroshan Sivathasan BSc, MBBS, MRCS (Eng)
Registrar in Plastic Surgery
Broomfield Hospital, Chelmsford

Sarah Slade BA (Hons), MIMI, RMIP
Clinical Photographer
Bradford Teaching Hospitals NHS Trust

Mr Mark S Soldin MB ChB, FCS (SA), FRCS (Plast)
Consultant Plastic & Reconstructive Surgeon
St George's Healthcare NHS Trust London

Mr M A Steward FRCS (Ed)
Consultant Colorectal & General Surgeon
Bradford Teaching Hospitals NHS Foundation Trust

Mr D N Sutton BDS, FRCDS (Ed), FRCS (Ed), FRCS (Eng)
Consultant Oral & Maxillofacial Surgeon
Bradford Teaching Hospitals NHS Foundation Trust

Mr Michael J Timmons MA, MChir, FRCS
Consultant Plastic & Reconstructive Surgeon
Bradford Teaching Hospitals NHS Foundation Trust

Professor Desmond J Tobin PhD, FRCPath, FIBiol
Director of the Centre for Skin Sciences
Professor of Cell Biology
Assoc. Dean of Research & Knowledge Transfer
University of Bradford

Mr David A L Watt MB ChB, FRCS (Plast)
Consultant Plastic & Reconstructive Surgeon
Bradford Teaching Hospitals NHS Foundation Trust

Professor Marc C Winslet MS, FRCS (Ed), FRCS (Eng), MEWI
Professor of Surgery, Head of Department
Chairman of Division of Surgery & Interventional Science
School of Medicine
Faculty of Biomedical Science
University College London

Dr A L Wright BMedSci (Hons), LRCP, MRCS, MB ChB, FRCP
Consultant Dermatologist & Lead Clinician
Bradford Teaching Hospitals NHS Foundation Trust

'The Anatomy Dissection Team'
Rachel Eyre, Rebecca Gayner, Emma Williams, James Davis, Lucy Collison, David Reynolds, Alexander, Morton, Gopigia Thana-Balasundaram, Timothy Chan, Oliver White, Zoya Georgieva, James Lewis, Brett Packham, Kevin Cao, Radoslaw Rippel, Donald Leith

ACKNOWLEDGEMENTS

*'Putting this MRCS OSCE revision guide book series together
has been one of our most challenging & rewarding experiences to date.*

*We could not have done it without the help of our teachers past & present,
our co-contributors – Professors, Consultants, other professional colleagues
or even our students...*

... BUT...

*In particular we would like to thank the following people in no particular order:
Mrs Gladys Miranda, Mr David Miranda, Dr Issa Asaad & Dr Lillian Asaad.*

Mums & Dads we thank you & will never forget your unconditional love & support.'

Ben & Kamil

PREFACE

The DrExam MRCS Part B OSCE revision guide series adopts an innovative approach which addresses the needs of candidates for the revised MRCS OSCE exam. The authors have tackled subjects that are common, complicated or important, according to the new syllabus. This was only achievable through the collaborative efforts of 6 professors, 26 consultants & 23 specialists from across the United Kingdom.

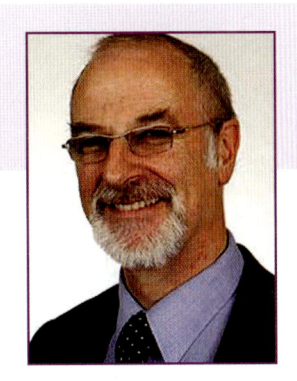

DrExam has several years of experience in teaching MRCS candidates on revision courses that have evolved & adapted to the changes in the exam. These highly successful courses (www.DrExam.co.uk) have become internationally attended & this book series has developed following high candidate success rates & positive feedback about the teaching quality, knowledge imparted & detailed course handouts provided.

What differentiates these books from others is that they are targeted specifically to the OSCE, in structured question-answer format throughout, illustrated by fantastic high-resolution colour images that were contributed by anatomists, radiologists, clinical photographers & medical illustrators. Each chapter, or sections within a chapter, has been written or verified by specialists within the field.

Topics covered in detail in Book 1 include: Radiology, Critical Care, Physiology, Anatomy, Surgical Pathology, Operative Surgery & Surgical Skills, Bones & Soft Tissues, Endocrinology, Oncology & Surgical Technology (Book 1).

Topics covered in detail in Book 2 include: Clinical Examination Protocols, Lumps 'n' Bumps, Head & Neck, Trunk & Thorax, Limbs Spine & Vascular, Neurosciences, Communication Skills, Ethics & History Taking. In addition, clinical examination is taught not only with written words & pictures, but also with a DVD containing all major examination routines. This allows the candidate to pick up 'nuances' of clinical examination that are not readily communicated through still images alone.

The Bradford Burns & Plastic Surgery Research Unit evolved following the Bradford City Football Club stadium fire disaster in 1985. Twenty five percent of the royalties from this series will be donated to the unit so that it may continue to make a valuable contribution to skin sciences research & future patient care. Ben Miranda & Kamil Asaad were Research Registrars at the unit & it is rewarding to see their continuing contribution.

The DrExam series is the most colourful, complete & structured MRCS OSCE revision guide to be released on the market to date & I thank all those who were involved in making this project a success. It will not only be of great value to any MRCS OSCE candidate, but also to training surgeons, doctors, medical practitioners & students who are required to revise these vital core subjects.

Professor David T Sharpe OBE

This book is dedicated to the memory of the 56 who died, 270 who were injured & thousands more who were affected by the Bradford City Football Club stadium fire disaster on 11th May 1985.

INTRODUCTION
(IMPORTANT – READ ME!)

BH Miranda
K Asaad

CONTENTS

How to Use this Book

Introduction to the MRCS OSCE

- OSCE Exam Overview
- OSCE Structure
- OSCE Disciplines
- OSCE Speciality Themes
- Point Scoring
- OSCE Domains
- What to Wear!

Approaching the OSCE Stations

Please read the following sections carefully, they provide the candidate with vital tips regarding the use of this book, accompanying DVD, how to approach the MRCS OSCE & maintain good clinical practice in the future.

HOW TO USE THIS BOOK

- The primary objective of this book is to present the most commonly asked, most complicated & most important topics that feature both **in the MRCS OSCE & in everyday clinical practice**. *Note: Additional clinical topics are covered in Book 2.*
- These topics are presented in **structured question-answer format throughout**, providing the candidate with tailored **revision material & model-answers** that have been **written by Professors, Consultants & Specialists** in their respective fields.
- Chapters are presented in **full colour throughout**, packed with **high-resolution radiological, anatomical & clinical images & illustrations**.
- An additional objective is to provide the candidate with model-answers that **optimise memory-recall** using a **system of classification & categorisation**. This not only **assists efficiency & accuracy of answers**, but also **improves the overall impression of the candidate by the examiner**.
- Candidates are advised to **learn & consistently practice these questions & answers**, so that they may be reproduced almost involuntarily, in order to successfully complete the OSCE & to become competent clinicians! This may be achieved via use of books, attendance at courses & on the wards / in clinic.
- **To cover the remaining half of the MRCS OSCE syllabus**, there is a sister volume: **DrExam Part B MRCS OSCE Revision Guide: Book 2** *Clinical Examination, Communication Skills & History Taking*. This is also accompanied with a clinical examination DVD.
- **There are two courses** also available to complement these books. Candidates can find these by visiting **www.DrExam.co.uk**.

INTRODUCTION TO THE MRCS OSCE

Note: The OSCE has recently changed format again & is likely to do so in the future. These changes are mostly to do with the format / marking scheme of the examination, however the knowledge & skill level required to succeed remains largely unaffected. The following information should be used as a general guide to the OSCE format, which should be confirmed by the candidate via contacting The Royal College of Surgeons.

OSCE Exam Overview

- Anatomy & surgical pathology
- Applied surgical science & critical care
- Clinical & procedural skills
- Communication skills

OSCE Structure
- 18 stations (possibility of several additional preparation stations)

OSCE Disciplines
Applied Surgical Science & Critical Care, Anatomy & Surgical Pathology, Surgical Skills & Patient Safety (DrExam Part B MRCS OSCE Revision Guide: Book 1)
- Applied surgical science & critical care
- Anatomy & surgical pathology
- Operative surgery & surgical skills
- Principles of surgery & patient safety

Clinical Examination, Communication Skills & History taking (DrExam Part B MRCS OSCE Revision Guide: Book 2)
- Clinical examination
- Communication skills
- History taking

OSCE Speciality Themes
The candidate will be required to have knowledge across the following:
- Head & neck
- Trunk & thorax
- Limbs & spine (including vascular)
- Neuroscience

Point Scoring

- Each station carries 20 marks
- The maximum achievable score for the 18 OSCE stations is 360
- An overall rating is additionally allocated by the examiner at each station as follows:
    1. *Fail*
    2. *Borderline fail*
    3. *Borderline pass*
    4. *Pass*
- A minimum pass mark will then be calculated based on the station marks & overall rating at each station.
- In addition to the minimum pass mark, the candidate must achieve a minimum level of competence in OSCE disciplines (see above) & OSCE domains (see below).

OSCE Domains

- 4 domains of knowledge, skill, competence & professional attributes are tested throughout the OSCE.
- These domains are intrinsic to good surgical practice.
- Domains may be tested throughout the 18 stations of the OSCE.
- It is therefore important to consider these 4 domains at every station throughout the OSCE.

Domain	Notes
Clinical Knowledge	Understand, process & apply knowledge in a clinical setting.
Clinical & Technical Skill	Apply knowledge, awareness & skill to generate differential diagnoses & aid investigation of a clinical problem. Perform surgical tasks that require manual dexterity, hand-eye coordination & visual-spatial awareness.
Communication	Process information, identify what is important & convey it to others clearly, by engaging a patient, carer or colleague during a consultation.
Professionalism	Demonstrate effective judgement & decision making by processing & addressing all appropriate information prior to formulating a plan. Identify rapidly deteriorating conditions & think laterally to maximise efficiency. Show awareness of limitations & seek help when appropriate. Accommodate changing information to manage a clinical problem. Anticipate & plan in advance. Prioritise effectively & demonstrate good time management.

What to Wear!

Modern infection control practices have precipitated a review of dress code for the OSCE as follows:

- Arms bare below the elbow
- No jewellery on hands or wrists except wedding rings / bands
- No ties or dangling clothing.

Female candidates may wish to present themselves as follows:

- Smart haircut with tied-back hair (if long)
- Smart blouse, sleeves rolled up to above the elbows
- Smart skirt / trousers
- Smart & comfortable shoes (not open)
- Minimal jewellery & makeup.

Male candidates may wish to present themselves as follows:

- Smart haircut
- Smart shirt, sleeves rolled up to above the elbows.
- No tie
- Smart trousers
- Smart & comfortable shoes
- No jewellery other than a wedding ring / band.

APPROACHING THE OSCE STATIONS

Clinical examination, history taking & communication skills stations are presented in detail in book 2.

The OSCE has already evolved & is likely to do so again. A greater emphasis is now being placed on basic surgical sciences topics & viva-style examination stations. The key throughout the OSCE is to produce a high volume of accurate & relevant information, as quickly & efficiently as possible. Your answers should be clear, concise, considered & classified in order to demonstrate knowledge & confidence to the examiner. This is often challenging, particularly during the high-stress examination scenario & it is here where candidates often stumble.

To help you prepare for this & practice your skills, continuous revision is vital, via active involvement within a hospital environment, use of books & attendance at courses. Further material is available in the sister volume **DrExam Part B MRCS OSCE Revision Guide: Book 2** *Clinical Examination, Communication Skills & History Taking. This is also accompanied with a clinical examination DVD. Revision courses are available by visiting www.DrExam.co.uk.* Remember, there is always enough time to pause for a few seconds, relax, take a few slow breaths & think about your answer. It is better to do this than to just deliver a poorly considered response quickly!

SECTION A: APPLIED SURGICAL SCIENCE & CRITICAL CARE

CHAPTER 1
RADIOLOGY

A Hameeduddin
BH Miranda
A Malhotra

CHAPTER CONTENTS

Radiography
- Systematic Interpretation of the Chest Radiograph
- Chest Radiograph OSCE Cases
- Systematic Interpretation of the Abdominal Radiograph
- Abdominal Radiograph OSCE Cases

Computed Tomography
- Systematic Interpretation of Computed Tomography Scans
- Computed Tomography OSCE Cases

Magnetic Resonance Imaging
- T1 & T2 Weighted Sequences
- Systematic Interpretation of Magnetic Resonance Imaging Scans
- Magnetic Resonance Imaging OSCE Cases

RADIOGRAPHY

X-rays are generated by an x-ray tube, positioned a fixed distance away from the patient, depending on the body part being imaged. An x-ray tube houses a tungsten metal plate which is bombarded by fast moving electrons. The kinetic energy produced by these electrons is converted into heat (99%) & x-rays (1%). The x-rays are absorbed differentially by different tissues in the body, such that the emerging x-rays are of varying intensity.

Conventional radiography involves a phosphor screen & film cassette positioned behind the patient. The emerging x-rays are absorbed by the intensifying phosphor screen & converted to light which exposes the film beneath. This is subsequently processed to form an image which can be viewed on a light box.

More departments are now using **digital radiography**. Instead of a film cassette, a flat panel detector is used. The x-rays are converted to an electron beam which in turn is converted to a digital output signal. This is then displayed on a video monitor & can be read straight away.

The pattern of x-ray attenuation by the body is represented by a grey-scale on the image. More x-rays are absorbed by bones which appear white, whilst air absorbs the least & is black on the film (Fig 1.1).

Fig 1.1: Key to radiograph densities:

Black	→	Air
Darker Grey	→	Fat
Grey	→	Soft Tissues
White	→	Calcium
Intense White	→	Metal

Systematic Interpretation of the Chest Radiograph

The CXR is an essential 1st line imaging modality for many clinical presentations. It may assist in diagnosing or excluding significant pathology. The CXR is also an invaluable component of trauma evaluation, pre & post-operative assessment. The candidate should therefore be familiar with normal CXR anatomy (Fig 1.2) & confident in the diagnosis of common conditions.

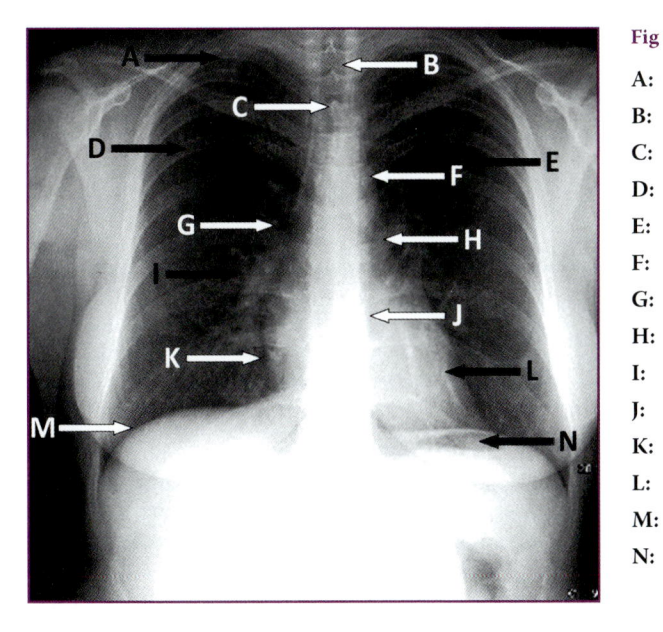

Fig 1.2: CXR Anatomy.

A:	1st Rib
B:	Trachea
C:	Spinous Process
D:	Posterior Rib
E:	Anterior Rib
F:	Aortic Knuckle
G:	Right Hilum
H:	Left Hilum
I:	Right Pulmonary Artery
J:	Descending Aorta
K:	Right Atrium
L:	Left Ventricle
M:	Right Hemi-Diaphragm
N:	Gastric Bubble

When presented with a CXR it is tempting to immediately look for pathology, however it is important to have a system which can be used to interpret the CXR.

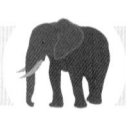

Memory: Pam Found Peter's Rubber In A CHEST

System	Explanation
Patient Details	Check that it is the correct patient's film, noting their name, hospital number, age, sex & ethnic background.
Film Details	Check the date & orientation of the film & describe the projection. The preferred projection for the CXR is posterior-anterior (PA). X-rays travel in a posterior-anterior direction. The plate is positioned close to the front of the patient with their arms elevated around the plate, thus removing the scapulae shadows from the film (Fig 1.2). An anterior-posterior radiograph (AP) is taken when the patient is too unwell or unable to stand. The plate is behind the patient & the x-rays travel in an anterior-posterior direction, thus magnifying mediastinal structures. The scapulae overlie the chest (Fig 1.3). Look for additional markers to indicate how the film has been taken e.g. supine, portable or semi-erect.
Penetration	The vertebral end-plates of the mid-thoracic vertebrae should be just visible behind the heart.
Rotation	The medial ends of the clavicles should be equidistant from the spinous processes of the vertebrae.
Inflation	Count 6–8 anterior ribs in the mid-clavicular line.
Air	Check for air under the diaphragm, pneumothoraces & subcutaneous emphysema.
CHEST	Examine both lungs (remember they extend behind the heart & diaphragms) & follow their contours, paying attention to the apices & costophrenic angles. Look for asymmetry & compare each side. Check that the domes of the diaphragm & heart borders are not obscured by adjacent lung pathology. Check for pleural effusions.
Cardiac & Vessels	Follow the structures of the cardiomediastinal contour (Fig 1.2). The heart borders should be easily traced & distinct. The cardiothoracic ratio should not be >50% (a measurement from the widest diameter of the heart to the widest diameter of the thoracic cage).
Hila	The left hilum is normally slightly higher than the right hilum. There is increased density at the hila with soft tissue masses, commonly lymphadenopathy e.g. lymphoma, sarcoid & TB.
External Devices / Objects	Chest drain, CVP line, ECG leads, ETT, foreign body, NGT, oxygen mask & tubing, pacemakers, penetrating object, pulmonary artery catheter, sternotomy wires, valve replacement etc.
Skeleton & Soft Tissues	Review the bones & soft tissues, checking for rib fractures & bony metastases. Follow the outline of both scapulae & evaluate both breast shadows in females.
Trachea	Check the trachea is central; it will be deviated towards a collapsed lung or tumour. It will be deviated away from a tension pneumothorax or large pleural effusion.

Chest Radiograph OSCE Cases

Case 1:
Study this radiograph & answer the following question:

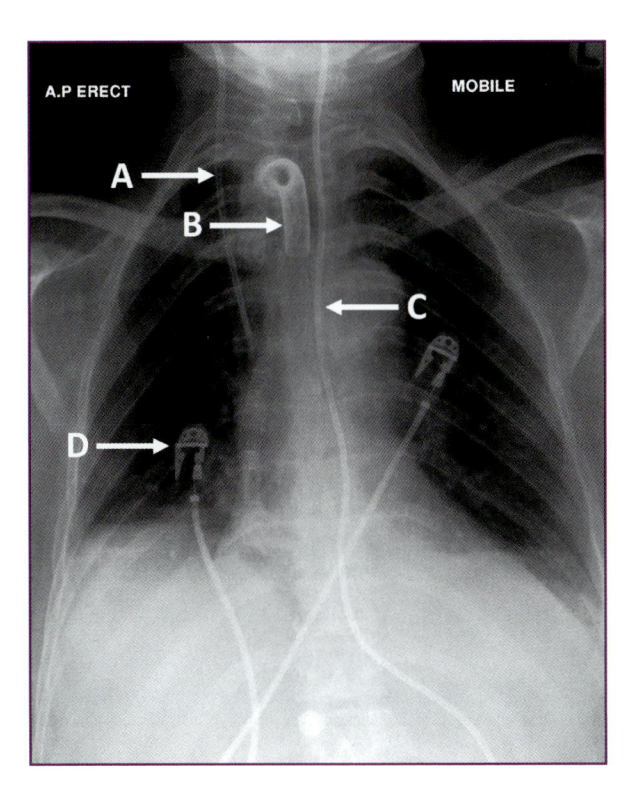

Fig 1.3: AP erect mobile CXR taken on ICU.

Q: What are the structures labelled A–D?

A: Right Internal Jugular Vein Line

B: Tracheostomy

C: Nasogastric Tube

D: ECG Electrode & Line

Case 2:

Study this radiograph & answer the following questions:

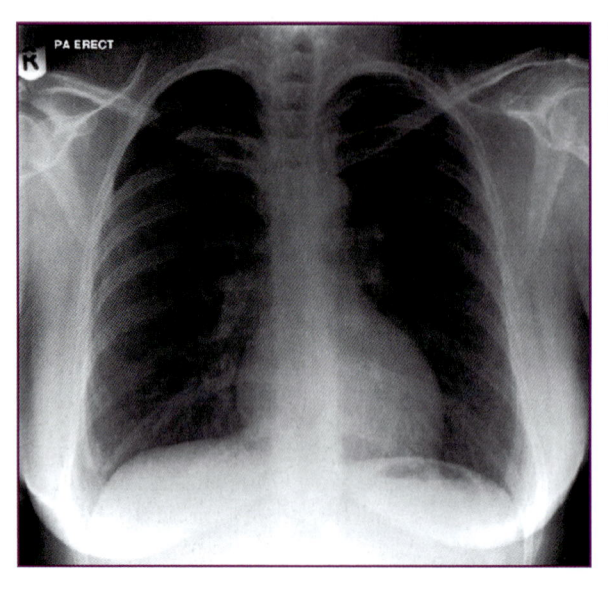

Fig 1.4: CXR of a 27-year-old woman who presented with right sided pleuritic chest pain & shortness of breath.

Q: What are the salient features?

There is a sharp line (the visceral pleura) outlining the superior edge of the right lung. There are no lung markings beyond this line.

Q: What is the diagnosis?

Right pneumothorax.

Q: What are the causes of this condition?

Cause	Explanation
Primary	Accounts for 80% of pneumothoraces, commonly affecting young, tall men. The underlying pathology is spontaneous rupture of an apical pleural bleb. The risk of recurrence is 30% on the same side & 10% on the contralateral side.
Secondary	This accounts for 20% of pneumothoraces. Causes include asthma, COPD, infection, malignancy & trauma.

Q: What is the management?

Type	Guidelines
Primary Pneumothorax	• A rim of air >2cm on the CXR requires simple aspiration & if successful the patient can be discharged. Failed aspiration requires insertion of an intercostal chest drain *(see operative surgery chapter)* & hospital admission. The drain may be removed & the patient discharged if the lung re-expands by 24 hours. • Referral to a chest physician is appropriate if the lung has not expanded by 48 hours. • Thoracic surgeon involvement is required if the lung has still not expanded by 5 days.
Secondary Pneumothorax	• A simple pneumothorax (air rim <2cm) in a patient aged <50 years who is not breathless, may be aspirated with hospital admission for 24 hours. Failed aspiration requires insertion of an intercostal chest drain *(see operative surgery chapter)* & hospital admission. • A breathless patient aged >50 years, with a rim of air >2cm, requires intercostal chest drain insertion & hospital admission. The drain may be removed & the patient discharged if the lung re-expands by 24 hours. • Referral to a chest physician is appropriate if the lung has not expanded by 48 hours. • Thoracic surgeon involvement is required if the lung has still not expanded by 3 days.

REMEMBER

- Shallow pneumothoraces are easily missed. Most occur at the apices so look carefully between the ribs for an 'extra line'. A PA erect film is required.
- In a supine patient, air will rise anteriorly, so check the bases of the lungs for increased blackening.
- In an intubated & ventilated patient, a pneumothorax may quickly develop into a life threatening tension pneumothorax. Look for signs of mediastinal shift away from the symptomatic side.
- Sometimes clothing artefact & skin folds may mimic a lung edge suggesting a pneumothorax. Check carefully to see if there are lung markings beyond these lines.

Case 3:

Study this radiograph & answer the following questions:

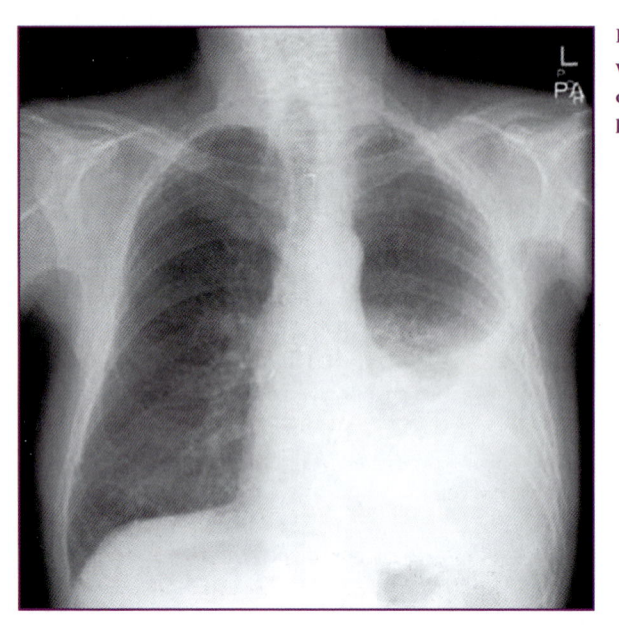

Fig: 1.5: PA CXR of 50-year-old woman, who presented with shortness of breath & decreased air entry on the left side.

Q: What abnormalities can you detect?

There is increased opacification of the left mid-lower lung with obscuration of the left hemidiaphragm & heart border. The left costophrenic angle is blunt & there is a meniscus at the superior border of the opacity.

Q: What is the diagnosis?

The features are consistent with a unilateral left pleural effusion.

Q: What would you do next?

It is always necessary to compare the CXR with a previous film to ascertain if changes are acute or chronic.

In this case the unilateral left pleural effusion was a new finding. Aspiration of the fluid +/- chest drain insertion is required to determine whether the fluid is a transudate or exudate. This will assist in guiding further management.

REMEMBER

- Always find out if there is a previous film for comparison.
- The Silhouette Sign:

Different structures absorb different amounts of x-rays depending on tissue density (Fig 1.1). Bone absorbs the most & appears white, whilst air absorbs the least & appears black. Other structures & fluids will appear on the spectrum of greyscale between white & black. This allows for clear outlining & identification of many different structures.

For example, the heart absorbs more x-rays than the adjacent lung, hence its silhouette is clearly demarcated under normal circumstances. The Silhouette Sign is an important concept that is demonstrated by this case. Obscuration of a normal anatomical silhouette indicates adjacent pathology. In this case, obscuration of the heart border & diaphragm is due to fluid in the pleural space.

Case 4:

Study this radiograph & answer the following questions:

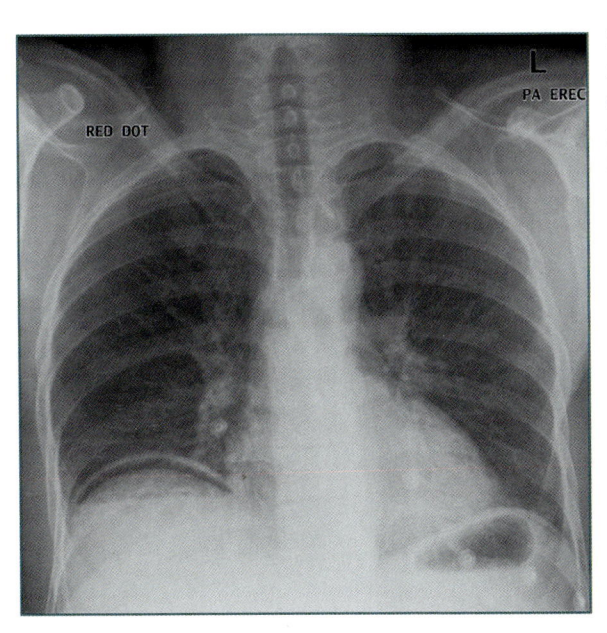

Fig 1.6: PA erect CXR of a 60-year-old male who presented with an acute abdomen. He had been discharged the previous day following a colonoscopy for suspected diverticular disease.

Q: What abnormality can be seen?

There is a crescenteric rim of air beneath the right hemidiaphragm.

Q: What does this signify?

This air is extraluminal & represents free intraperitoneal air. The cause is most likely due to iatrogenic perforation of the sigmoid colon at colonoscopy.

Q: What is the immediate treatment?

Immediate management involves ALS resuscitation, patient stabilisation & (IV) antibiotics. In this case the cause of perforation is known & the patient should be taken directly to theatre. **Note: Small perforations may be treated conservatively.**

> **REMEMBER**
> - If a perforation is suspected, erect CXR & AXR are required. If the CXR is taken supine & free air cannot be detected, a lateral decubitus AXR should be performed.
> - CT of the abdomen & pelvis is highly sensitive in the detection of free air. It is useful when searching for sealed perforations.

Case 5:
Study this radiograph & answer the following question:

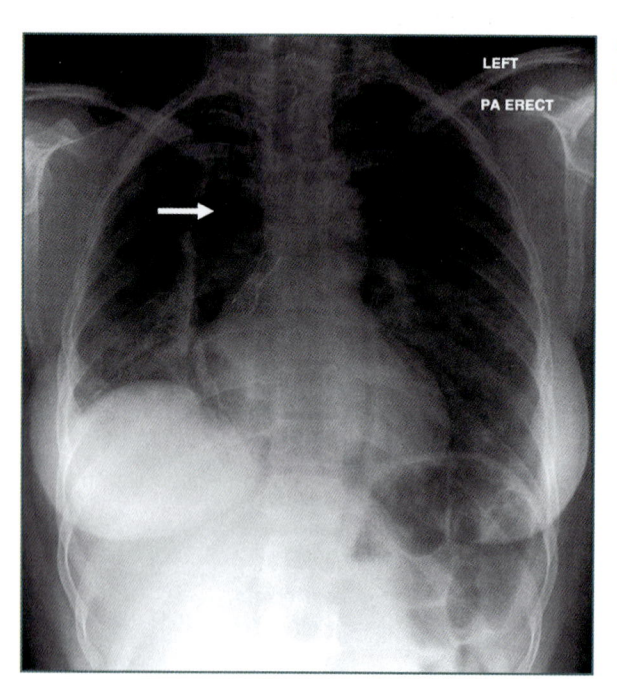

Fig 1.7: A middle aged woman has this PA erect CXR taken post-operatively.

Q: What are the salient findings & can you explain them?

There is bilateral surgical emphysema in the subcutaneous tissues of the neck.

In addition there is a right pneumomediastinum (arrowed).

There is a stent situated in the right main bronchus & this accounts for the post-operative leak of air into the mediastinum & subcutaneous tissues.

Case 6:

Study this radiograph & answer the following questions:

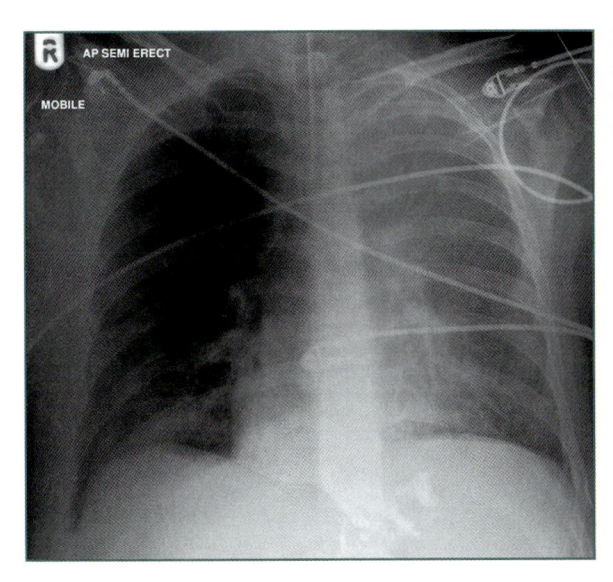

Fig 1.8: AP semi-erect mobile CXR of a 50-year-old alcoholic who presented with haematemesis & haemodynamic instability.

Q: What are the salient features?

This is a mobile AP film suggesting the patient is unwell.

There is a veil-like opacity throughout the left hemithorax, consistent with left upper lobe collapse. There is an ET tube in situ with the tip appropriately positioned above the carina.

High density material is seen in the region of the gastro-oesophageal junction, consistent with sclerotherapy for bleeding varices. There are also ECG electrodes & tubing present.

Q: What is the most likely cause for the features in the left hemithorax?

Iatrogenic due to intubation. The ET tube can be positioned incorrectly in the left or right main bronchus causing collapse. In this patient the ET tube was correctly withdrawn prior to the radiograph.

Case 7:

Study this radiograph & answer the following questions:

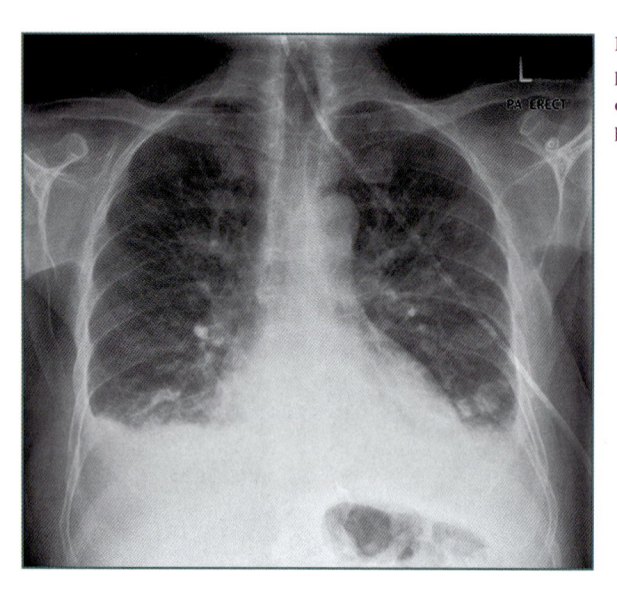

Fig 1.9: This is a PA erect CXR of a patient who presented with shortness of breath 12 hours post surgery for a knee replacement.

Q: What are the salient features?

There is bilateral 'fluffy' shadowing throughout the lung fields. There are bilateral pleural effusions with upper lobe venous congestion. The heart is enlarged & oxygen tubing traverses the left side of the chest.

Q: What is the diagnosis?

Pulmonary oedema.

Q: What other signs can be present on the radiograph in pulmonary oedema?

- Septal lines due to interstitial oedema
- 'Bat wing' perihilar shadowing
- Left atrial enlargement
- Splaying of the carina
- Upper lobe blood diversion.

Systematic Interpretation of the Abdominal Radiograph

The most common indication for an AXR is to exclude bowel obstruction or perforation. Other significant pathology may also be diagnosed, so a systematic approach to interpretation is crucial. Remember that an AXR carries approximately 35X the radiation dose of a CXR & should only be requested in specific circumstances (Fig 1.10). Always consider normal anatomy when interpreting the AXR (Fig 1.11).

Fig 1.10: Indications for AXR, based on The Royal College of Radiologists' guidelines.

- Acute Abdominal Pain: Erect CXR rules out perforation or obstruction.
- Acute SBO & LBO.
- Acute IBD Exacerbation: To monitor toxic dilation of the colon.
- Acute & Chronic Pancreatitis.
- Suspected Urinary Tract Stones: Unenhanced CT is more sensitive for detection of calculi.
- Haematuria.
- Renal Failure.
- Sharp / Poisonous Foreign Body.
- Blunt / Penetrating Abdominal Trauma.
- Palpable Mass.*
- Constipation.**
- Foreign Body in Upper Oesophagus / Pharynx.***
- Smooth & Small Foreign Body.****

* This is a non-routine investigation & should only be ordered to assist further management.

** Only in geriatric or psychiatric populations to show the extent of faecal impaction.

*** A low threshold for laryngoscopy or upper endoscopy should be maintained.

**** Only if the smooth foreign body has not passed in 6 days. This is useful for localisation.

Fig 1.11: Normal AXR (left) with anatomy delineated (right).

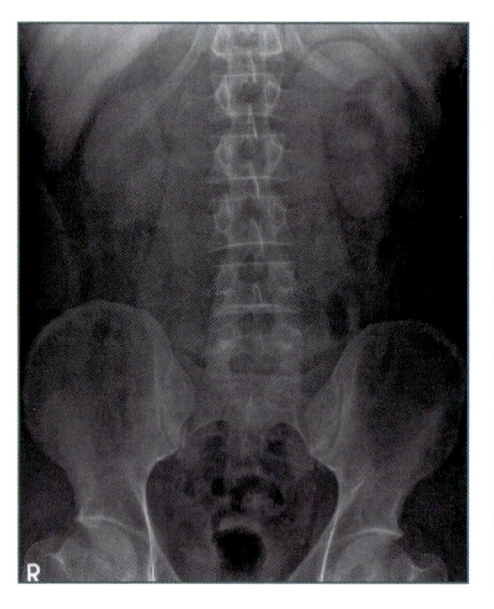

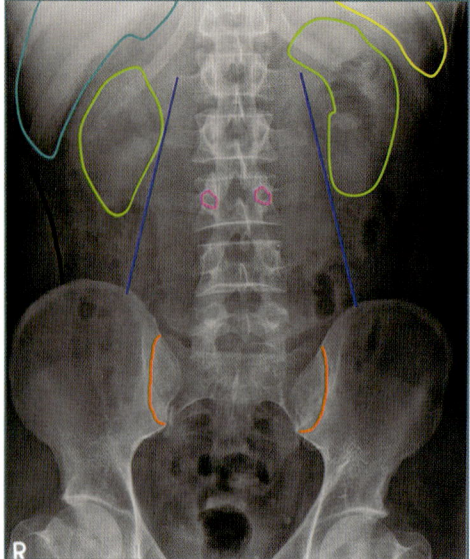

Key:

Light Blue	→	Liver
Yellow	→	Spleen
Green	→	Kidneys
Dark Blue	→	Psoas Shadows
Purple	→	Pedicles
Black	→	Properitoneal Fat Plane
Orange	→	Sacroiliac Joints

When presented with an AXR it is tempting to immediately look for pathology, however it is important to have a system which can be used to interpret the AXR.

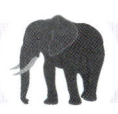

Memory: Penny Found Alan Growing Oranges But Couldn't Replicate One

System	Explanation
Patient Details	Check that it is the correct patient's film, noting their name, hospital number, age, sex & ethnic background.
Film Details	Check the date & orientation of the film & describe the projection.
	The standard AP projection is taken supine with the patient lying on their back. Occasionally an erect film may be taken to demonstrate an air-fluid interface, or a lateral decubitus film to demonstrate free air. Look for additional markers that indicate how the film has been taken.
Adequacy	Ensure the film demonstrates the symphysis pubis, hernial orifices, properitoneal fat & lung bases.
Gas pattern	Discussed below.
Organs	Discussed below.
Bones	Discussed below.
Calcification	Discussed below.
Review Areas	Discussed below.
Objects	Drains, lines & foreign objects

GAS PATTERN:

Intraluminal & extraluminal gas must be considered as follows:

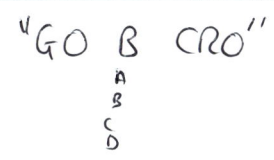

Intraluminal Gas:

Consider the extent of bowel involvement & the distribution of bowel gas patterns. Remember there is a large spectrum of normal variation. The stomach bubble is normally present in the left upper quadrant.

Table 1.1: Important differences between small & large bowel.

Difference	Small Bowel	Large Bowel
Location	Central	Peripheral (although the transverse colon can hang down to occupy the central portion of the film).
Calibre	<3cm	Transverse Colon: <6cm
		Caecum: <9cm
Mucosal Markings	**Valvulae conniventes** markings appear to extend across the entire lumen & are closer together than haustra (Fig 1.12).	**Haustra** markings incompletely extend across the lumen & are wider apart than valvulae conniventes (Fig 1.12).

Fig 1.12: Valvulae conniventes of the small bowel (left) & haustra of the large bowel (right).

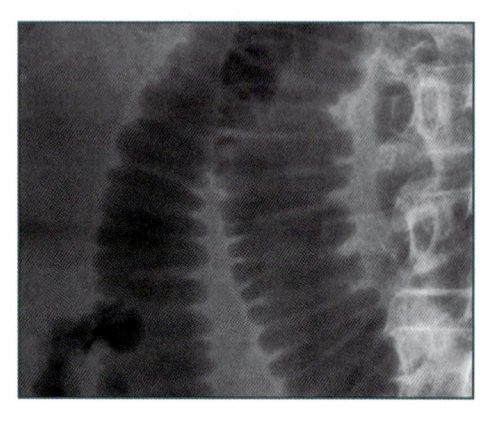

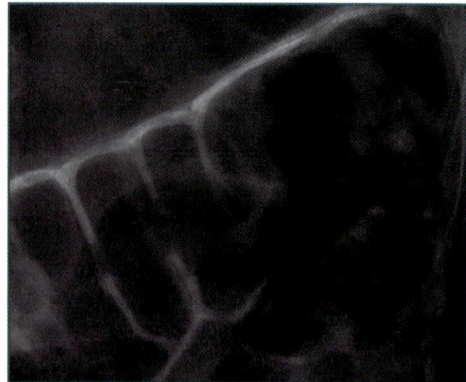

Extraluminal Gas:

This is always abnormal, either iatrogenic or pathological, so remember to check the *3 x Bs* of extraluminal gas on the AXR. Pneumoperitoneum is a common OSCE case, so pay particular attention to the relevant radiological signs (Table 1.2).

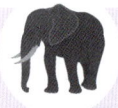

Memory: Remember to check the 3 x Bs of extraluminal gas.

- **B**eneath the Diaphragm: Perforation at endoscopy, post-operative or perforated viscus.
- **B**iliary System: Look for free air in a branching pattern in the RUQ.
- **B**owel Wall: Ischaemic bowel & necrotising enterocolitis.

Table 1.2: Radiological signs of pneumoperitoneum.

Sign	Explanation
Rigler's Sign	Both sides of the bowel wall are seen. This occurs when the bowel wall is outlined by abnormal free gas in the peritoneum lying against the extraluminal wall, with normal intraluminal gas on the other side. **PITFALL: A false Rigler's Sign may result from 2 bowel loops overlapping each other.**
Falciform Ligament Sign.	The falciform ligament connects the liver to the anterior abdominal wall & may be seen when surrounded by free gas from perforation. (Silver's sign)
Continuous Diaphragm	When there is massive pneumoperitoneum, the right & left hemi-diaphragms appear as 1 continuous line.

Note: Properitoneal fat planes can mimic free air when lying adjacent to organs.

ORGANS:

The outlines of the intra-abdominal organs should be traced. This is usually possible, although sometimes these outlines are obscured by overlying bowel gas. When tracing organ outlines, if they become obscured, consider adjacent pathology (Fig 1.11).

BONES:

Check for the following features:

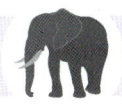

Memory: 'A B C D'

Feature	Explanation
Alignment	Look at the lumbosacral spine, checking for scoliosis & degenerative changes. Look at all the pedicles, as bony metastases often cause erosion here.
Breaks	Check for hip & pelvic fractures, particularly pubic rami fractures which are easily overlooked. Check the hip joints for OA or replacements.
Crohn's	Check the sacroiliac joints are not sclerotic or fused, associated with inflammatory bowel disease & sero-negative arthritides.
Density	Look at the bone density & ensure the bones are not osteoporotic, look for sclerotic or lytic lesions associated with bony metastases.

CALCIFICATION:

Some calcification may be normal e.g. costal cartilages & vasculature (Table 1.3). Pathological calcification may cause symptoms e.g. ureteric calculi, or it may be abnormal but asymptomatic e.g. gallstones. It may be the primary disease process e.g. nephrocalcinosis, or a sequela of chronic disease e.g. pancreatitis (Table 1.3). It is therefore vital to consider the patient's medical history when evaluating calcification.

Table 1.3: Classification of radiological calcification.

Normal Calcification	Pathological Calcification
Costal Cartilages	Gallstones
Mesenteric Lymph Nodes	Pancreas
Phleboliths (small rounded calcific densities in veins)	Vascular*
	Fibroid Uterus & Ovarian Dermoid Cyst
	Nephrocalcinosis
	Renal Tract Calculi**
	Prostate

* An aortic aneurysm may calcify & this can be seen on a plain film.

** When searching for ureteric calculi, remember the course of the ureters along the psoas shadows. Calculi are often seen just adjacent to the tips of the transverse processes.

REVIEW AREAS:

- Check the hernial orifices for bowel gas. When seen in the presence of dilated loops of small bowel, this may indicate SBO due to a strangulated or incarcerated hernia.
- Check the lung bases for consolidation & pleural effusions.
- Look carefully at the outline of the sacrum. There are many overlying structures here so pathology is easily overlooked.

Abdominal Radiograph OSCE Cases

Case 8:
Study this radiograph & answer the following questions:

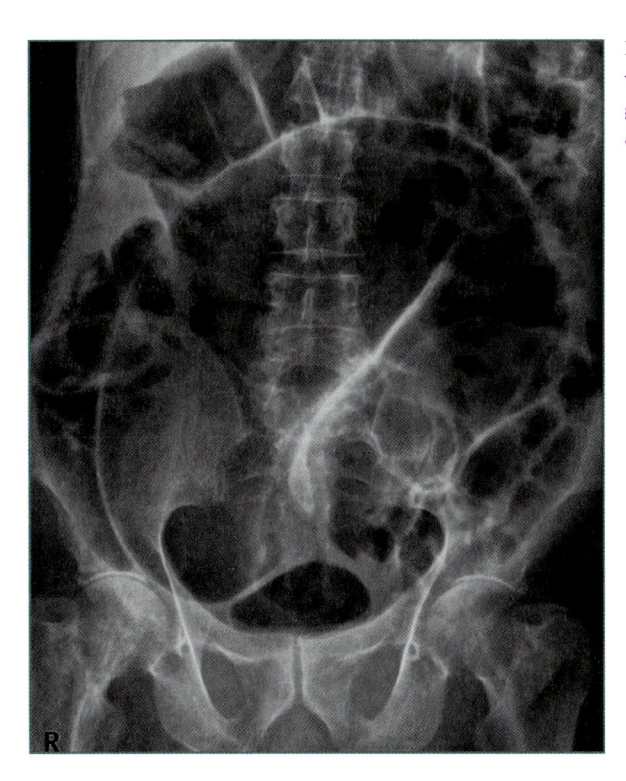

Fig 1.13: AXR of a 70-year-old man who presented with a history of gradual onset colicky abdominal pain & distension.

Q: What are the radiological signs?

There is a grossly dilated loop of large bowel extending from the pelvis towards the diaphragm. Two loops of bowel are closely opposed, with an oblique white line giving the appearance of a **coffee bean**. There is loss of haustra in the affected bowel.

Gas is seen in the rest of the large bowel except for the rectum.

Q: What is the diagnosis?

The signs are consistent with a sigmoid volvulus. Volvulus accounts for approximately 10% of the causes of LBO.

Q: What would you do next?

Insertion of a rectal tube alleviates symptoms in 90% of cases, avoiding bowel wall ischaemia & perforation.

Q: What are the differences between sigmoid & caecal volvulus?

Difference	Sigmoid Volvulus	Caecal Volvulus
Epidemiology	Accounts for 8% of LBO.	Accounts for 1–3% of LBO.
Patient Factors	Elderly & psychiatric populations.	20–40yrs.
Features	A loop of sigmoid colon twists on its mesenteric axis, resulting in closed loop obstruction.	A mobile caecum twists around the terminal ileum & ascending colon, causing complete obstruction.
Radiological Signs	Bowel loop typically resides in the RUQ, but can lie in the LUQ.	Bowel loop typically resides in the LUQ, but can lie anywhere in the abdomen.
	Coffee bean shape.	Kidney bean shape.
	>1 air-fluid level.	Only 1 air-fluid level (usually).
	Loss of haustra.	Haustra are maintained.
	The large bowel dilates proximal to the sigmoid 'twist' whilst the rectum empties. There may be faecal loading in the remainder of the colon as chronic constipation is a risk factor.	The large bowel collapses distal to the caecal 'twist'. There may be associated SBO.

Case 9:

Study this radiograph & answer the following questions:

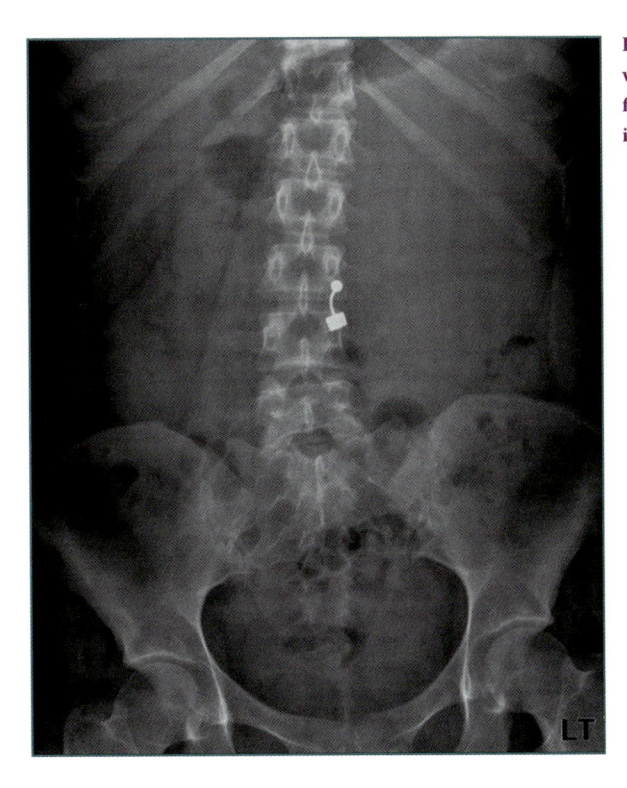

Fig 1.14: AXR of a 20-year-old woman who presented with left flank tenderness & markedly raised inflammatory markers.

Q: What are the important radiological observations?

There is increased opacification in the LUQ. The key features are obscuration of the left psoas muscle shadow & left renal outline, however the splenic outline may still be traced. This important sign indicates pathology in the left side of the abdomen. There is also a belly-button ring present in the centre of the radiograph. It is important to note if additional items are internal or external.

Q: What further imaging would you request?

In this young woman the next investigation should be USS as it is non-invasive & avoids radiation. This will demonstrate where the pathology arises from & if it is cystic or solid.

After USS, CT would be the next investigation of choice. This demonstrated a large cystic mass compressing the left kidney (Fig 1.15).

The patient was taken to theatre & histology was consistent with an infected gastrointestinal duplication cyst.

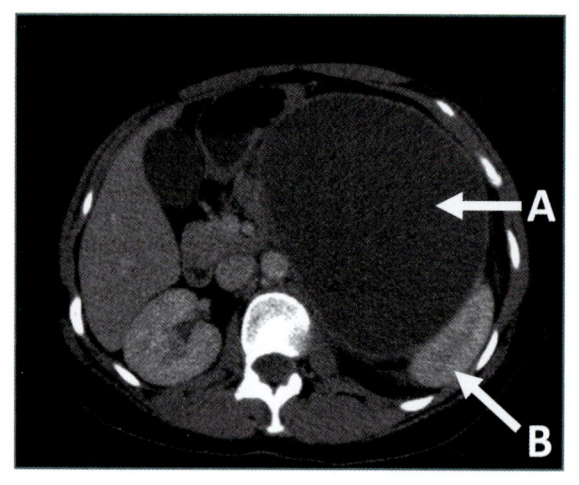

Fig 1.15: Enhanced CT at the level of L1 showing duplication cyst.

Key:

A: Low Attenuating Cystic Mass

B: Compressed Left Kidney

Case 10:

Study this radiograph & answer the following questions:

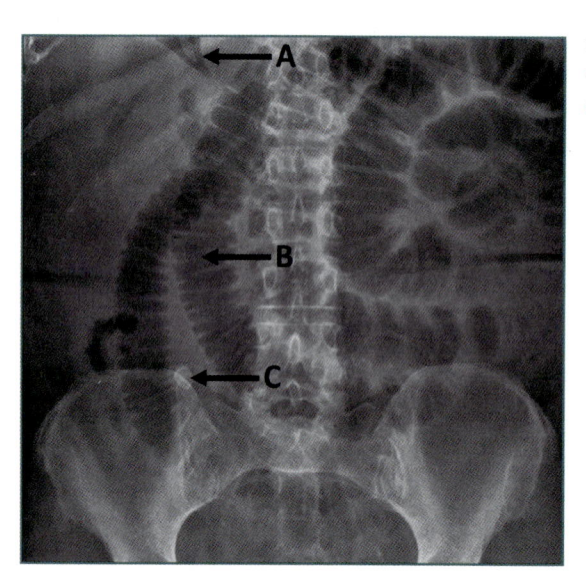

Fig 1.16: AXR of an 80-year-old woman who presented to A&E with vomiting & abdominal distension.

Q: What are the 3 salient radiological features labelled A– C?

A: There is extraluminal air in the RUQ, within the biliary tree (pneumobilia).

B: There are multiple dilated loops of small bowel with a diameter >3cm, consistent with obstruction. There is associated large bowel decompression (not labelled).

C: A calcified lesion is also seen above the right sacro-iliac joint.

Q: What is the diagnosis?

The features of **SBO, pneumobilia & ectopic gallstone** represent **Rigler's Triad.** This triad is consistent with gallstone ileus.

Q: What would you do next?

A CT will demonstrate the site of the fistulous connection in the GI tract & site of the impacted gallstone.

> **REMEMBER**
>
> Gallstone Ileus:
>
> This accounts for approximately 25% of intestinal obstruction in patients aged >65 years & is more common in women. It is associated with high mortality so early diagnosis is essential.
>
> The gallstone erodes through the gallbladder & adjacent bowel, forming a cholecystoduodenal fistula in 60% of cases (others include cholecystocolonic or cholecystogastric).
>
> Gallstones >2.5cm in diameter become impacted, usually at the distal ileum.
>
> Remember to look specifically for the features of Rigler's Triad on the AXR.

Case 11:

Study this radiograph & answer the following questions:

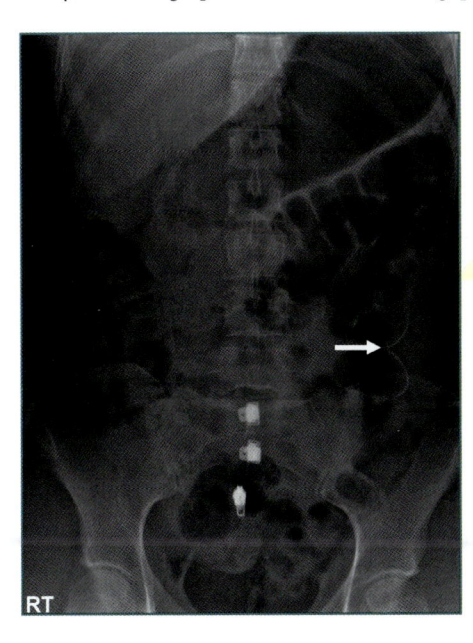

Fig 1.17: AXR of a 45-year-old male who presented to A&E with an acute abdomen.

Q: What is the arrowed salient feature?

Both sides of the bowel wall of the descending colon are visualised. This is consistent with Rigler's Sign & diagnostic of pneumoperitoneum.

Q: What is the management?

Initial management follows ALS resuscitation. A full history & thorough clinical examination will help delineate the patient's risk factors for perforation. After the patient is stabilised & appropriate investigations are requested, arrangements for emergency surgery must be made. In some stable cases, CT is useful to help localise the site of perforation.

Case 12:

Study this radiograph & answer the following questions:

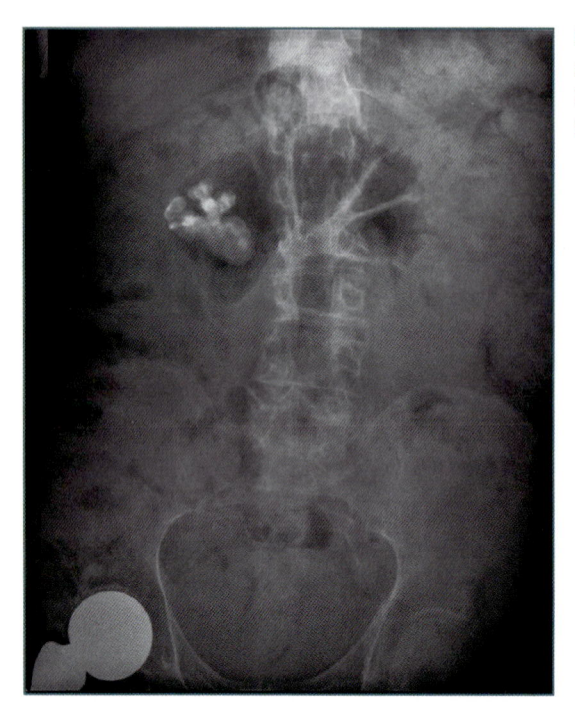

Fig 1.18: KUB radiograph of a 35-year-old male who presented to A&E with acute left loin to groin pain & urine positive for haematuria on dipstick.

Q: What are the salient features & the cause of the patient's symptoms?

There is a large calculus projected over the right renal outline consistent with a **staghorn calculus**. The patient has also had a right hip hemiarthroplasty.

Q: What percentage of renal calculi are radio-opaque?

Approximately **90%** of renal calculi **are radio-opaque**.

Q: What is the optimal imaging technique for suspected renal colic?

A low dose **unenhanced CT KUB** generates a similar radiation dose as a conventional IVU. CT KUB is also **more sensitive & specific than IVU** in the detection of renal calculi.

Furthermore a CT KUB can **assist diagnosis** of alternate pathology such as a **leaking AAA or appendicitis** (Fig 1.19).

Most centres perform CT KUB as a 1st line investigation, but USS & IVU are still performed where this facility is not available.

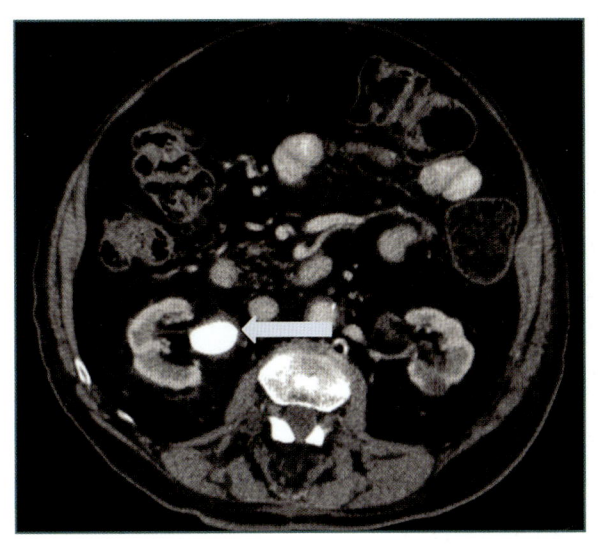

Fig 1.19: CECT demonstrating a right renal staghorn calculus.

> ### REMEMBER
> Remember that there are 3 common sites where renal calculi cause obstruction, so take care to analyse them carefully:
>
> - Pelvic-uretric junction.
> - Site where ureters cross the pelvic brim.
> - Vesico-ureteric junction.
>
> Remember that 10% of renal calculi are radio-lucent.

Case 13:

Study this radiograph & answer the following questions:

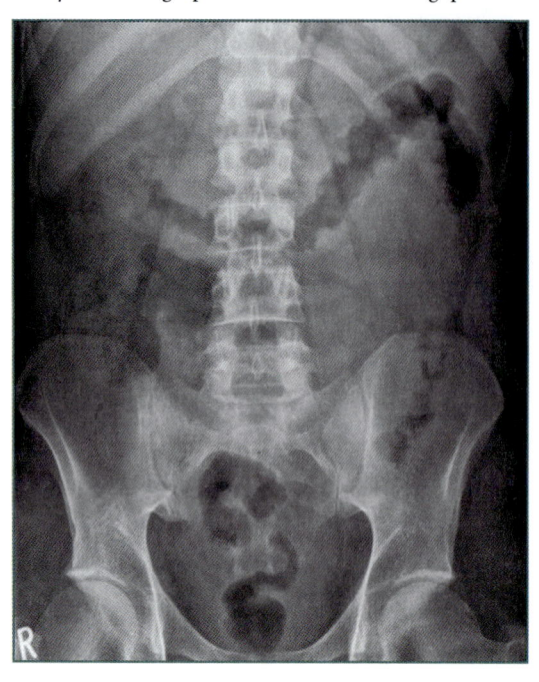

Fig 1.20: AXR of a 25-year-old female admitted to the ward with a tender abdomen & raised inflammatory markers.

Q: What are the salient features?

The transverse colon & descending colon are thick walled with identations consistent with 'thumb printing'. There is no evidence of obstruction or perforation.

Q: What is the significance of this?

Thumb printing indicates that the bowel wall is oedematous. This is commonly due to:
- IBD (usually UC) as in this case.
- Ischaemia.
- Pseudomembranous colitis.

In cases of IBD, it is important to look for radiological features that indicate associated intestinal & extra-intestinal complications e.g. gallstones, renal stones, sacroiliitis & toxic megacolon.

Q: What further imaging should be performed?

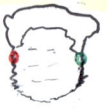

Whilst the patient is symptomatic, serial AXRs should be performed to monitor the possible development of toxic megacolon. This is a complication of UC that requires emergency surgery to prevent bowel perforation. CECT may also be performed in some circumstances to exclude localised perforation.

COMPUTED TOMOGRAPHY

CT allows tomograms (slices through the body) to be acquired & processed to generate 3D representations. Modern multidetector helical CT scanners are comprised of a gantry, which houses thousands of detectors positioned in a stationary ring, an x-ray tube, sliding table & computer. The patient is positioned in the gantry & the relevant body part is then 'scanned'. As the patient moves through the scanner, the x-ray tube rotates 360° around the patient in a continuous manner. The x-ray beam is attenuated differentially by body tissues & the emerging x-rays are detected by the detectors within the gantry. Data are acquired in the form of a continuous ribbon of contiguous slices collected by each detector. These data are then integrated by the computer & reconstructed for viewing as familiar images. Helical scanning allows for volumes of data to be acquired rapidly, in a single breath-hold. These data may be reconstructed, allowing sagittal, coronal & axial views.

Advances in CT technology have been significant. CT angiography has replaced invasive arterial catheterisation & virtual colonoscopy allows effective screening for colorectal cancer. Staging of malignancies are routinely performed, biopsies, nerve blocks & drainage procedures may also be performed with CT guidance. The main disadvantage is the high dose of ionising radiation required to produce such high quality images (Table 1.4).

Table 1.4: CT radiation doses for common body sites.

CT Site	Typical Effective Dose (mSV)*	Equivalent Number of CXRs	Equivalent Natural Background Radiation Dose
Head	2	100	10 months
Chest	8	400	3.6 years
Abdomen / Pelvis	10	500	4.5 years

* Most diagnostic medical exposures are expressed in millisieverts (mSV).

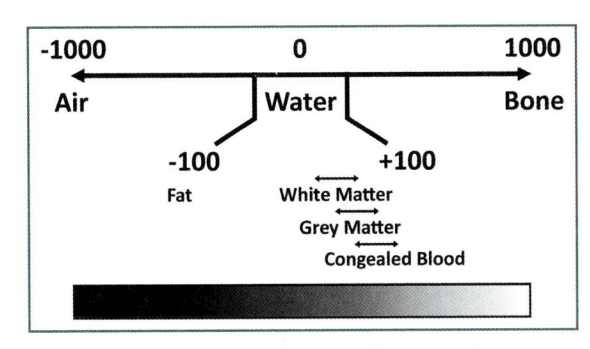

Fig 1.21: Windowing & the Hounsfield Scale.

The dataset acquired is displayed on a monitor, in a greyscale that reflects the densities of body organs & tissues. The density of an object is compared to water & allocated a **Hounsfield Unit (HU)**. The Hounsfield Scale (Fig 1.21) defines water as 0HU, air as -1000HU & cortical bone at +1000HU. Most soft tissues lie between -100HU & +100HU. The greyscale on the display monitor can resolve up to 256 shades of grey, however the human eye can only decipher up to 30. For this reason, images are 'windowed' to narrow or widen the scale depending on the region of interest. For example to demonstrate bony abnormalities, a range of +400HU to +1000HU is chosen & the greyscale accordingly adjusted. Changing the window allows differentiation of the tissues of interest, by altering image brightness & contrast. Window settings therefore include:

Window Setting	Indication
Lung	Parenchymal abnormalities, pneumothoraces & pleural disease (Fig 1.22).
Mediastinal	Assessment of mediastinal structures including lymph nodes (Fig 1.22).
Bone	Focal bony deposits, fractures & degenerative changes (Fig 1.22).
Abdomen	Assessment of solid viscera (Fig 1.22).

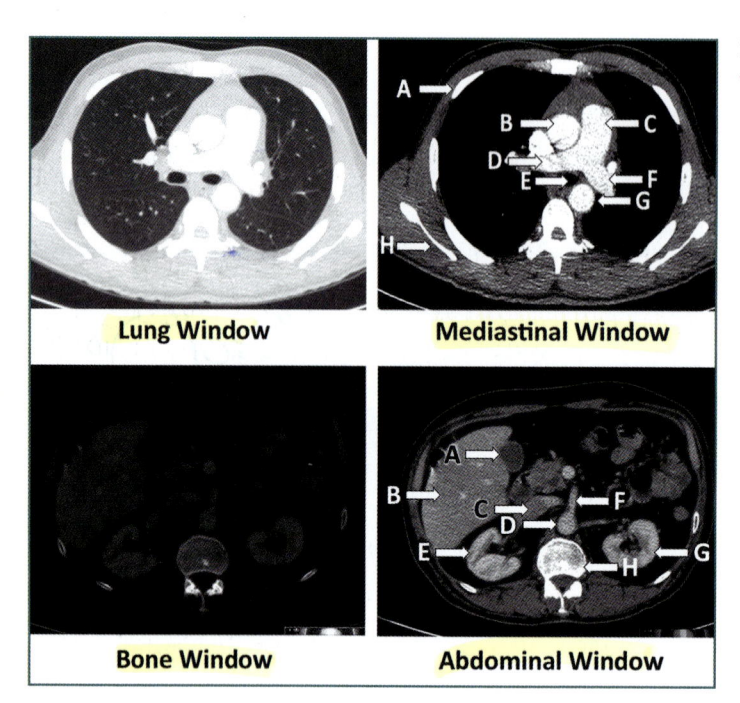

Fig 1.22: Example CT window settings.

Q: What are the structures labelled in the mediastinal & abdominal windows (Fig 1.22)?

Label	Mediastinal	Abdominal
A	Rib	Gallbladder
B	Ascending Aorta	Liver
C	Pulmonary Artery Trunk	IVC
D	Right Pulmonary Artery	Aorta
E	Trachea	Right Kidney
F	Left Pulmonary Artery	SMA
G	Descending Aorta	Left Kidney
H	Right Scapula	L2 Vertebra Body

Protocols:

Depending on the clinical concern, a number of CT protocols may be used (Table 1.5). Most CT scans require IV contrast to assess solid organs & oral contrast for stomach & bowel. Unenhanced scans (no contrast medium) are obtained primarily to look for abnormal calcification, commonly in the renal tract. Unenhanced scans are also used in patients with impaired renal function when contrast is contraindicated. Diabetic patients should stop metformin for 48 hours after contrast due to the risk of lactic acidosis. The only absolute contraindication to CT is pregnancy.

Table 1.5: Common CT protocols for corresponding clinical concerns.

- Arterial phase 30s
- Portal venous phase 90s
- Collecting/ureters/bladder 15min.

Clinical Concern	Protocol
Renal Colic	Unenhanced low dose CT KUB.
Pulmonary Embolus	CT Pulmonary Angiography.
Perforation, Appendicitis, Diverticulitis & Collections	CECT: Obtained 90 seconds after contrast in the portal venous phase. If the patient is well & not NBM, oral contrast may also be useful.
Aortic Aneurysm Rupture & Dissection	CT Angiography.
Trauma	CECT: Obtained in the arterial phase (30 seconds after contrast) to assess vascular injury & in the portal venous phase to assess organ injury.
Colonic Neoplasm	CT Pneumocolon: The bowel is prepared as for colonoscopy & inflated with air through a rectal catheter.
Renal Tract Pathology	CT IVU: Initial unenhanced images (essentially a KUB) are taken to look for calcification. These are followed by contrast enhanced images in the portal venous phase to assess the kidney parenchyma for focal lesions. Finally, an image is taken 15 minutes later to highlight the collecting system, ureters & bladder.

Systematic Interpretation of Computed Tomography Scans

System	Explanation
Patient Details	Check that it is the correct patient's images, noting their name, hospital number, age, sex & ethnic background.
CT Details	Check the date of the film & describe the projection.
Protocol	The protocol is specific to the clinical question. Check whether the patient has had IV or oral contrast, look at the phase of the scan. Decide if the scan is unenhanced or enhanced. Abdominal CECT scans in the portal venous phase will fill & brighten the IVC, portal & hepatic veins, renal veins, SMV & IMV. Abdominal CECT scans in the arterial phase will fill & brighten the aorta more than the veins.

Handwritten annotations at top: Protocol/projection → Organs → Bowel → Free air/fluid/collect → Vessels + LN, OTHER: Bone, Lung, Q.

System	Explanation
Organs	Scroll through each solid organ systematically. With CECT images, ensure that all organs enhance uniformly with no hypoattenuating lesions or solid masses. Check that each organ has clean fat around it. 'Stranding' of fat adjacent to an organ implies inflammation.
Bowel	It is useful to follow bowel starting from the rectum. Check the calibre of the bowel for obstruction. If the bowel is abnormally dilated look for a **'transition point'** or cause for obstruction e.g. mass / stricture. Sometimes a transition point can't be found, but the level of obstruction is still useful e.g. RIF / pelvis. Small bowel is difficult to follow, note if it is dilated or fluid filled. Check the bowel wall thickness for oedema or the presence of gas (pneumotosis intestinalis – best seen on lung windows).
Free Air	Changing to a lung window also allows visualisation of air throughout the abdomen & thorax. Look for small locules of extraluminal gas indicating bowel perforation. Check carefully around the liver & falciform ligament. Check In the thorax for a pneumothorax.
Free Fluid & Collections *(handwritten: Serous 0-20, Blood 30-45, Clot 60-100)*	Check for fluid around the liver, in the paracolic gutters & pelvis. Check the density of any fluid for haemoperitoneum. Serous fluid will be approximately 0-20HU, acute blood 30-45HU & coagulated blood 60-100HU. Check for abscesses or walled-off collections.
Vessels	Check the phase of the CECT scan. Check for filling defects consistent with thrombus. With arterial phase CECT scans, check for contrast extravasations e.g. leaking AAA.
Lymph Nodes	In the thorax check the axillae, mediastinum & hila for lymphadenopathy >1cm in the short axis of the lymph node. In the abdomen, check along the aorta, coeliac axis, porta hepatis & inguinal regions.
Bones	Always change to the bone window to look for fractures or metastatic deposits.
Lungs	If the abdomen has been imaged, the lung bases are usually included. Always change to a lung window to look at the lung parenchyma for basal nodules. Check for pleural effusions & consolidation. If the entire chest has been imaged, look for cavities, masses & consolidation. Use the soft tissue window to assess for lymph nodes & pleural disease.
Clinical Question	Always remember the clinical indication for the CT scan. If there is concern regarding perforation look carefully at the abdomen, using the lung window, for locules of gas. If the concern is appendicitis, check the appendix for stranding or a calcified appendicolith. Always provide the radiologist with as much clinical information as possible.

REMEMBER

- Always remember the clinical question that requires answering.
- Remember to use the bone, soft tissue & lung windows in each scan.
- Once you have found an abnormality don't stop searching, keep looking systematically!

COMPUTED TOMOGRAPHY OSCE CASES

Case 14:
Study this image & answer the following questions:

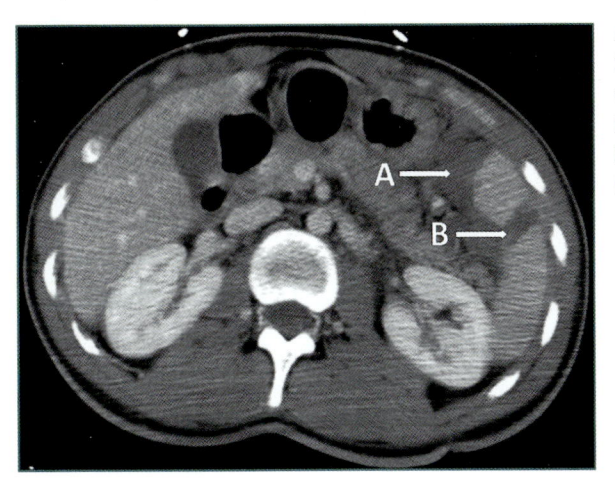

A 27-year-old man was involved in a high speed road traffic accident & brought to A&E. He is haemodynamically stable with bruising over the abdomen (Fig 1.23).

Q: What type of investigation is shown here?

A CECT axial image of the abdomen at the level of L2. The image has been acquired in the portal venous phase as the contrast in the IVC is equal or brighter than the contrast in the aorta. In an arterial phase CECT, the contrast is brighter in the aorta.

Q: What are the salient abnormalities labelled A & B?

There is a hypoattenuating region in the lower pole of the spleen, consistent with a complete laceration (B). There is associated free fluid surrounding the spleen, consistent with subcapsular haematoma (A).

Q: How is this injury graded?

Splenic injury is graded I–V (Table 1.6). Grades I–III are classified according to the extent of parenchymal injury & associated haematoma. Grades IV–V are classified according to the extent of parenchymal injury only. This case is a grade III injury. Remember that the true extent of any pathology may never completely assessed on a single image.

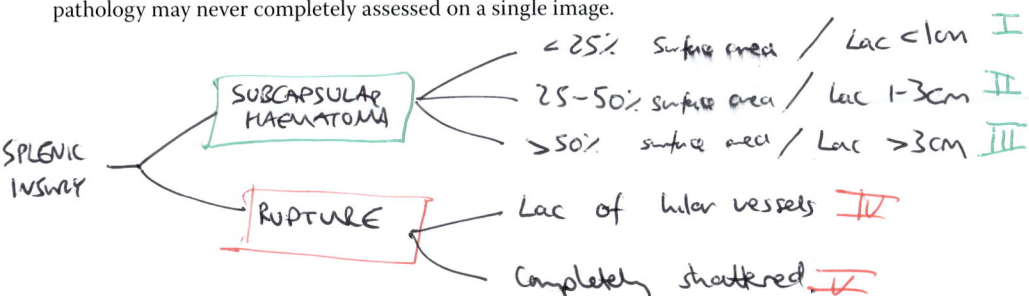

Table 1.6: Splenic injury grading.

Grade	Haematoma	Parenchymal Injury
I	Subcapsular <25% of Surface Area	Laceration <1cm Deep
II	Subcapsular 25–50% of Surface Area	Laceration 1–3cm Deep
III	Subcapsular >50% of Surface Area	Laceration >3cm Parenchymal Depth
IV	-	Laceration Involving Hilar Vessels >25% Devascularisation
V	-	Completely Shattered Spleen

Q: What are the treatment options for splenic injury?

The patient first requires ATLS resuscitation & stabilisation. Grades I–II are more likely to be treated conservatively, whilst grades IV–V require surgery. Up to 90% of stable patients can be managed conservatively or with arterial embolisation. Treatment options therefore include:

- Clinical Observation.
- Arterial Embolisation.
- Splenorrhaphy.
- Splenectomy.

REMEMBER

- The spleen is the most frequently injured intraperitoneal organ in blunt abdominal trauma.
- There is a high association with additional injury:
    - Lower Rib Fractures   45%
    - Solid Viscera / Bowel Injury   30%
    - Left Kidney   10%
    - Left Hemidiaphragm   5%
    - Other   10%
- 25% of left rib fractures have an associated splenic injury.
- 25% of left renal injuries have an associated splenic injury.
- CECT is diagnostically accurate in 95% of cases.
- A high attenuation area adjacent to the spleen, which is isodense to arterial blood, is likely to represent active haemorrhage.

Case 15:

A young man is assaulted, sustaining injuries to his head & neck. On admission to A&E he is intubated with a GCS of 6. After the patient is ATLS resuscitated & stabilised, an urgent CT scan of the head is obtained.

Study this image & answer the following questions:

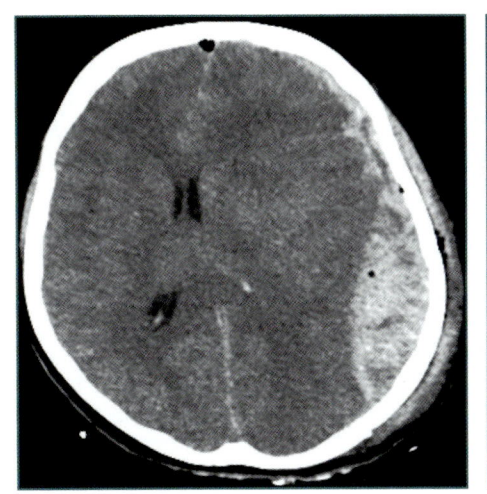

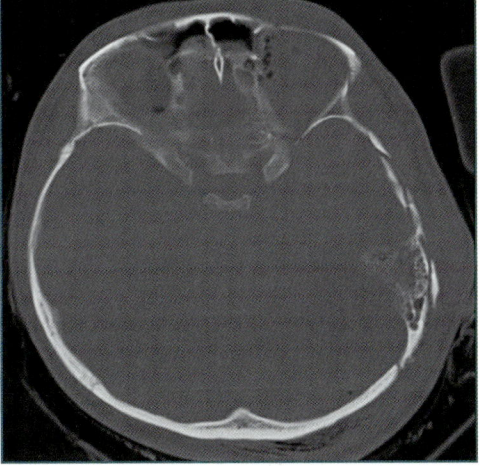

Fig 1.24: CT scans of a young man who sustained head injuries after being assaulted.

Q: What do the above CT images demonstrate?

Left Image: There is a lentiform area of high attenuation situated in the left frontoparietal region. This is consistent with an acute extradural haemorrhage. A further rim of subdural blood is seen extending anteriorly. There is mass effect with midline shift & left lateral ventricle compression. There are small locules of gas within the collection. There is associated soft tissue swelling.

Right Image: This is an axial CT image viewed on a bone window. There is an extensive comminuted fracture through the left temporal bone, extending to the skull base through the mastoid air cells.

Q: What would you do next?

This patient requires urgent neurosurgical input. Evacuation of the extradural haematoma will avoid a rapid increase in ICP & subsequent brain herniation.

Case 16:

Study this image & answer the following questions:

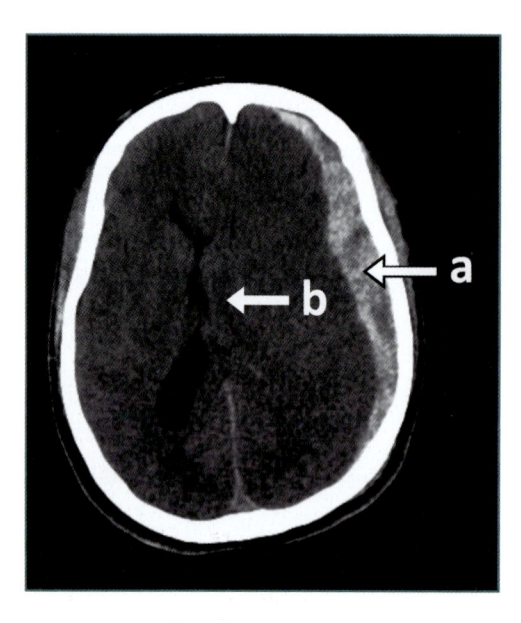

An elderly female is brought into casualty with a reduced GCS & headache. There is a clinical history of a fall 3 weeks earlier (Fig 1.25).

Q: What are the salient features?

There is crescenteric high attenuation overlying the left cerebral hemisphere, consistent with left subdural haematoma (a). There is mass effect with midline shift & effacement of the left lateral ventricle (b).

Q: What is the prognosis?

Acute subdural haemorrhage is associated with a high mortality (35–50%). Although the haemorrhage is venous & collects more slowly than extradural haemorrhage, there is greater underlying parenchymal injury associated with the mechanism of injury.

Q: What are the differences between an extradural & subdural haemorrhage?

These may be classified as follows:

Classification	Extradural	Subdural
Cause	Trauma to the middle meningeal artery (90%) or resulting in a venous bleed (10%).	Trauma to bridging veins due to shearing forces. This is commonly seen in elderly patients with a history of falls. It may also be seen in infants due to non-accidental injury.
Location	Blood fills the extradural space between the inner skull & tight dura mater.	Blood fills the space between the dura & arachnoid mater.
Shape	• Lentiform. • Blood may cross the midline but not a suture line (unless a diastatic fracture is present through the suture).	• Cresenteric. • Blood may cross suture lines but not the midline.
Fracture	>85% associated with skull fracture.	<1% associated with a fracture.
Prognosis	With urgent evacuation, even a large bleed may have a better outcome than a subdural haemorrhage.	Mortality is higher than extradural haemorrhage due to the varied clinical presentation & damage to underlying brain parenchyma. Furthermore, the rate of haematoma formation may be more rapid than subdural haemorrage.

REMEMBER

Acute blood on a CT head is bright white. As blood ages it becomes darker & this may be seen in subdural haemorrhage as follows:

Acute Subdural Haematoma	< 1 week	Bright White
Subacute Subdural Haematoma	1–3 weeks	Isodense to Brain Parenchyma
Chronic Subdural Haematoma	> 3 weeks	Hypodense to Brain Parenchyma

Case 17:

Study this image & answer the following questions:

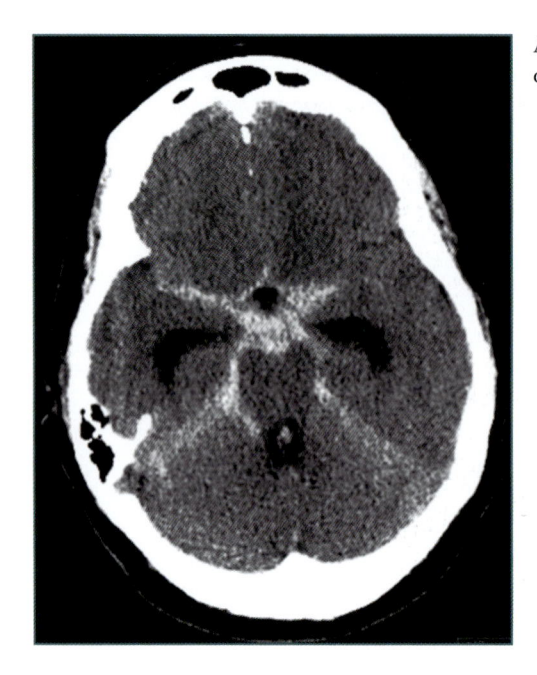

A 35-year-old man presented with a sudden onset headache & collapse (Fig 1.26).

Q: What are the 2 salient findings?

There is **acute haemorrhage** present in the **subarachnoid spaces**. There is associated **dilatation of the temporal horns of the lateral ventricles**, indicating the development of **obstructive hydrocephalus**.

Q: What are the causes of subarachnoid haemorrhage?

Approximately **80% are due to rupture of an aneurysm**. The remaining causes may be classified as follows:

- **Congenital aneurysm** rupture e.g. berry aneurysm.
- **Aquired aneurysm** rupture e.g. arteriosclerotic, infective, inflammatory & traumatic.
- **Arteriovenous malformation**.
- **Hypertensive haemorrhage**.
- **Bleeding diasthesis** e.g. warfarin.
- **Tumour.**

Case 18:

Study this image & answer the following questions:

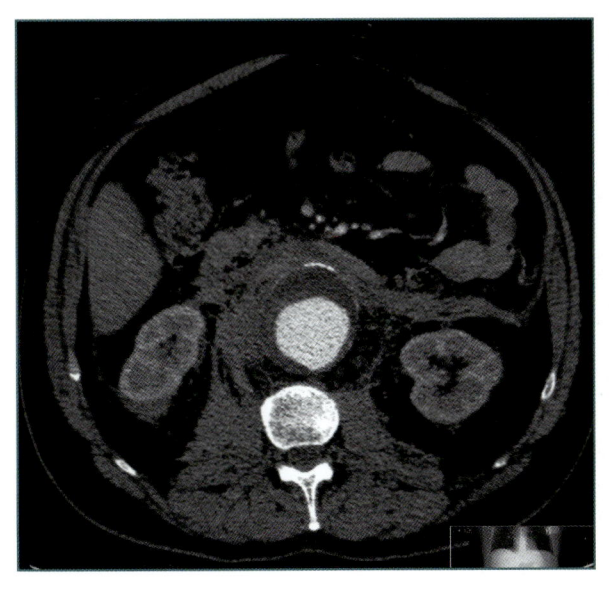

A 70-year-old gentleman was admitted with abdominal pain & hypotension (Fig 1.27).

Q: What are the salient CT imaging findings?

This is an axial arterial phase CECT image, showing an aneurysmal abdominal aorta. The contrast is high density in the aorta, which is surrounded by thrombus & a high density calcified wall. There is mixed density fluid surrounding the aorta consistent with rupture of the aneurysm.

Q: What are the repair options?

After ALS resuscitation & stabilisation of the patient, there are 2 repair methods:

1. **Open Repair:** This involves a GA & laparotomy (*see operative surgery chapter*).
2. **Endovascular Repair:** This involves a femoral venous cut-down & insertion of a stent graft under radiological guidance. As this may be performed without a GA, there is a reduced intensive care stay, quicker recovery & shorter hospital stay.

Case 19:

Study this image & answer the following questions:

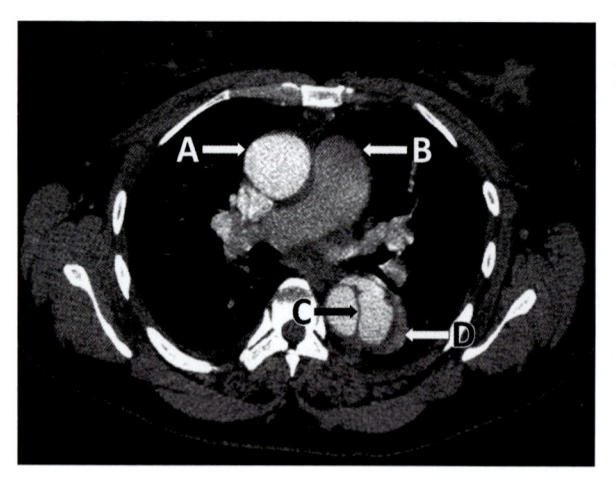

A 45-year-old male presented with central chest pain radiating to the back (Fig 1.28).

Q: What is the study above?

This is an axial image from a CT angiogram through the thorax at the level of the main pulmonary artery trunk (B). Contrast is present in both the ascending (A) & descending aorta.

Q: What are the salient findings?

There is a hypoattenuating 'line' through the descending aorta (C). This represents a dissection flap & is consistent with acute aortic dissection. Further soft tissue density is seen lateral to the wall of the descending aorta consistent with haematoma (D).

Q: What are the risk factors for aortic dissection?

- **Hypertension** (80% are associated with hypertension).
- **Collagen disorders** e.g. Marfan's & Ehlers-Danlos Syndrome.
- **Pregnancy** (50% of dissections in young patients are in pregnant women).
- **Aortic coarctation**.
- **Trauma**.

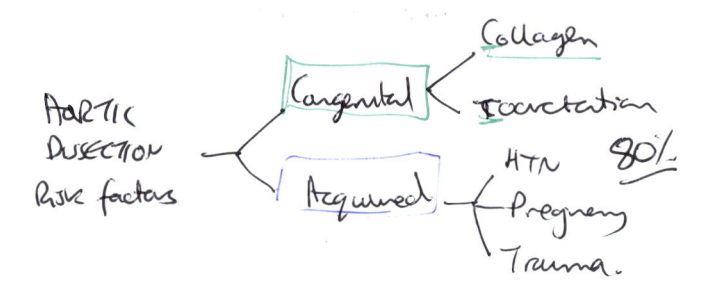

Q: How is aortic dissection classified?

There are 2 commonly used classifications i.e. **DeBakey (types I–III)** & **Stanford (Type A & B)**. The Stanford classification is more commonly used & is described below:

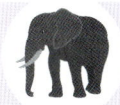

Memory: **Type A** — Affects Ascending Aorta & Arch
Type B — Begins Beyond Brachiocephalic vessels.

Type	Location	Preferred Management
Type A	Affects the ascending aorta & arch (within the initial 4cm of the ascending aorta in 90% of cases)	Surgical
Type B	Descending aorta	Medical

* In both Type A & B it is important to control hypertension.

MAGNETIC RESONANCE IMAGING

MRI works on the principle that hydrogen atoms, ubiquitous in body tissues, will resonate when placed within a strong magnetic field. A brief radio-frequency (RF) gradient is then applied which displaces the proton alignment such that differing amounts of energy are absorbed. When the RF wave is stopped, protons re-align with the magnetic field & emit different levels of radio-wave energy. This energy signal is detected & processed by a computer algorithm, similar to CT, in order to generate cross-sectional images.

MRI is the imaging modality of choice for musculoskeletal, neurological, some vascular & pelvic imaging. MRI is always preferable to those investigations that carry a high radiation hazard, although it is still uncertain as to the effects of MRI during the 1st trimester of pregnancy.

Contraindications for MRI include:

- Cardiac Pacemakers
- Cochlear Implants
- Neurostimulators
- Some Cerebral Aneurysm Clips
- Metal Shrapnel
- Metallic Heart Valves
- Some Surgical Prostheses (require a 6 week post-operative period for reinforcing fibrosis prior to scanning).

As with CT imaging, contrast can be injected to highlight blood vessels, inflammation & malignancy.

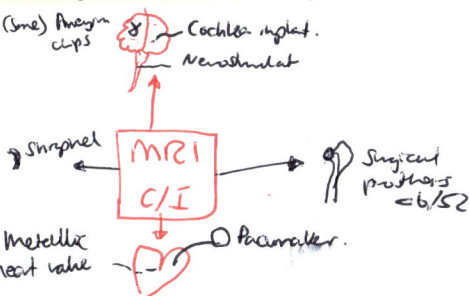

The advantages & disadvantages of MRI include:

Advantages	Disadvantages
No Ionising Radiation	Long Scan Times
Excellent Contrast Resolution	Patients May Experience Claustrophobia
Multiplanar Capabilities	Noisy Scanners
MR Angiography / Venography	Expensive
(do not require arterial cannulation)	Availability

T1 & T2 Weighted Sequences

Most tissues are differentiated by their T1 & T2 relaxation times. T1 measures the speed that protons exchange energy with their surrounding structures. T2 measures the speed that tissues lose their magnetisation.

In general: T1 sequences allow for anatomy delineation.

T2 sequences characterise pathology.

Depending on the clinical circumstance, many other additional sequences may be used e.g. fat-suppression or fluid suppression. The ability of MRI to characterise soft tissues so well is due to the differences in proton densities between different tissues & the differences in the amount of fat & water content that tissues have.

T1 & T2 weighted sequences accentuate the properties of protons in different tissues, assigning a high, intermediate or low signal on the final processed image.

A pulse sequence consists of 2 main components:

- **TR** (Repetition Time): The time from the application of 1 RF pulse to the application of the next RF pulse.
- **TE** (Echo Time): The time from the application of the RF pulse to the peak of the signal returned after the RF pulse is stopped.

Weighting	TE	TR	Fat	Fluid
T1	Short	Short	Bright	Dark
T2	Long	Long	Bright	Bright

Systematic Interpretation of Magnetic Resonance Imaging Scans

MRI does not easily lend itself to systematic interpretation in the same manner as the previously discussed imaging modalities. Here is a simple guide:

System	Explanation
Patient Details	Check that it is the correct patient's images, noting their name, hospital number, age, sex & ethnic background.
Image Details	Check the date of the film.
Weighting	Decide if the image is T1 or T2 weighted (Table 1.7 & Fig 1.29).
Anatomy	Systematically identify anatomy in a similar manner to that described for CT. Comment on associated abnormalities.

Table 1.7: Differences in tissue appearance between T1 & T2 weighted images.

Weighting	High Signal (Bright)	Low Signal (Dark)
T1	Fat Bone Marrow *High on both* Protein Some Blood Products Melanin Heavy Metals (including gadolinium)	Fluid Collagen Ligaments *Low on both* Tendons Cortical Bone
T2	Fluid Protein *High on both* Fat	Flowing Blood (flow voids) Collagen Ligaments *Low on both* Tendons Cortical Bone Air

Note: Ligaments, tendons & cortical bone are low signal on all pulse sequences. This is because their hydrogen ions are fixed & cannot resonate, therefore they cannot produce any signal.

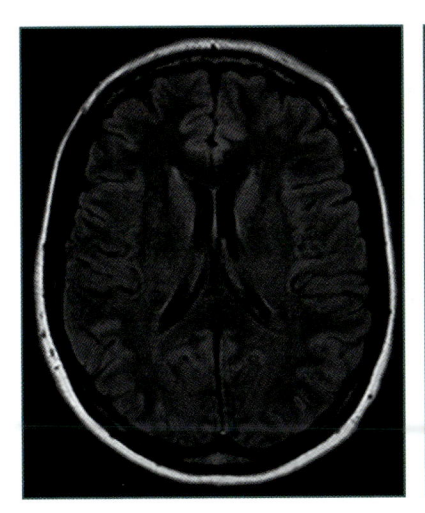

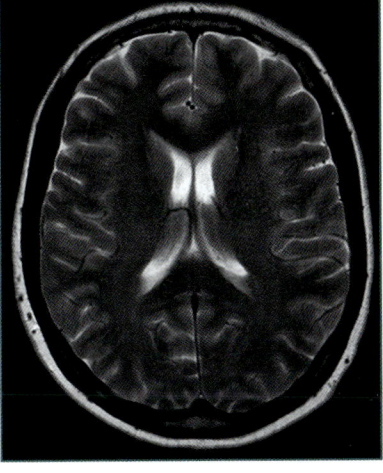

Fig 1.29: MRI brain. Left = T1 weighted (CSF = dark, fat = bright). Right = T2 weighted (CSF & fat = bright).

Magnetic Resonance Imaging OSCE Cases

Case 20:

Study this image & answer the following questions:

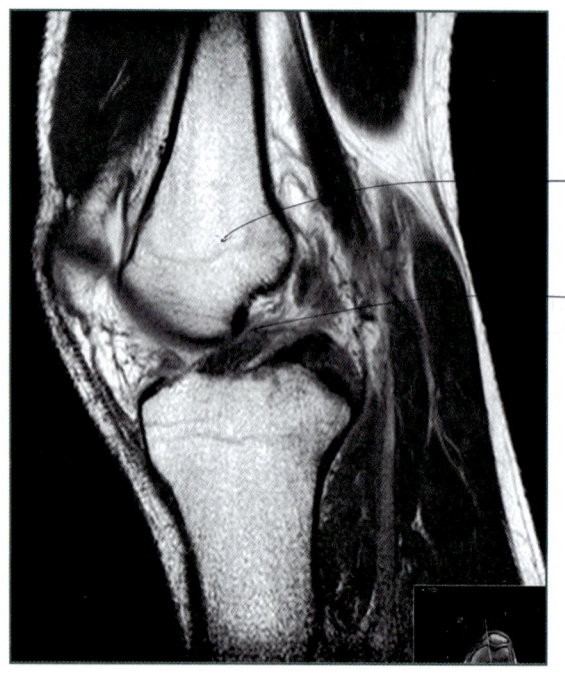

A 19-year-old man sustained a knee injury whilst playing football (Fig 1.30).

Q: What are the salient features?

This is a T1 weighted sagittal MRI of the knee showing disruption of the ACL fibres, consistent with a tear.

Note: The fatty marrow is bright on this T1 weighted image

Q: What is the mechanism of injury?

An ACL tear is the most common ligamentous injury of the knee.

There is usually a history of twisting, valgus impaction, internal rotation & hyperextension of the knee. The patient may describe an audible 'pop' & the knee giving way.

Q: What other radiological signs may be present in this injury?

- Haemarthrosis
- Bone Contusion
- Meniscal Tear (65% are lateral) — *65% ACL tears assoc. c̄ Lateral meniscal tear*
- Medial Collateral Ligament Tear.

REMEMBER (Fig 1.31):
Cruciate ligaments are imaged best via MRI. Left = intact ACL. Middle = intact PCL. Right = PCL tear.

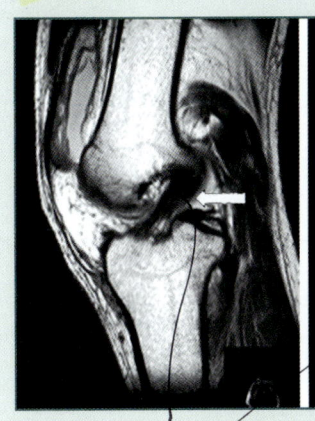

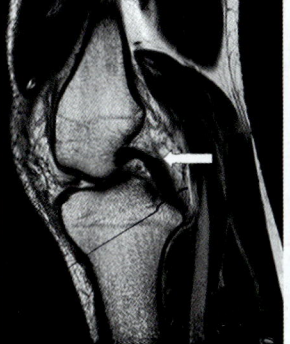

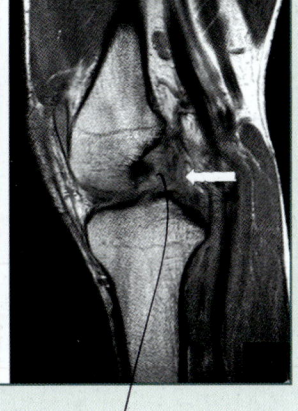

Continuous low signal — *Disrupted low signal.*

Case 21:

Study this image & answer the following questions:

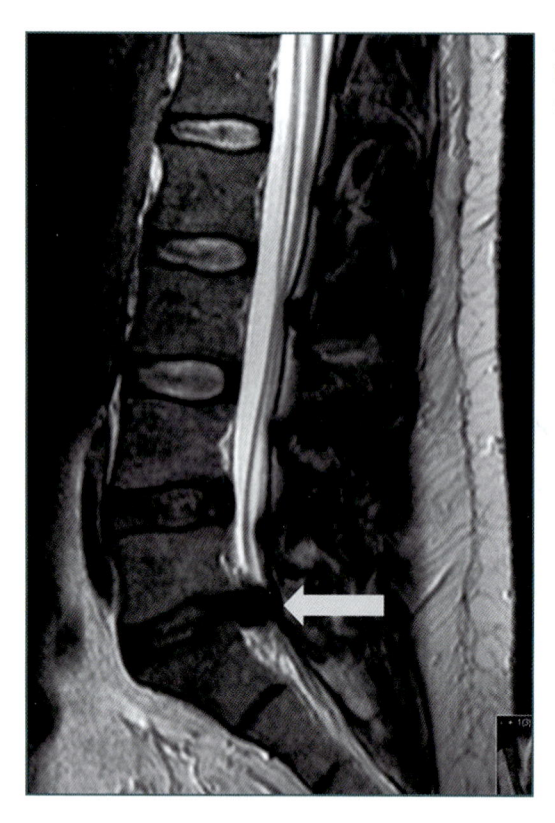

A 50-year-old male presented to A&E with bilateral leg weakness & urinary retention (Fig 1.32).

Q: What investigation is shown?

This is a T2 weighted sagittal MRI of the spine. Note that the CSF is bright.

Q: What are the salient features?

There is herniation of the lumbar intervertebral disc at the level of L5/S1, causing compression of the cauda equina.

Q: What would you do next?

This is a surgical emergency requiring urgent decompression of the spinal canal, usually within 48 hours. In the case of a herniated lumbar disc laminectomy & discectomy may be performed.

Case 22:

Study this image & answer the following questions:

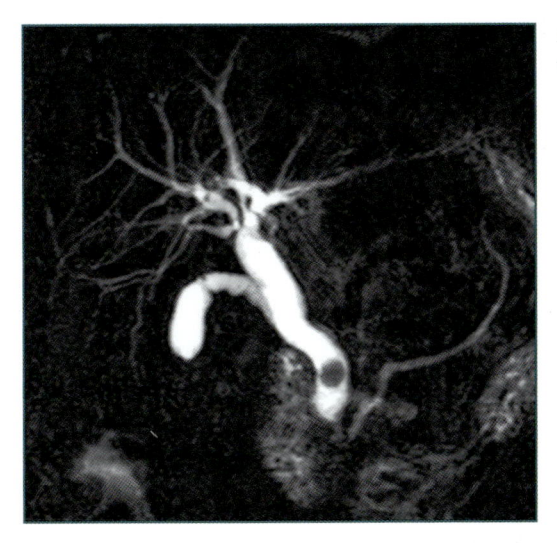

A 45-year-old woman presented to A&E with RUQ pain (Fig 1.33).

Q: What investigation is shown?

This is a magnetic resonance cholangiopancreatogram (MRCP). This study requires the patient to fast for 6 hours prior to the study, no contrast is injected as this is a heavily weighted T2 sequence designed to delineate the intra & extra-hepatic biliary system.

Q: What are the salient features?

There is a rounded filling defect in the distal common bile duct consistent with an impacted gallstone.

Case 23:

Study this image & answer the following questions:

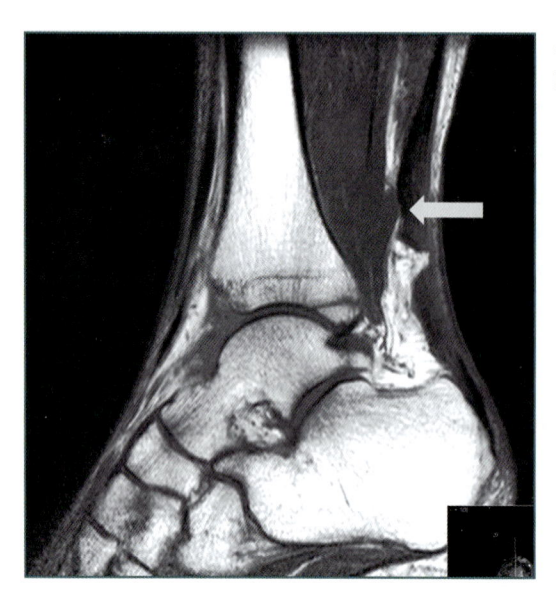

A 38-year-old man presented with acute pain around his ankle (Fig 1.34).

Q: What are the salient features?

This is a T1 weighted sagittal MRI of the ankle. There is discontinuity of the Achilles tendon (arrowed) consistent with complete rupture.

Q: What are the treatment options?

Achilles tendon rupture may be treated non-surgically or surgically depending on the size of the gap between the 2 ruptured ends. Both treatments require months of immobilisation with a plaster cast, positioning the foot in plantar flexion. Serial casts may also be required to gradually reposition the foot, depending on the pattern of injury. Physiotherapy is also required.

Case 24:

Study this image & answer the following questions:

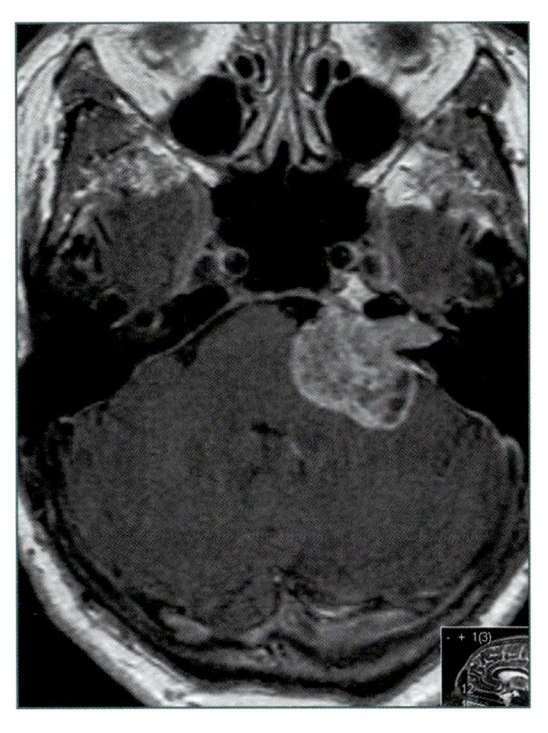

A 65-year-old male presents with progressive hearing loss (Fig 1.35).

Q: What investigation is shown?

This is a dedicated internal auditory meatus protocol MRI.

Q: What are the salient findings?

There is an enhancing mass in the left internal auditory meatus, consistent with an acoustic neuroma.

Case 25:

Study this image & answer the following questions:

A young man presents to A&E with a decreased level of consciousness & history of progressive headaches (Fig 1.36).

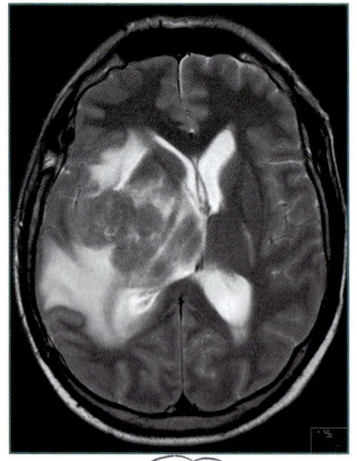

Image A: T2

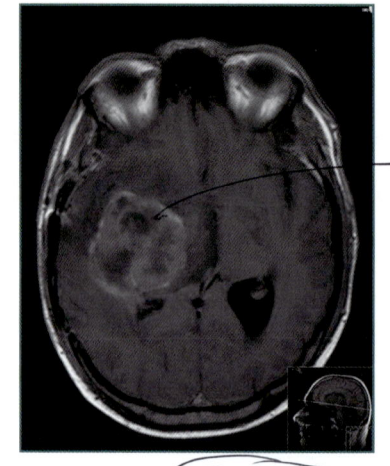

Image B: T1 + GAD

- Large mass R frontoparietal which enhances c̄ contrast
- significant mass effect
- marked oedema

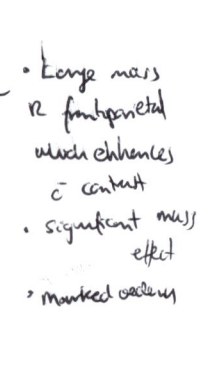

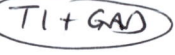

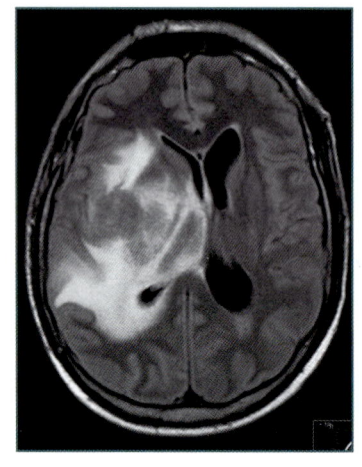

Image C: FLAIR

Q: What MRI sequences are shown?

A: T2 MRI (CSF is bright).

B: T1 MRI with gadolinium.

C: FLAIR sequence (fluid suppression results in the CSF signal being suppressed, hence the bright signal represents true oedema).

Q: What is the likely diagnosis?

There is a large mass in the right frontoparietal region which enhances with contrast. There is significant mass effect with midline shift & compression of the right lateral ventricle. There is marked oedema surrounding the mass. The most likely diagnosis is a glioblastoma multiforme.

FLAIR = fluid attenuation inversion recovery
→ v. long TE + TR times → suppresses CSF so as to bring out periventricular lesions.

CHAPTER 2
CRITICAL CARE

BH Miranda
N Sivasathan
BS Ghoorun

CHAPTER CONTENTS

Anaesthetics

Arterial Blood Gases

Burns

Pulmonary Artery Catheters

Cardiopulmonary Bypass

Head Injury & Cerebral Autoregulation

Nutrition

Renal Failure

Renal Replacement Therapy

Fluids

Respiratory Failure

ALI & ARDS

Oxygen Therapy & Mechanical Ventilation

Pancreatitis

SIRS, SEPSIS & MODS

ICU Admission

Brainstem Death

ANAESTHETICS

Q: What is anaesthesia? What is an anaesthetic?

- **Anaesthesia** is a noun, meaning total / partial loss of sensation.
- **Anaesthetics** are agents that induce anaesthesia.

Q: What different types of anaesthesia do you know of?

Type	Explanation
Topical	Render part of a body surface insensitive to noxious stimuli e.g. cornea, nasal passages & throat. Preparations include creams, ointments & sprays.
Local (LA)	A small area of the body is rendered insensitive to noxious stimuli without loss of consciousness e.g. field block for lumps & bumps.
Regional	A larger area of the body is rendered insensitive to noxious stimuli without loss of consciousness. For example, a brachial plexus block may be used to operate on the upper limb. Other examples include Bier's Block & spinal anaesthesia.
General (GA)	Considered to have 3 primary goals. The patient is rendered **insensitive to noxious stimuli – reversible loss of consciousness – muscle relaxation.**

Q: What factors influence the type of anaesthetic to be used?

- Procedure duration i.e. long procedures are likely to require GA.
- Procedure location e.g. extensor tendon repair (LA / Regional) v. oesophagogastrectomy (GA).
- ASA status.
- Surgeon / anaesthetist preference.
- Patient preference.

Q: How do local anaesthetic agents work?

- LAs may be classified as amides e.g. lidocaine, bupivacaine & prilocaine, or esters e.g. cocaine & procaine.
- They cause **reversible** inhibition of cell membrane **Na$^+$-channels**, hence preventing the generation & propagation of action potentials. As Na$^+$-channels are proteins, the greater the protein affinity of the LA, the greater its efficacy. Furthermore, LAs with greater lipid solubility are more potent & have a longer duration of action.
- LAs exist in 2 forms, namely cationic & ionised base, **affected by the pH of their surroundings**. In an acidic environment, LA molecules are unable to penetrate the cell membrane & this is why they are ineffective in abscesses.
- NaHCO$_3$⁻ may be added to LA preparations to increase pH & therefore increase LA efficacy.

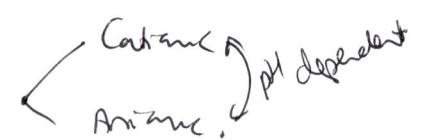

Q: What are the possible complications associated with using LA?

All are consequential to membrane destabilisation; hence the nervous system is primarily affected. At higher doses, the cardiovascular system may be affected. Complications are commonly related to errors of dose or accidental intravascular administration (hence it is important to aspirate prior to injection to ensure that a vessel has not inadvertently been entered).

Complications may therefore be classified as neurological or cardiovascular as follows:

Classification	Examples
Neurological *Low Dose*	Perioral & Glossitic Paraesthesia, Light-Headedness, Dizziness, Drowsiness, Seizures, Tinnitus, Tremors, Confusion & Coma.
Cardiovascular *HIGH Dose*	Bradycardia, Hypotension, Ventricular Fibrillation & Asystole.

Q: You suspect that a patient on the ward has lidocaine toxicity. How would you manage this?

An ALS approach is required. Specific management is primarily supportive. Measures include: securing airway, ensuring adequate oxygenation, IV access & hydration. Seizure control may be achieved with diazepam / midazolam (phenytoin is ineffective). ECG & cardiac monitoring may be necessary as arrhythmias such as ventricular fibrillation will require defibrillation.

Q: Can you discuss the use of adrenaline with local anaesthetic agents?

Adrenaline produces localised vasoconstriction, decreasing absorption of local anaesthetic from the site of infiltration & improving duration of anaesthesia. It may also be used to reduce blood loss intraoperatively. Furthermore, the skin pallor induced by adrenaline may assist in indicating those areas that have been successfully infiltrated.

Adrenaline should not be used in tissues with end-arteries e.g. digits & penis. It must be used with caution around degloving or flap injuries. This is because vasoconstriction may result in ischaemic necrosis.

Adrenaline is contraindicated in haematoma blocks (for reduction of Colles' Fracture), for which the only acceptable LA is plain prilocaine. Prilocaine undergoes faster hepatic metabolisation & has lower direct neurotoxicity than lidocaine. Beware however, prilocaine may produce methaemoglobinaemia which is of particular concern in children.

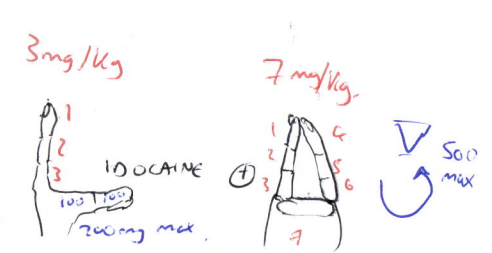

Q: What are the safe maximum doses of LA?

Anaesthetic		Dose (mg / kg)	Maximum Adult Dose (mg)
Lidocaine	Plain	3	200
(short acting)	With Adrenaline	7	500
Bupivacaine	Plain	2	150
(long acting)	With Adrenaline	3	150

Q: What is a Bier's Block, when should it be used & what are important considerations?

This is a type of intravenous regional anaesthesia. It is indicated for limb surgery lasting <1 hour, e.g. carpal tunnel decompression & Dupuytren's Fasciectomy, or when a GA or brachial block cannot be used.

A cannula is first placed in a distal limb vein. The limb is then exsanguinated & a double-cuffed tourniquet is inflated to at least 50mmHg above the $P_{syst.}$. Finally, prilocaine is injected via the cannula.

Systemic toxicity may arise if the tourniquet is released early (i.e. <20 mins). Contraindications for use include patients with sickle cell anaemia or Raynaud's Disease.

Q: What is spinal anaesthesia? What is caudal epidural anaesthesia?

These are types of regional anaesthesia that involve injection into one of the meningeal spaces surrounding the spinal cord. They are useful for surgery below the umbilicus (pelvis, perineum, lower limb) & in children for whom emergency surgery is required, e.g. reduction of incarcerated hernia, but with a contraindication for a GA. Instillation site & duration of action are as follows:

Classification	Instillation Site	Duration of Action
True Spinal / Intrathecal	Subarachnoid Space CSF	Short–Medium
Caudal Epidural	Extradural Space	Potentially Long

Q: In what circumstances would a spinal anaesthetic be useful?

- When GA is contraindicated e.g. patients with severe respiratory disease.
- To reduce the risk of aspiration.
- To achieve patient satisfaction e.g. Caesarean section.
- To achieve localised muscle relaxation e.g. pelvic surgery.
- To provide post-operative analgesia. Epidurals may be left in-situ for around 5 days.
- To prevent anaesthetic drugs crossing the placental circulation. Babies born to mothers having spinal anaesthesia may be more alert that those born to mothers having GA.

Handwritten annotation (mind map):
Complications of spinal
- Insertion: Bleeding/haematoma, infection, neural injury
- Catheter: Block, dislodgement, infection
- Drug: ↓BP, urinary retention
- Removal: haematoma (cord comp/paralysis), headache ∴ Stop LMWH 12h pre-removal

Q: Aside from hypotension & urinary-retention, what are other possible complications of spinal anaesthetics?

Mechanism	Complications
During Insertion	Direct Neural Injury, Bleeding, Haematoma & Headaches.
Due to Catheter	Block, Dislodgement, Infection & Chronic Fibrosis.
During Removal	Haematoma, Cord Compression & Paralysis. Anticoagulants should be stopped prior to removal e.g. LMWH is stopped at least 12 hours prior to removal.

ARTERIAL BLOOD GASES

Q: How is pH calculated?

$pH = -\log_{10}[H^+]$

Q: What processes generate the bulk of the body's H^+?

- Aerobic cellular respiration produces CO_2 as a by-product. This then dissolves in blood via the bicarbonate system & enzyme carbonic anhydrase as follows:

$$CO_2 + H_2O \leftrightarrow H_2CO_3 \leftrightarrow H^+ + HCO_3^-$$

- Anaerobic cellular respiration producing lactic acid.
- Ketone body production e.g. acetone, acetoacetate & β-hydroxybuterate.
- Metabolism of cysteine & methionine (sulphur-containing amino acids).

Q: How does the body cope with alterations in $[H^+]$?

There are a number of mechanisms that are involved:

Mechanism	Explanation
Respiratory	Hyperventilation blows of CO_2 & increases pH. Hypoventilation blows off less CO_2 & decreases pH.
Metabolic	Kidneys may retain or excrete H^+ & HCO_3^-. The liver is involved in the metabolism of ammonia, lactate, ketones & amino acids.
Intracellular	Proteins in cytoplasm.
Extracellular	Bicarbonate system, phosphate system & plasma proteins.

Q: Why are ABGs clinically useful?

They allow assessment of:
- Acid-base balance.
- Oxygenation.
- Removal of by-products e.g. CO_2.
- Electrolytes.

Accordingly, they facilitate the evaluation of efficiency of ventilation, sepsis & organ-failure.

Q: Where would you take an ABG from?

- Radial artery (after doing Allen's Test).
- Brachial artery.
- Ulnar artery.
- Dorsalis pedis.
- Femoral artery.
- Arterial line.

It is better to use a distal artery e.g. radial so that complications e.g. thrombus & aneurysm will not compromise the whole limb. The commonest complication is haematoma, so elevation & pressure are required after the procedure, especially if the patient is on anticoagulants.

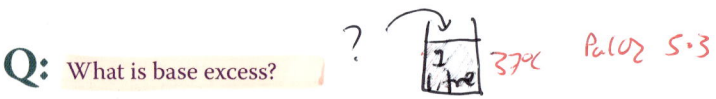

Q: What is base excess?

Base excess is defined as the amount of acid or alkali required to return 1L of blood to a normal pH at 37°C with a P_aCO_2 of 5.3kPa. It is useful as it helps to assess metabolic involvement of acid-base imbalances. The reference range is -2 to +2 mmol/L. A value below this normal range is compatible with metabolic acidosis. A value above this normal range is compatible with metabolic alkalosis.

Q: How would you interpret an ABG?

There are 3 components in the description:
1. Acidosis or alkalosis.
2. Respiratory or metabolic.
3. Partial, complete or no compensation. Complete compensation can only have occurred if the pH is within normal limits.

Method:
1. Look at the **pH** & decide if there is an acidosis or alkalosis. Remember that if the pH is normal, this could indicate complete compensation.
2. Look at the P_aCO_2 that may be high, indicating a respiratory acidosis **or** compensation of a metabolic alkalosis. If it is low, this may indicate a respiratory alkalosis **or** compensation of a metabolic acidosis.

3. Look at the **HCO₃-** that may be high, indicating a metabolic alkalosis **or** compensation of a respiratory acidosis. If it is low, this may indicate a metabolic acidosis **or** compensation of a respiratory alkalosis.
4. Look at the **base excess** to complete assessment of the metabolic component.
5. Look at the P_aO_2 & F_iO_2 to complete assessment of the respiratory component, particularly checking for respiratory failure.

Q: Can you describe the acid-base disturbances (A–F) below?

Parameter & Reference Range	pH (7.35-7.45)	P$_a$CO$_2$ (4.5-6kPa)	HCO$_3$- (22-28mEq/L)	Base Excess (-2 to +2)
A	↓	↓	↓	↓
B	↓	↑	↑	Normal
C	↑	↑	↑	↑
D	↑	↓	↓	Normal
E	↓	↑	↓	↓
F	↑	↓	↑	↑

Key: ↓ = below normal reference range. ↑ = above normal reference range.

A: Metabolic acidosis with respiratory compensation (if the P_aCO_2 were normal, this would indicate no compensation).

B: Respiratory acidosis with metabolic compensation (if the HCO$_3$- were normal, this would indicate no compensation).

C: Metabolic alkalosis with respiratory compensation (if the P_aCO_2 were normal, this would indicate no compensation).

D: Respiratory alkalosis with metabolic compensation (if the HCO$_3$- were normal, this would indicate no compensation).

E: Mixed respiratory & metabolic acidosis.

F: Mixed respiratory & metabolic alkalosis.

Q: What are the common causes of acidosis & alkalosis in a surgical patient?

Metabolic Acidosis	Respiratory Acidosis	
Shock	**Pulmonary:**	**Neurological:**
Sepsis	LRTI	Benzodiazepines
DKA	COPD	Head Injury
Aspirin	Pulmonary Embolism	Myasthenia Gravis
Diarrhoea	Pulmonary Oedema	Myopathy
	Fractured Ribs / Flail Chest	

Memory: 'If the fluid comes down, then the pH comes down'.

Metabolic Alkalosis	Respiratory Alkalosis
Diuretics	Anxiety
Hepatic Failure	Pain
Vomiting	Meningitis

Memory: 'If the fluid is comes up, then the pH comes up'.

BURNS

Q: What is a burn injury?

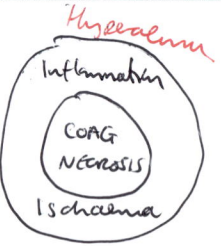

Jackson's Burn Model describes burns as *'tri-zone injuries'* with:
- A central area of *coagulative necrosis* ...
- surrounded by a static area of *inflammation & ischaemia*, ...
- further encircled by an area of *hyperaemia*.

Burn **injury severity** is determined by the:
- **Cause** of the burn.
- **Duration** of exposure.
- **Temperature** (if appropriate) of the burn.

The effects of the burn are **local** & **systemic**, the latter being due to release of inflammatory mediators. Burn injuries may be associated with internal damage either as a direct consequence of the burn (electrical burn), or as part of additional trauma.

Q: How would you classify burn injuries?

Depth	Cause
Superficial	Flash / Flame
Partial Thickness	Contact e.g. Hot / Cold
Full Thickness	Friction
	Chemical
	Electrical
	Radiation

Q: How do you assess burn size?

[handwritten: PALM / WALLACE'S RULE OF 9'S / LUND (+) BROWDER (age adjusted)]

Assessment	Explanation
The Patient's Palm	The patient's palm may be used to estimate 1% of the TBSA.
Wallace's Rule of Nines	In an adult; the entire head = 9%, entire arm = 9%, anterior leg = 9%, posterior leg = 9%, anterior trunk = 18%, posterior trunk = 18% & perineum = 1%.
Lund & Browder Chart	This is the most accurate clinical assessment method & is adjusted for age (see additional OSCE questions chapter).

Q: What fluid regime would you use to treat a burn injury?

The **Parkland Formula** is in greatest use. Hartmann's or CSL is the fluid of choice & is given as follows:

[handwritten: %·Kg × 4]

%TBSA x weight (kg) x 4ml in 24 hours.

50% of this given in the 1st 8 hours post burn injury.

Note: Fluid resuscitation is required in burns with TBSA 15% in adults or 10% in children. Children also require additional maintenance fluid with dextrose-saline adjusted for weight in kg. the formula & indications are a guide only & the patient must be reassessed for adequacy of resuscitation.

[handwritten: eg   10% × 60 Kg × 4 / 1000 = 2.4 L in 24hr ↓ 1.2 Ltre over first 8h.]

Q: You are the burns CT2 & are called to see a patient who has sustained a flame burn in a confined space. Aside from the mechanism & degree of the burn injury, what else in particular would you be concerned about?

Burns involving smoke, noxious gases or facial injuries, particularly when sustained in confined spaces, are associated with an increased risk of **inhalational injury**. This may lead to airway obstruction, such that prophylactic intubation must be considered. Bronchoscopy & carboxyhaemoglobin levels may be useful in aiding diagnosis although diagnosis is primarily clinical. **If in doubt, intubate!** Features may include the following:

- Injury in Confined Space
- Perinasal / Perioral Soot Deposits
- Carbonaceous Sputum
- Burnt Facial Hairs e.g. Eyebrows
- Loss of Consciousness
- Facial Swelling
- Hoarse Voice
- Wheezing & Signs of Respiratory Distress.

Q: Which burn injuries should be referred to a burns unit?

- Full Thickness TBSA >5%
- Partial Thickness TBSA >10% in Patients <10yrs / >50yrs
- Face, Eyes, Ears, Hands, Feet, Genitalia & Perineum
- Joints
- Inhalation, Chemical & Electrical
- Circumferential.

Q: How would you calculate the prognosis of a patient with a burn injury?

The **Bull Chart** (1971) estimates chance of survival based on age & %TBSA. As a general rule, if the patient's age + %TBSA is >100, the survival prognosis is poor (approximately 20%).

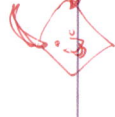

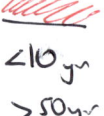

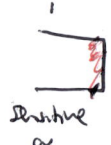

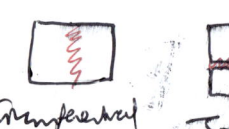

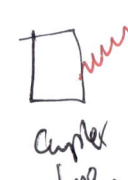

PULMONARY ARTERY CATHETERS

Q: How is a CVP line used to measure left atrial pressure?

- A central venous pressure line is inserted into the lower SVC / right atrium to record right atrial pressure.
- Right atrial pressure is assumed to be equal to left atrial pressure, allowing extrapolation of left ventricular pressure & filling.

Note: If the left side of the heart is asynchronous with the right side, the assumption that left atrial pressure is equal to right atrial pressure is no longer valid.

Q: What is a PAC?

- A pulmonary artery catheter / Swann Ganz / pulmonary artery flotation catheter, is a multi-lumen balloon-tip catheter, used most commonly to achieve central access.
- The catheter is passed using the Seldinger technique, via an internal jugular route, through the SVC & into the right atrium.
- Balloon inflation allows for the catheter to be 'floated' through the right ventricle, such that it may be 'wedged' into the pulmonary artery.
- A connected transducer measures pressure along this course, indicating the position of the catheter (Fig 2.1).

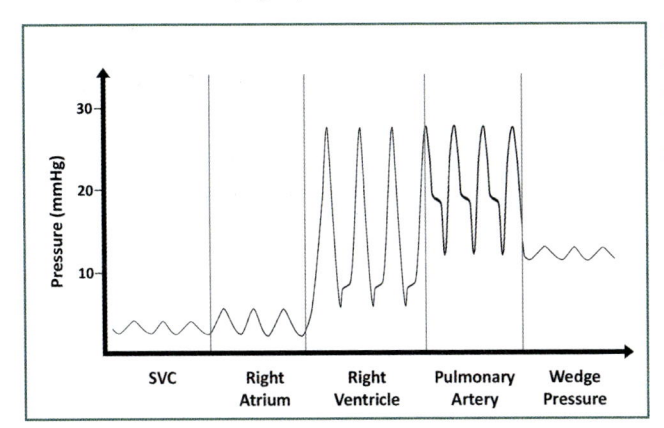

Fig 2.1: Pulmonary artery catheter pressure recordings along its course of insertion. The pulmonary artery wedge pressure is also shown.

Q: What is the significance of 'wedge' pressure?

Once in the pulmonary artery, the PAC balloon may be inflated, allowing it to become 'wedged' in position. As there are no valves between the pulmonary artery & left atrium, the pulmonary artery wedge / occlusion pressure is considered to be representative of left atrial pressure.

DIRECT: HR, MAP, venous blood sat + temp, ejection %, CO

DERIVED: Pulmonary & Systemic vascular resistance, stroke volume

Q: What direct & derived measurements are obtainable using a PAC?

Direct	Derived
Cardiac Output	Cardiac Index
Ejection Fraction	O_2 Delivery & Consumption
Heart Rate	Pulmonary Vascular Resistance
Mean Arterial Pressure (MAP)	Systemic Vascular Resistance (SVR)
Mean Pulmonary Artery Pressure	Stroke Volume
Mixed Venous Blood Temperature	
Mixed Venous O_2 Saturation	
Pulmonary Artery Wedge / Occlusion Pressure	

Q: What are the complications of PAC insertion?

Immediate	Late
Arrhythmia	Catheter Block / Knot
Air Embolism	Catheter Migration / Dislodge
Haematoma	Sepsis
Pneumothorax	
Pulmonary Artery Rupture	
Pulmonary Infarction	
Valve Injury	

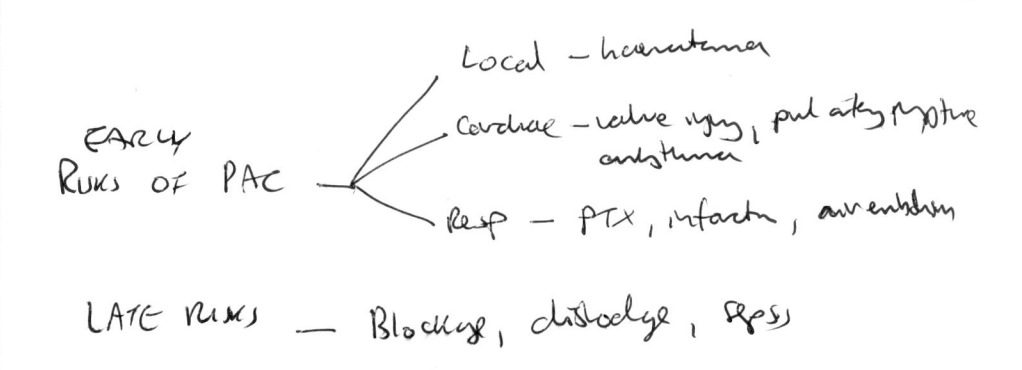

EARLY RISKS OF PAC
- Local – haematoma
- Cardiac – valve injury, pul artery rupture, arrhythmia
- Resp – PTX, infarction, air embolism

LATE RISKS – Blockage, dislodge, sepsis

CARDIOPULMONARY BYPASS

Q: What is cardiopulmonary bypass & how does it work?

This technique temporarily maintains the circulation & oxygenation of blood throughout the body. The system works according to the following principles:

- Right Atrium Cannula Insertion
- Gravitational Drainage of Venous Blood into Reservoir
- Blood Heparinisation
- Membrane Oxygenator Adds O_2 & Removes CO_2
- Heat Exchanger Controls Blood Temperature
- Oxygenated Blood is Passed Through a Bubble Trap & Microemboli Filter
- Blood is Returned to Aortic Circulation.

Q: What are the clinical indications for cardiopulmonary bypass?

Indication	Examples
Cardiothoracic Surgery	• Aortic Surgery • Coronary Artery Bypass Graft • Cardiac Valve Repair / Replacement • Lung Transplant • Pulmonary Thrombectomy
Neurosurgery	• Basilar Artery Aneurysm Repair • Glomus Jugulare Tumour Excision • Haemangioblastoma Excision
Supportive	Critically ill patients: • Drug Overdose • Hypothermia

Q: What are the complications of cardiopulmonary bypass?

Immediate	Early	Late
Air Embolism (circuit disruption)	ARDS	Coma
Coagulopathy (heparin)	Arrhythmia	Focal Neurological Deficit
Hypothermia	Acute Renal Failure	Mesenteric Ischaemia
Inflammatory Response (foreign surface contact)		Pancreatitis
Thrombocytopaenia		Seizures

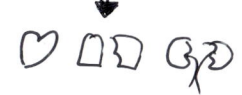

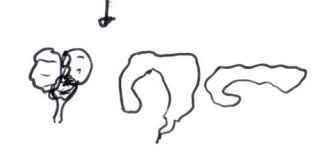

HEAD INJURY & CEREBRAL AUTOREGULATION

Q: What is the difference between primary & secondary brain injury?

Brain Injury	Explanation
Primary	Occurs at the time of injury i.e. direct brain cortex injury.
Secondary	Occurs after the injury & may be due to: **Memory:** The 4 x H's of secondary brain injury. • **H**ypoxia • **H**ypotension • **H**ypercarbia • **H**igh ICP

Q: What is the Monro-Kellie doctrine?

The Monro-Kellie doctrine describes the intracranial pressure-volume relationship as governed by the following 3 components (Fig 2.2):

- Brain Tissue
- Blood
- CSF.

These 3 components occupy space within a closed & rigid box (the skull) that has a fixed volume. Change in 1 component must result in a compensatory change in another component(s) in order to prevent a rise in ICP (Fig 2.3).

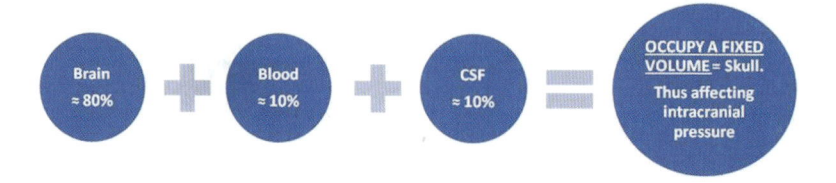

Brain ≈ 80% + Blood ≈ 10% + CSF ≈ 10% = OCCUPY A FIXED VOLUME = Skull. Thus affecting intracranial pressure

Fig 2.2: Diagrammatic representation of the Monro-Kellie doctrine.

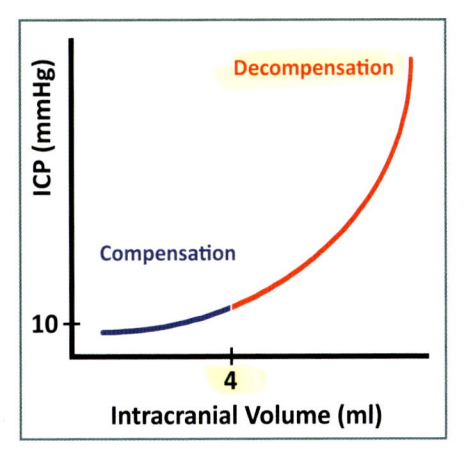

Fig 2.3: Graph representing the relationship between intracranial volume & ICP.

If the volume of 1 component increases, there must be a decrease in another component(s) to maintain ICP (**compensation**).

When the intracranial volume passes a critical point (approximately 4mls), compression occurs, such that any further increase in intracranial volume, results in a rapid increase in ICP (**decompensation**).

Q: What are the causes of increased intracranial pressure?

These may be broadly classified as medical or surgical as follows:

Classification	Cause	Explanation
MEDICAL	Electrolyte Imbalance	Effective increase in brain size due to resulting oedema.
	Infection	Effective increase in brain size due to inflammation or mass-effect & compression e.g. cerebral abscess & meningitis.
	Stroke	Effective increase in brain size due to inflammation. Haemorrhagic stroke may have additional mass-effect & compression.
SURGICAL	Haemorrhage / Haematoma	Mass-effect & compression e.g. extradural, subdural & subarachnoid. Subarachnoid haemorrhage may result in additional decrease in CSF resorption.
	Oedema	Effective increase in brain size due to e.g. contusions & DAI.
	Tumour	Mass-effect & compression.

Q: What is cerebral perfusion pressure (CPP) & how does it relate to intracranial pressure (ICP)?

CPP represents the pressure gradient that drives cerebral blood flow, O_2 delivery & metabolite clearance. The normal range for CPP is approximately 70–90mmHg. CPP is dependent on the mean arterial pressure (MAP) (normal range approximately 60–150mmHg) & ICP (normal range approximately 5–15mmHg) as follows:

$$CPP = MAP - ICP$$

Q: How is cerebral blood flow autoregulated?

The brain autoregulates to ensure constant cerebral blood flow across a range of MAP (Fig 2.4). Consequently, P_aCO_2 has a crucial role by controlling the degree of intracranial vasodilation.

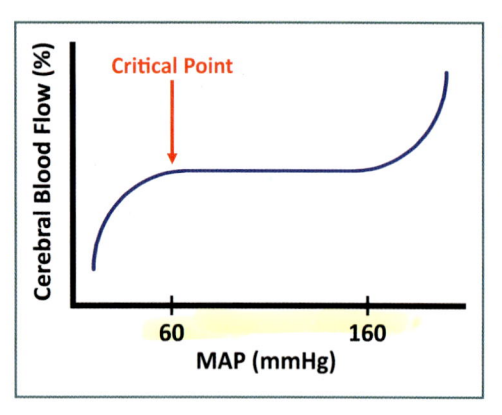

Fig 2.4: Graph representing the relationship between MAP & cerebral blood flow.

Cerebral blood flow is regulated between a MAP range. Below a **critical point** (approximately 60mmHg), cerebral blood flow decreases dramatically.

Q: What is the clinical relevance of a dilated pupil in a patient with a head-injury & what would other relevant signs & symptoms be?

High ICP may cause distortion & pressure on cranial nerves & vital neurological centres. If this progresses, fatal internal or external brain herniation may occur. An acutely dilated pupil that is unreactive to light suggests ipsilateral oculomotor (III) nerve palsy as it runs through the tentorium cerebellum. Similarly, ipsilateral abduction may be lost due to abducens (VI) nerve palsy. These nerves may also be affected as part of a serious traction injury.

Other unfavourable signs include; headache, nausea & vomiting, drowsiness, loss of consciousness & papilloedema.

Q: How would you clinically decide if a head injury patient had an associated base of skull fracture?

The following features may be present:
- Panda / raccoon eyes indicating periorbital ecchymosis.
- Subconjunctival haemorrhage obscuring the white of the eyes.
- CSF rhinorrhoea.
- CEF otorrhoea.
- Battle's Sign, indicating mastoid ecchymosis, is a late sign.

Q: What are the principles of head injury management?

Management follows ATLS principles. The primary goals are to prevent secondary brain injury, cerebral ischaemia & herniation. A rise in ICP results in a fall in CPP with a reduction in O_2 supply (resulting in ischaemia) & CO_2 clearance (resulting in vasodilation). This precipitates a vicious cycle that worsens the brain injury & increases the ICP further. Management principles therefore include:

Management	Explanation
ATLS	• This is a traumatic event so follow ATLS guidelines.
Airway & C-spine	• Maintain airway. • Be highly suspicious of an associated C-spine injury by immobilising the neck. • Avoid neck vessel compression to prevent reduced cerebral venous outflow.
Breathing & Ventilation	• Induce hyperventilation to 'blow off' CO_2 (aim for a P_aCO_2 <4.5kPa) & optimise P_aO_2. 'Blowing off' CO_2 helps to reduce intracranial vasodilation.
Circulation	• Control MAP to ensure an adequate CPP. • Strict fluid balance to avoid cerebral oedema.
ICP Monitor	• Allows measurement of ICP. • Allows therapeutic tapping of CSF.
Drugs	• Mannitol may be used under neurosurgical guidance. This is an osmotic diuretic that helps to reduce cerebral oedema. • Sedatives & barbiturates prevent an increase in basal metabolic rate that would otherwise result in an increased O_2 demand. Decreasing the O_2 demand also decreases cerebral blood flow & therefore also decreases ICP. • Steroids may be used for tumours with associated oedema.
General	• Head up tilt reduces venous congestion e.g. 30°. • Nutritional management. • Antibiotics may be used as prophylaxis or treatment.

Q: Is it safe to perform a lumbar puncture in a patient with a head injury?

There would normally not be a need for this unless a concomitant CNS infection is suspected. Remember that if the ICP is raised, coning may occur upon performing a lumbar puncture. For this reason a CT scan of the head should be undertaken to exclude lesions that may be associated with a raised ICP.

NUTRITION

Q: Why is an understanding of nutrition vital in a surgical patient?

Nutritional support should be considered in patients who may be unable to fulfil dietary requirements. An understanding of basic nutritional concepts is vital for the following reasons:

1. To fulfil basal energy requirements (approximately 30kcal/kg).
2. To compensate for malnutritional states or disease e.g. intestinal fistulae & Crohn's Disease.
3. To compensate for catabolic states e.g. post-operative & sepsis.
4. To enhance wound healing.
5. To enhance immune responses.

Q: What are the normal nutritional requirements of a healthy adult?

Nutritional requirements are only based on guidelines & vary between sexes & individuals. The recommended daily calorific intake for males is 2500kcal/day & for females is 2000kcal/day. In practice, particularly with critically ill & surgical patients, dietary advice & assessment should be obtained from a dietician. The following should be considered as **approximate guidelines** only & do not include vitamins or minerals.

Nutrient	Energy Provision	Requirement	% of Daily Total Calorific Intake
Carbohydrate	4.2 kcal/g	3.5 g/kg/day	50–60%
Fat	9.1 kcal/g	1 g/kg/day	25–35%
Protein	4.2 kcal/g	0.9 g/kg/day	10–20%
H_2O	–	40 ml/kg/day	–

Q: How would you assess a patient's nutritional status?

Assessment	Examples	Assessment	Examples
Clinical	• General Appearance	Anthropometric	• Height & Weight
	• Hand Grip Strength		• BMI = Weight (kg) / Height (m^2)
	• Pulmonary Function Tests		• Fat e.g. Skin Fold Thickness
Hydration Status & Fluid Balance	• Skin Turgidity		• Muscle e.g. Arm Circumference
	• Peripheral Oedema	Biochemical	• FBC e.g. Hct
	• Pulmonary Oedema		• U&Es e.g. Na^+ & Urea
	• Input / Output Charts		• LFTs e.g. Albumin
Calculation	• Based on Sex, Weight & Catabolic State e.g. Burns		• Other e.g. Mg^{2+} & Zn^{2+}
			• 24h Urinary Creatinine

Q: What forms of nutritional supplementation do you know of?

These may be broadly classified as enteral (delivered via the gastrointestinal tract) or parenteral (delivered via a peripheral vein).

Classification	Administration	Pre-Requisites	Considerations
ENTERAL	• Oral • Nasogastric • Nasojejunal	Functional gastrointestinal tract with no risk of aspiration.	• Psychologically more satisfying for patient than TPN. • Maintains bowel mucosa integrity, preventing bacterial translocation & MODS. • Relatively cheap.
	• Gastrostomy • Jejunostomy	Gastrointestinal stasis.	• Better if required for prolonged use e.g. 6 weeks. • Maintains bowel mucosa integrity, preventing bacterial translocation & MODS. • Planned as part of elective procedure e.g. oesophagectomy or gastrectomy. • Site leakage & irritation may occur. • Infection & peritonitis may occur. • Tube migration may cause bowel obstruction.
PARENTERAL	• PICC Line • Hickman Line	Compromised gastrointestinal tract or hypercatabolic state.	• Does not maintain bowel mucosa integrity. • Requires regular blood monitoring e.g. trace elements. • Fluid imbalances may occur. • Metabolic derangements may occur. • TPN-associated jaundice may occur. • Risk of 'line sepsis'. • Relatively expensive.

Q: What are the key constituents of TPN?

TPN is prepared specifically for each patient to take into account individual requirements. The chief components are:

- Carbohydrate >50%
- Fat >30%
- Amino Acids (Protein breakdown)
- Water
- Electrolytes
- Trace Elements
- Vitamins.

RENAL FAILURE

Q: What are the key differences in solute between blood plasma & urine in a healthy adult?

Solute	Total amount in blood plasma (g)	Total amount in urine per day (g)
Urea	4.8	25g (= 5x)
Creatinine	0.03	1.6g (= 50x)
Protein	200 (= 2000x)	0.1
Bicarbonate	4.6	0
Glucose	3	0

Q: What are oliguria & anuria?

Terminology	Definition
Oliguria	Oliguria is the decreased production of urine (<0.5ml/kg/h). This indicates renal-impairment & occurs in up to 25% of critically ill patients.
Anuria	Total absence of urine production. Surgically, this should be considered to be due to obstruction of the lower urinary tract until proven otherwise.

Q: How would you define acute & chronic renal failure?

Failure Type	Definition
Acute	Sudden, usually reversible impairment of functioning nephrons, resulting in reversible (usually) kidney function impairment.
Chronic	Progressive, permanent loss of functioning nephrons, resulting in irreversible kidney function impairment. CRF lies on a spectrum of CKD, the latter being classified into 5 stages according to the severity of GFR reduction. CRF = advanced stage 4 / 5 CKD.

* Remember that acute-on-chronic renal failure may also occur.

Q: What are the markers of renal failure?

- That of the cause e.g. pyelonephritis.
- Decreased urine output.
- Deranged U&Es e.g. creatinine >125μM. **Note: Creatinine rises with age, so an acceptable 'rule of thumb' upper limit for adult creatinine is 90 + age.**
- Urine osmolality.

Q: How is renal failure classified & what are the common causes?

Classification	Causes	Examples
PRE-RENAL 'inadequate renal perfusion'	Hypovolaemia	• Inadequate Fluid Management (extremely common) — ↓ Intake • Haemorrhage • Burns • Diarrhoea & Vomiting } Losses
	Decreased Cardiac Output	• Heart Failure • Pulmonary Embolus Pump.
	Hypotension	• Sepsis • Anaphylaxis Distribution
	Vascular	• Renal Artery or Vein Obstruction Renal flow
INTRINSIC RENAL 'parenchymal disease'	Drugs	• Gentamicin • NSAIDs } Nephrotoxics
	Glomerular	• Glomerulonephritis • Antibody Mediated e.g. Wegener's Granulomatosis & Goodpasture's Syndrome
	Interstitial	• Pyelonephritis Infection. • Sarcoid • Lupus } Autoimmune.
POST-RENAL 'outflow obstruction'	Ureteric	• Calculus • Carcinoma
	Cystic	• Calculus • Carcinoma
	Prostatic	• BPH • Carcinoma
	Urethral	• Blocked Catheter (extremely common) • Calculus • Stricture • Carcinoma

Q: You are asked to see a patient 12 hours post right hemicolectomy. The nurses are concerned that he has not passed urine for the last 2 hours. How would you manage this patient?

Take a full history & perform a thorough examination. Check fluid balance & observations charts. Check blood results, imaging & the operation note. The most common causes are inadequate fluid management (pre-renal) & blocked catheter (post-renal). A blocked catheter is likely if the patient suddenly becomes anuric. Continue to proceed with this patient as follows:

1. Flush & reposition catheter to assess for blockage. If the patient has no catheter, consider insertion. This may solve the problem, negating the requirement of some of the points below.
2. Check observations & perform a fluid challenge, hence ensuring the patient is not hypovolaemic. Consider inserting a CVP line for closer monitoring.
3. Run an appropriate set of blood tests, including U&E.
4. Review patient immediately after all of the above are complete.
5. Implement fluid resuscitation as appropriate.
6. Manage hyperkalaemia as appropriate.
7. Rationalise medication e.g. Gentamicin & NSAIDS.
8. Consider further imaging & medical referral if the above do not improve the problem.

Note: Furosemide is often used to improve urine output but is seldom appropriate! Although it may improve oliguria, it 'squeezes the kidneys dry' & masks the true clinical picture of renal failure.

RENAL REPLACEMENT THERAPY

Q: What is renal replacement therapy?

RRT is a life-saving intervention that may be required acutely or chronically e.g. Stage 5 CKD = ESRF. It may be administered in a continuous or intermittent manner, either via the vasculature (using an arteriovenous or venovenous circuit) or via the peritoneum. There are 4 types of RRT:

RRT Type	Explanation	Continuous	Intermittent
Haemodialysis	A selectively permeable membrane is utilised. This removes small molecules that pass through the membrane along a diffusion gradient. Fluid passes across via osmosis.	Y	Y
Haemofiltration	Continuous convection of molecules occurs across a membrane. This is suitable for removing a large volume of fluid that is then replaced with a physiological solution. It is not useful for removing small molecules.	Y	N
Haemodiafiltration	Combination of the above, either simultaneously or sequentially, removing urea more efficiently.	Y	N
Peritoneal Dialysis	Utilises the peritoneum & its capillary network as a selectively permeable membrane. Dialysis fluid is introduced into the peritoneum, via a Tenckhoff Catheter. Fluid, ions & waste products diffuse from the blood into the dialysate, which is then drained off several hours later. This is mainly used in ambulatory CRF patients & is less efficient than the above.	Y	N

Q: What are the indications for renal replacement therapy?

- Severe derangement of U&Es e.g. refractive hyperkalaemia >6mmol/L or urea >35mmol/L.
- Severe acidosis e.g. pH ≤7.0.
- Severe fluid overload e.g. pulmonary oedema resistant to standard treatment.
- Complications of uraemia e.g. encephalopathy & pericarditis.
- ESRF.
- Creatinine clearance <10ml/min.
- Removal of toxic drugs e.g. aspirin overdose.

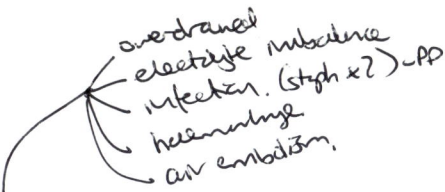

Q: What are the complications associated with RRT?

- Hypotension due to acute hypovolaemia.
- Dysequilibrium syndrome due to an acute change in plasma osmolality resulting in fluid shift & cerebral oedema.
- Line Sepsis
- Immune reactions due to extracorporeal circuit activating complement cascade.*
- Air embolism & haemorrhage due to disconnection from circuit.*
- Infection. This is more common with peritoneal dialysis & the characteristic microorganisms are gram positive e.g. *Staphylococcus aureus* & *epidermidis*. *

* These may cause SIRS.

Q: Should you transfuse a surgical patient who has CRF?

Not without discussing with a nephrologist. CRF patients usually have a degree of anaemia. Altering their haematocrit alters their blood viscosity & flow patterns, which in turn may impair renal function. Consider the need for transfusion in light of their usual Hb level. If transfusion is required, this should be done slowly.

FLUIDS

Q: What are the different fluid compartments in the body?

Approximately ⅔ of the body-mass is due to fluid, so a 70kg adult would have 45kg of fluid. Water has a density of 1kg/L, so since the bulk of body fluid is water, 45kg = 45L. Note that an adult requires 30-40mL/kg of fluid every day.

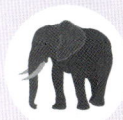

> **Memory:** 'Rule of Thirds' (Fig 2.5)
> - Body fluid is distributed in extracellular (ECF) & intracellular (ICF) & compartments in the ratio ⅓ : ⅔.
> - ECF is then subdivided into intravascular & interstitial compartments, in the ratio of ⅓ : ⅔.

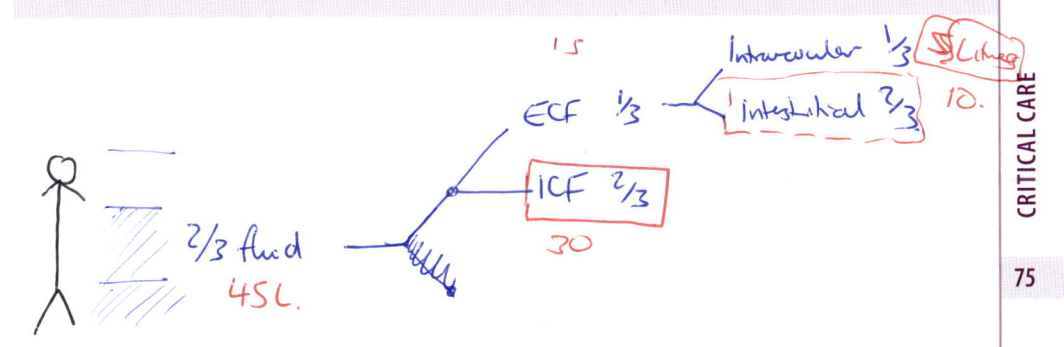

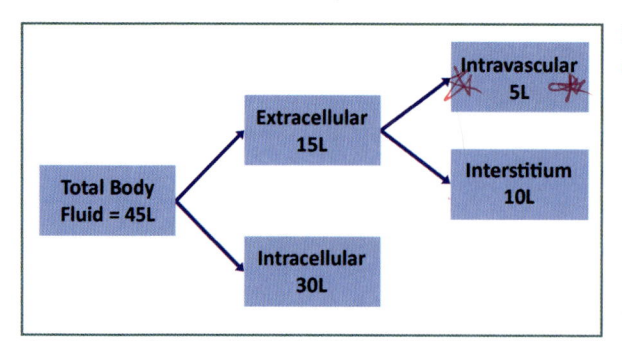

Fig 2.5: Body fluid distribution (rule of thirds).

Q: Can you discuss the factors relating to use of colloids?

- Classification:

Natural	Synthetic
Blood	Gelatin-Based (Gelofusine™)
FFP	Starch-Based (Voluven™)
Human Albumin	

Note: There is a risk of anaphylaxis with all of the above. Coagulopathy may be more common with starch-based colloids than with gelatin-based colloids.

- Colloids remain in the intravascular fluid compartment, at-least initially, since their large molecules do not pass through the vascular endothelium freely.
- Choice of fluid for resuscitation is determined by the compartment facing the greatest loss, so major haemorrhage would be initially managed by replacement with colloids. Note: Starch-based colloids may be less effective for major haemorrhage resuscitation than gelatin-based colloids.
- Colloids are routinely used, as part of a fluid challenge, to assess adequacy of fluid resuscitation.
- Colloids are more expensive than crystalloids.

(handwritten top right):
Sodium
0.9% SALINE — 150 mM
HARTMANN'S — 131 mM
DEX/SALINE — 30 mM

Q: Can you briefly outline the composition of Hartmann's Solution, normal saline & dextrose-saline?

Composition	Hartmann's (mmol/L)	Normal Saline (mmol/L)	Dextrose-Saline (mmol/L)
Na⁺	131	150	30
Cl⁻	111	150	30
Lactate*	29	-	-
K⁺	5	-	-
Ca²⁺	2	-	-

(handwritten): → HCO₃⁻ ; ACIDOSIS BUFFER

*Lactate is hepatically metabolised to HCO₃⁻ (29mmol/L) which can buffer any acidosis that may be present e.g. post-operative, infection, shock. Ringer's lactate is similar, but not identical, to Hartmann's Solution.

Q: Can you briefly discuss the distribution of normal saline & 5% dextrose throughout the body fluid compartments during resuscitation?

- Normal saline distributes throughout the ECF compartment, according to the rule of thirds (Fig 2.5).
- 5% Dextrose distributes throughout the ECF & ICF compartments, according to the rule of thirds (Fig 2.5).
- Crystalloids would suffice for the majority of scenarios necessitating fluid resuscitation.
- During major haemorrhage, colloids are initially required for fluid resuscitation, as more crystalloid would be required (according to the rule of thirds) in order to adequately replace intravascular volume.

Q: Can you briefly discuss the fluid requirements of an average 70kg male over 24h?

Fluid replacement may be achieved in a number of ways e.g. oral, IV, enteral, TPN. Per day, the average 70kg male requires replacement of the following:

- **Maintenance:** 2.5L H₂O, 120–140mmol Na⁺, 70mmol K⁺
- **Insensible Losses:** 600ml (from skin), 400ml (from lungs), 100ml (from faeces)

Q: What would a suitable IV fluid replacement regime be for an average 70kg male over 24 hours?

- 1L Dextrose-Saline   +20mmol KCL
- 1L Dextrose-Saline   +20mmol KCL
- 1L Normal Saline   +20mmol KCL

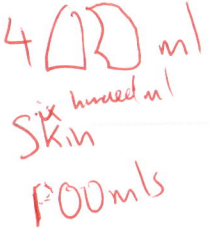

(handwritten): 400 ml six hundred ml Skin 1200 mls

RESPIRATORY FAILURE

Q: What is respiratory failure?

This is characterised by impaired pulmonary gas exchange with or without hypercapnia. Hypoxemia is therefore also characteristic (P_aO_2 <8kPa). It may be confirmed by ABG measurements & may be acute or chronic. There are 2 types of respiratory failure:

Respiratory Failure	Problem	ABG Finding
Type I	Hypoxia due to a V/Q mismatch.	• P_aO_2 <8kPa. • P_aCO_2 may be normal or low.
Type II	Hypoxia & Hypoventilation	• P_aO_2 <8kPa • P_aCO_2 >6.7kPa

Q: What are the normal reference ranges for P_aO_2 & P_aCO_2?

At sea-level, the reference range for P_aO_2 is 10–14kPa, however this varies according to altitude & F_iO_2. The reference range for P_aCO_2 is 4.5–6kPa.

Q: How would you classify the causes of hypoxaemia?

Cause	Explanation
Hypoxic	Due to respiratory failure as described above.
Anaemic	Suboptimal O_2 carriage of blood due to a reduction or alteration in Hb.
Histotoxic	Mitochondrial respiration is impaired e.g. due to CN^- poisoning.
Stagnant	Due to poor tissue perfusion e.g. cardiac failure & arterial obstruction.

Q: What are the causes of respiratory failure?

Causes may be classified according to the type of failure, although some overlap may occur.

Type I	Type II	
Asthma	*Anatomical:*	*Neurological:*
Pneumonia	Chest Wall Trauma	Head Injury
Pulmonary Oedema	Chest Wall Deformity	CVA
Pulmonary Embolism	Pneumothorax	Myasthenia Gravis
ARDS	Pleural Effusion	Guillain Barré
	Pharmacological:	Motor Neurone Disease
	Opiates	*Disease:*
	Sedatives	COPD

Q: What is 'mixed-defect' respiratory failure?

If a patient is tachypnoeic & trying to optimise oxygenation, such as in Type I respiratory failure, exhaustion will eventually ensue. Exhaustion results in the patient hypoventilating which reduces CO_2 excretion & oxygenation, such that Type II respiratory failure ensues. Hence, a mixed Type I & II respiratory defect has occurred.

ALI & ARDS

Q: What is ALI & ARDS?

Acute lung injury & the acute respiratory distress syndrome represent a spectrum of disease where ARDS is the most severe form. They have an identifiable aetiology & are characterised by:

1. Non-cardiogenic pulmonary oedema seen as diffuse pulmonary infiltrates on the CXR.
2. Progressive hypoxaemia.
3. Reduced lung compliance.

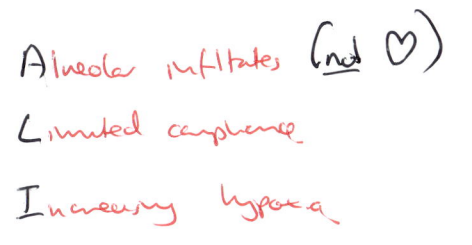

Q: Can you list some of the **causes** of ALI & ARDS?

Memory: **'FAT HIPS'**
- **F**at Embolus
- **A**spiration Pneumonia
- **T**rauma & Burns
- **H**eart Bypass
- **D**IC
- **P**ancreatitis
- **S**epsis.

Handwritten notes: CAUSES — 1° LUNG: Fat embolus, Asp pneumonia. SECONDARY: Cardiac – bypass, Haem – DIC, GI – pancreatitis, Sepsis, Trauma/burns.

Q: How would you **diagnose** ALI & ARDS?

- They must be of **acute** onset.
- Diffuse pulmonary **infiltrates** are seen on the CXR.
- Pulmonary artery **wedge pressure** <18mmHg.
- P_aO_2/F_iO_2 <40kPa = ALI.
- P_aO_2/F_iO_2 <26.6kPa = ARDS.

Handwritten notes: Δ ① Acute onset ② CXR ③ Wedge <18 (Ali laks <18). ALI ⊥ ARDS PaO_2/FiO_2 <40   <26.6

Q: What **pathological changes** occur in ALI & ARDS? What are the **treatment principles?**

The pathological changes that occur may be classified according to phase & time of onset as follows:

Phase	Onset	Pathology	Treatment Principles
Inflammation / Exudation	1–2 days	Mediated by macrophages & neutrophils via release of cytokines, proteases & formation of free radicals. Interstitial alveolar oedema occurs & hyaline membranes are formed.	• Primarily Supportive • Treat Cause • PEEP Ventilation • Inverse Ventilation (Inspiration:Expiration Ratio = 2:1) • Ventilate Prone
Proliferation	1–2 weeks	Proliferation of type II pneumocytes & fibroblasts. Granulation tissue is produced that narrows alveoli & vessels.	Inhaled NO may help via vasodilation at ventilated areas of lung to improve V/Q mismatch.
Fibrosis	2–4 weeks	Significant pulmonary fibrosis may occur in some patients.	Steroids may be useful here.

Handwritten notes: IPF — 1-2 days, 1-2 weeks, 2-4 weeks

OXYGEN THERAPY & MECHANICAL VENTILATION

Q: What methods of O_2 delivery do you know of?

Method	Maximum Achievable F_iO_2
Nasal Cannula	30–40%
Face Mask	50%
Venturi Mask	60%
Reservoir Bag	100%
Mechanical Ventilation	Highly variable depending on set parameters

Q: What modes of ventilation do you know of?

Mode	Driven By	Explanation	Indications
IPPV *Intermittent Positive Pressure Ventilation*	Ventilator	The ventilator forces cyclical delivery of gas mixture into the lungs. This also generates +ve intrathoracic pressure during inspiration (normally this is –ve) & decreases venous return to the heart.	• Respiratory Failure • Reduce Work of Breathing • Optimise Intracranial Pressure • LVF
PEEP *Positive End Expiratory Pressure*	Ventilator	The ventilator delivers gas during expiration, 'splinting' alveoli open & preventing collapse. This improves shunting & overcomes decreased lung compliance.	• ARDS
CPAP *Continuous Positive Airways Pressure*	Patient	The patient ventilates spontaneously, while the ventilator is set to ensure delivery above a minimum level & below a maximum level of pulmonary pressures. This 'splints' alveoli open, preventing collapsing during respiration, but may not regulate tidal volume.	• Respiratory Failure • Sleep Apnoea • LVF
SIMV *Synchronised Intermittent Mandatory Ventilation*	Patient & Ventilator	The patient ventilates spontaneously, with ventilator 'kick-in' as required if an inhalation is missed. This allows respiratory muscles to rest during mandatory breaths.	• IPPV Weaning
PSV *Pressure Support Ventilation*	Patient & Ventilator	The patient ventilates spontaneously, combined with ventilator pressure support if the patient is unable to generate adequate pulmonary pressure. This ensures an adequate tidal volume.	• IPPV Weaning

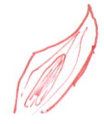

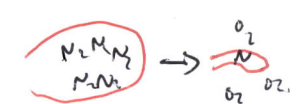

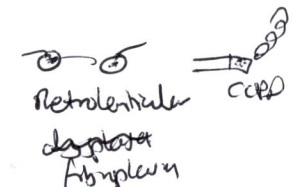

Q: What are the complications of O₂ therapy?

- **Reduced Hypoxic Ventilatory Drive:** This may occur in COPD patients who may rely on hypoxia to stimulate respiration. If the patient is severely hypoxic however, this must be considered over the risk of reducing hypoxic ventilatory drive.

- **Pulmonary Toxicity & Pulmonary Fibrosis:** These may occur as a consequence of O₂ free radical generation.

- **Absorption Atelectasis:** Delivery of O₂ flushes out N₂, resulting in a decrease in alveolar 'splintage'.

- **Retinopathy:** This occurs due to rentrolenticular fibroplasia.

- **Fire:** O₂ is flammable.

PANCREATITIS

Q: What is pancreatitis & what are the classical clinical features?

Inflammation of the pancreas, which may be an acute process, or develop into a chronic condition. Clinical features include severe epigastric pain that radiates through to the back, nausea & vomiting.

Q: What are the causes of acute pancreatitis?

Memory: **I GET SMASHED**

Idiopathic	Steroids
	Mumps
Gallsones	Autoimmune
Ethanol	Scorpion Venom
Trauma	Hyper-calcaemia / lipidaemia
	ERCP
	Drugs e.g. azathioprine / furosemide

Q: How would you manage a patient with acute pancreatitis?

- **ALS Approach** & **Fluid Resuscitation**
- Full **History**
- Thorough Clinical **Examination**
- Prognostic **Blood Tests** & **ABG** (Modified Glasgow Criteria):

> Memory: **PANCREAS** for Modified Glasgow Criteria
>
> | | |
> |---|---|
> | P_aO_2 | <8kPa |
> | Age | >55 |
> | Neutrophils | >15 x 10⁹/L |
> | Corrected Calcium | <2mmol/L |
> | Raised Urea | >16mmol/L |
> | Enzymes (LDH) | >600U/L |
> | Albumin | <32g/L |
> | Sugar (Glucose) | >10mmol/L |

Day 0, 1, 2.

Note: Presence of the above criteria should be assessed on admission, then daily for at least 48 hours. Presence of ≤2 criteria = severe pancreatitis unlikely. Presence of ≥3 criteria = severe pancreatitis more likely. Mortality rates are; 1–2 criteria = <1%, 3–4 criteria = 15% & >4 criteria = approaching 100% mortality.

- **USS:** Assessment of causal **gallstones** (may require emergency ERCP & sphincterotomy).
- **CT:** Performed between 3–10 days after onset, to delineate severity e.g. ischaemia, necrosis.

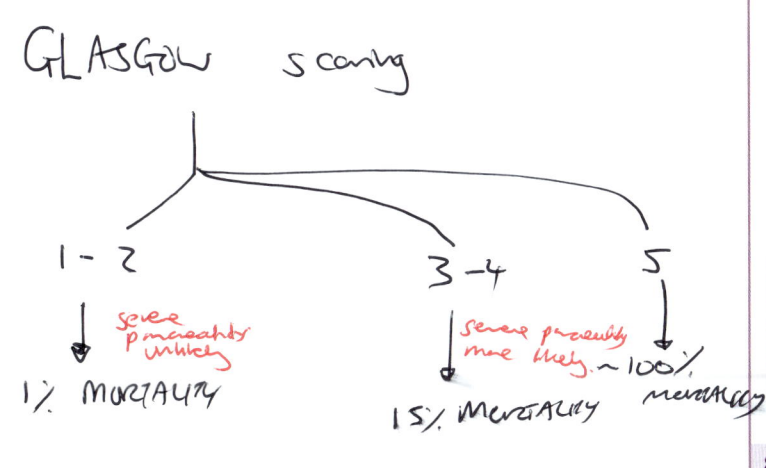

[Handwritten annotations:]

GLASGOW scoring
- 1-2 → severe pancreatitis unlikely → 1% mortality
- 3-4 → severe presumably more likely → 15% mortality
- 5 → ~100% mortality

1x USS - urgent ?gallstones
CT @ D3-10 - ?ischaemia ?necrosis (i.e. early)

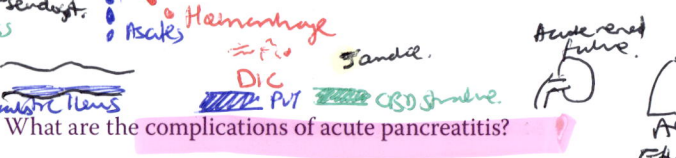

Q: What are the complications of acute pancreatitis?

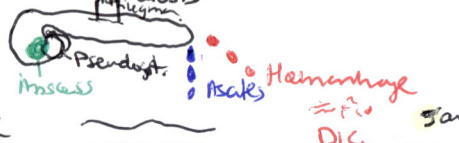

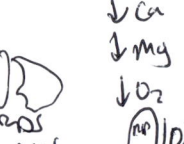

Classification	Complications
Local	Abscess, Ascites, Haemorrhage, Necrosis, Phlegmon, Pseudocyst
Gastrointestinal	Paralytic Ileus
Haematological	DIC
Hepatobiliary	CBD Stricture, Jaundice, Portal Vein Thrombosis
Metabolic	Hypoalbuminaemia, Hypocalcaemia, Hypomagnesaemia, Hypoxaemia Hyperglycaemia
Renal	Acute Renal Failure
Respiratory	ARDS, Pleural Effusion
Other	Chronicity (more common if ETOH is the cause) Overall Mortality =10%

SIRS, SEPSIS & MODS

Q: What is SIRS? What are the features of SIRS?

The systemic inflammatory response syndrome is defined when ≥2 of the following criteria are met:

Criteria	Value
Temperature	<36°C or >38°C.
Respiratory Rate	>20/min or P_aCO_2 <4.3kPa.
Heart Rate	>90/min.
WCC	<4x10⁹/L or >12x10⁹/L or >10% neutrophils / immature forms.

Q: What causes SIRS? What processes lead to its development?

Progression of inflammation throughout the body, principally haematogenously, results in SIRS. Causes may be thought of as 'triggers' of development & may be classified as infective or non-infective & by system involvement as follows:

Cause	Non-infective	Infective
Cardiovascular	Ruptured AAA / Major Haemorrhage*	Central Line Colonisation
Gastrointestinal	Pancreatitis*	Bowel Anastomosis Leak
Genitourinary	Acute Tubular Necrosis	UTI
Respiratory	Aspiration Pneumonia	LRTI
Soft Tissues	Embolus → Ischaemia	Necrotising Fasciitis
General	Burns* & Trauma*	Sepsis*

* These are more common triggers of SIRS.

A trigger results in an over-exaggerated, progressively increasing, inflammatory response. This is mediated by release of cytokines, mediators & vasoactive agents (e.g. bradykinin, histamine, NO & prostaglandins). These become systemically distributed throughout the body resulting in vasodilation, increased vascular permeability & features of SIRS. Organ failure may ensue (Fig 2.6).

Trigger of Progressive Inflammatory Response ⇒ Release of Cytokines, Mediators & Vasoactive Agents ⇒ Vasodilation, Increased Vascular Permeability & Negative Inotropy ⇒ Organ Failure May Ensue

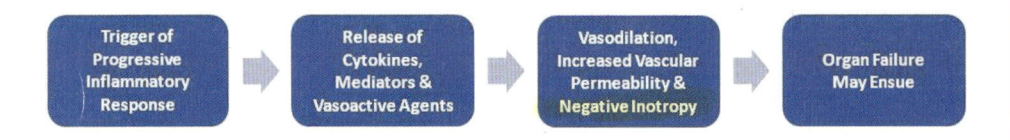

Fig 2.6: Schematic representation of the processes leading to SIRS & organ failure:

Q: What are the roles of cytokines & mediators in the progression of SIRS?

The progressive inflammatory response is governed by a balance between pro- & anti-inflammatory cytokines & mediators. Positive feedback propagates the pro-inflammatory state, primarily causing endothelial cell breakdown. Common cytokines & mediators may therefore be classified according to their effect as follows:

Effect	Examples
Pro-Inflammatory	IL-1, IL-6, TNF-α. Also IL-8 & PAF
Anti-Inflammatory	IL-10 & TGF-β

Q: Can you define infection, bacteraemia, septicaemia, sepsis, severe sepsis, septic shock & septic syndrome?

Terminology	Definition
Infection	Invasion of a sterile organ or tissue by pathogens.
Bacteraemia	Presence of circulating viable bacteria within the blood stream. This may be transient e.g. after brushing teeth.
Septicaemia	Active multiplication of microbes in the bloodstream, resulting in a serious & overwhelming infection.
Sepsis	SIRS in the presence of documented infection.
Severe Sepsis	Sepsis with organ or tissue dysfunction.
Septic Shock	Sepsis with hypotension (P_{syst} <90 or fall by ≥40 mmHg) or tissue hypoperfusion that is **refractory to IV fluid replacement**. This may lead to organ or tissue dysfunction.
Septic Syndrome	SIRS with end-organ hypoperfusion. This is similar to severe sepsis but there is no identifiable infective aetiology.

Q: What is MODS & how does the 'multiple hit hypothesis' relate to it?

Multiple organ dysfunction syndrome is potentially reversible & defined by the presence of ≥2 dysfunctioning organs. Mortality rises with increasing severity & increasing numbers of compromised systems. Mortality is approximately 50–60% for 2 affected organs & >80% for 3 affected organs.

Intensive intervention is required to prevent the development & outcomes of MODS due to the 'multiple hit hypothesis'. This hypothesis describes that, in an already critically ill patient, exaggerated immune-responses occur to relatively trivial insults. In such circumstances, organ failure & rise in mortality may occur more easily.

Q: What treatment strategies should be employed in SIRS or MODS?

Early, goal-directed treatment strategies are required to improve oxygenation & tissue-perfusion. These may be classified as follows:

Strategy	Specific Examples
General	Position the patient in semi-recumbent position, DVT & gastric stress ulcer prophylaxis. Steroids may be required depending on the aetiology.
Antimicrobial	Broad spectrum antibiotics followed by specific treatment when sensitivities known.
Cardiovascular	IV fluids, inotropes / vasopressors & PAC. MAP should be >65 mmHg.
Renal	IV fluids, diuretics & RRT e.g. haemofiltration, haemodialysis, peritoneal dialysis or haemodiafiltration. Urine output should be >0.5ml/kg/hr.
Respiratory	O_2 & ventilation. Venous oxygen saturation should be >70%.
Nutritional	Enteral or parenteral feeding to meet increased energy-requirements.
Surgical	Reduce infective load e.g. drain abscess.

Q: What is MOFS, & state some of its unfavourable predictive factors?

The progression of MODS to an irreversible state is multi-organ failure syndrome. Mortality is higher at the extremes of age, in immunocompromised patients (e.g. DM, HIV, steroids & immunosuppressants), in sepsis, with associated foreign materials (e.g. prosthetic heart valves) or with burn injuries.

ICU ADMISSION

Q: When would you consider patient admission to an ICU?

- Homeostatic Failure — e.g. electrolytes / thermoregultation
- High Risk of MODS — e.g. pancreatitis
- High Risk Procedure — e.g. AAA repair
- Intensive Monitoring Required — e.g. cardiovascular / neurological
- Mechanical Support Required — e.g. ventilation
- Preoptimisation — e.g. pre-operative
- Severe Condition — e.g. head injury / septicaemia.

Q: What are the major differences between an ICU & HDU?

HDU (high dependency unit)	ICU (intensive care unit)
1 Nurse : 2 Patients	1 Nurse : 1 Patient
Ward / On-Call Doctor(s)	Specific Doctor(s) Without Other Commitments
No Requirement for Patient Ventilation	Patients May Require Ventilation

BRAINSTEM DEATH

You are called to the surgical ward, by a nurse, to see a patient who is brainstem dead.

Q: What important conditions must be confirmed prior to diagnosing brainstem death?

- Patient Comatosed / Ventilated
- Coma Cause Known
- Irreversible Brain Damage
- Reversible Causes of Coma Excluded: Alcohol
  Drugs
  Endocrine Disturbance e.g. Hypothyroidism
  Hypothermia
  Metabolic Disturbance e.g. Hypoglycaemia
  Recent Circulatory Arrest.

Q: How would you diagnose brainstem death?

This must be performed by 2 doctors (1 who is a consultant), both registered ≥5 years & not part of the transplant team. The following are tested & should be ABSENT:

- **Pupillary Light Response:** (cranial nerve II)
- **Occulovestibular Reflex:** (cold caloric stimulation – cranial nerves III & VI)
- **Corneal Reflex:** (cranial nerves V & VII)
- **Occulocephalic Reflex:** (doll's eye movements – cranial nerve VIII)
- **Gag Reflex:** (cranial nerves IX & X)
- **Motor Response to Pain:** (grimacing to pain)
- **Ventilatory Effort Following Apnoea Testing:** (P_aCO_2 rises to 6.65kPa).

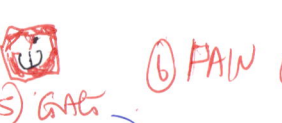

CHAPTER 3
PHYSIOLOGY

BH Miranda
BS Ghoorun

CHAPTER CONTENTS

Calcium Homeostasis

Peripheral Nerves

Nerve Action Potential

Neuromuscular Junction & Muscle Relaxants

Blood Pressure Regulation

Arterial Waveform & Cardiac Cycle

Cardiac Action Potentials

Cardiac Output

Shock

Lung Function

Oxygen Transport

Thermoregulation

Renal Function

CALCIUM HOMEOSTASIS

Q: How is calcium distributed throughout the body?

Distribution	Explanation
Bone	99% forms the mineral hydroxyapatite in bone.
Extracellular	1% is extracellular & distributed as follows: • 55% free as Ca^{2+} (this is physiologically important). • 40% bound to plasma proteins e.g. albumin & globulin. • 5% as a complex with e.g. phosphate, citrate & lactate.

Q: What hormones are responsible for calcium homeostasis?

Hormone	Body Calcium Effect	Explanation
PTH	Increase	• Increased resorption from bone. • Increased reabsorption in kidneys. • Increased 1α-hydroxylase activity.
1,25-Dihydroxycholecalciferol	Increase	Vitamin D_3 is synthesised from cholesterol in the skin with UV light. This is converted in the liver to 25-hydroxycholecalciferol. This is converted in the kidney to 1,25-dihydroxycholecalciferol via 1α-hydroxylase activity. The effects include: • Increased reabsorption in kidneys. • Increased absorption in bowel.
Calcitonin	Decrease	• Decreased resorption from bone. • Increased excretion in kidneys.

Q: Can you classify the functions of Ca^{2+}?

Function	Examples
Cellular	Enzyme Cofactor & 2nd Messenger
Cardiovascular	Cardiac Action Potential
Haematological	Clotting Cascade Factor IV
Muscular	Cardiac, Skeletal & Smooth Muscle Contraction
Skeletal	Constituent of Bones & Teeth

Q: What are the causes & clinical features of hypercalcaemia & hypocalcaemia?

The main causes of hypercalcaemia include hyperparathyroidism (1° & 3°) & cancer. With respect to cancer the causes include 1° malignancy e.g. myeloma, 2° metastases to bone & paraneoplastic syndromes e.g. small cell lung carcinoma resulting in PTHRP release. The causes of hypercalcaemia may therefore be remembered as follows:

Calcium State	Causes	Clinical Features
HYPERCALCAEMIA	Memory: Harry Caught Sally Twanging Mark's Fiddle.	
	Hyperparathyroidism (1° & 3°)	• BONES e.g. Bone Cysts
	Cancer (1°, 2° & Paraneoplastic)	• STONES e.g. Renal Calculi
	Sarcoid	• GROANS e.g. Abdominal Pain, Constipation & PUD
	Thyrotoxicosis	• MOANS e.g. Psychosis
	Milk-Alkali Syndrome	• Cardiac Arrhythmias
	Familial Hypocalciuric Hypercalcaemia	
HYPOCALCAEMIA	Lack of Sunlight Exposure	• Circumoral Paraesthesia
	Malnutrition	• Muscle Cramps & Tetany
	Pancreatitis	• Convulsions
	Hypoparathyroidism e.g. Post Thyroid Surgery	• Clotting Delay (Factor IV)
		• Chvostek's & Trousseau's Signs

Q: What are the treatment options for hypercalcaemia?

- Treat cause.
- IV fluids ± furosemide (may help to eliminate calcium).
- Bisphosphonates.
- Steroids for sarcoid.
- Calcitonin rarely used.

PERIPHERAL NERVES

Q: What is the structure of a peripheral nerve?

- An **epineurium** surrounds **groups of fascicles**.
- Groups of fascicles are **surrounded by perinurium**.
- Fascicles consist of **nerve fibres surrounded by endoneurium**.
- **Nerve fibres consist of axons** that may be myelinated with Schwann Cells.

Q: What are the important physiological principles relating to nerve injuries?

1. **Wallerian Degeneration:** The proximal end of the nerve undergoes regression to the next proximal Node of Ranvier. The distal end of the nerve undergoes regression distally to form a 'hollow' neural tube.
2. **Increased Gene Expression:** Occurs in the nerve cell bodies, to upregulate growth.
3. **Axon Generation:** The proximal axon begins to grow at a rate of 1mm/day.
4. **Schwann Cells:** Assist guidance of the growing proximal axon towards the distal neural tube.

Q: What types of nerve injury are there?

Classification	Explanation	Examples	Prognosis
Neurotmesis	Complete Nerve Transection	Complete Laceration Injury	Poor / Variable
Axonotmesis	Axon & Myelin Sheath Partial Division with Epineurium Undamaged	Partial Laceration	Moderate
Neuropraxia	Nerve 'Bruising' with Minimal Damage	Stretch / Compression Injury	Good

NERVE ACTION POTENTIAL

Q: Can you draw a nerve action potential & explain the events that occur?

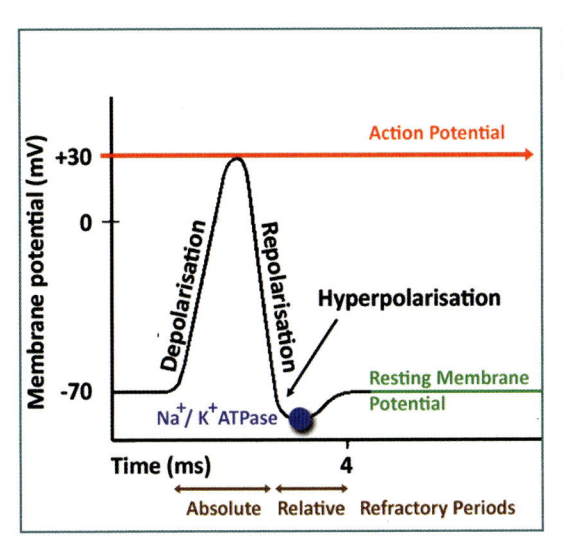

Fig 3.1: Diagram showing a nerve action potential.

Action Potential

Na⁺ / K⁺ ATPase

Resting Membrane Potential

Refractory Periods

Event	Notes
Resting Membrane Potential	This is the membrane potential at rest. The concentration gradient of intracellular & extracellular ions (Na⁺, K⁺ & Cl⁻) results in a resting membrane potential of -70mV.
Threshold Potential	This is the membrane potential to which a membrane must be depolarised in order to induce an action potential.
Depolarisation	Strong stimuli result in the opening of fast voltage gated Na⁺ channels, such that there is Na⁺ influx into the cell. If stimuli evoke a response above the threshold potential, an **all or nothing response** of depolarisation occurs. This is the beginning of the **action potential** that is then propagated along the axon.
Repolarisation	Once depolarisation has reached a membrane potential of 30mV, Na⁺ channels close. Voltage gated K⁺ channels open, such that K⁺ now moves out of the cell.
Hyperpolarisation	This occurs as K⁺ channels close & the **Na⁺/K⁺ ATPase** pump pumps Na⁺ OUT & K⁺ IN to the cell again. This results in the return to & maintenance of the resting membrane potential.
Absolute Refractory Period	This is the period of time where no further stimuli can precipitate a response.
Relative Refractory Period	This is the period of time where only strong stimuli can precipitate a response.

Q: What is saltatory conduction?

Myelinated axons are surrounded by Schwann cells that are interrupted by unmyelinated gaps called the Nodes of Ranvier. Current is generated at these nodes only, quickly jumping between them, hence reducing the signal propagation time.

NEUROMUSCULAR JUNCTION & MUSCLE RELAXANTS

Q: Using a diagram, can you briefly outline the electrophysiological events that occur at the neuromuscular junction?

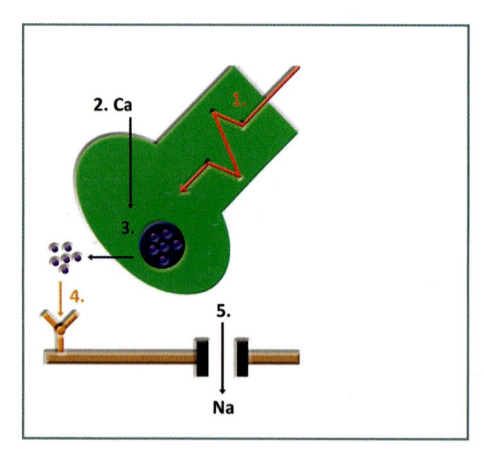

Fig 3.2: Diagram of events occurring at the neuromuscular junction.

- Action Potential
- Axon & Synaptic Knob
- ACh Vesicle
- ACh Molecules
- ACh Receptor
- Muscle Motor End Plate
- Na^+ Channel

Step	Notes
1. Action Potential	The action potential propagates down the **axon**, resulting in depolarisation.
2. Calcium Influx	Calcium influx occurs in response to depolarisation.
3. ACh Vesicles	**Storage vesicles** release **ACh** in response to calcium influx.
4. ACh Receptor Binding	ACh diffuses from the **synaptic knob**, across the synaptic cleft, then binds to **nicotinic cholinergic receptors** on the **muscle motor end plate**.
5. Sodium Channels	Sodium channels open & influx of sodium into the motor end plate occurs. Depolarisation, known as the **end plate potential**, occurs. If this depolarisation is large enough, an **action potential** is generated & muscle contraction ensues.

Note: Bound ACh is hydrolysed by acetylcholinesterase. The choline produced by this process is taken up by the presynaptic membrane & re-used to form ACh.

Q: What muscle relaxants may be used as part of anaesthesia & how do they work?

Category	DEPOLARISING	NON-DEPOLARISING
Example	Suxamethonium	Tubocurarine & Atracurium
Action	Mimics effect of ACh but is not rapidly hydrolysed by acetylcholinesterase. **Note: May precipitate hyperkalaemia, so beware e.g. in burns.**	Competitive inhibitor of ACh at postsynaptic nicotinic receptors. Reversed by Neostigmine. They also have action on presynaptic membrane receptors, interfering with calcium influx, hence reducing further ACh release from storage vesicles.
Effect	Results in an initial contraction, followed by paralysis.	Gradual paralysis occurs.

Q: What condition is characterised by the presence of IgG Ab against ACh receptors & what are the clinical features?

Myasthenia Gravis. Clinical features range from mild symptoms to myasthenic crisis that may result in terminal respiratory failure. The basic hallmark feature is muscle FATIGABILITY. Bulbar features are also typical & include dysarthria & dysphagia. Clinical features may be classified according to level of involvement & include:

Involvement	Clinical Features
Face	Facial expression muscle weakness e.g. expressionless face & myasthenic snarl.
Ocular	Diplopia, decreased eye movements & FATIGABLE ptosis.
Mastication	Mastication muscle weakness resulting in decreased ability to chew.
Deglutition	Deglutition muscle weakness resulting in dysphagia.
Speech	Muscle weakness resulting in poor phonation & articulation (dysarthria).
Neck & Limb	FATIGABLE neck & limb muscle weakness.
Respiratory	Respiratory muscle weakness & loss of cough reflex results in retained secretions & pneumonia. In a myasthenic crisis, muscle paralysis may occur, such that assisted ventilation is required to sustain life.
Thymus	Associated thymus pathology, of any type, affects 75% of patients e.g. thymoma, hyperplasia & atrophy. Associated thymoma is found in 25% of patients.
Autoimmune	Associated autoimmune disease may be present e.g. Graves' Disease, Hashimoto's Disease & rheumatoid arthritis.

Q: What specific investigations may help assist a diagnosis of myasthenia gravis?

A full work up, including **full history**, **thorough clinical examination** & **appropriate investigations** is vital for diagnosis. Specific investigations however include:

1. **ACh Receptor Ab:** Present in 85% of patients.
2. **EMG:** Specific muscle fibre electrical patterns are found in myasthenia gravis.
3. **Tensillon Test:** (IV) edrophonium, a short acting anticholinesterase, is given to temporarily inactivate acetylcholinesterase. Temporary symptom improvement confirms myasthenia gravis.
4. **Striated Muscle Ab & CT:** May indicate thymus pathology & mediastinum extension.
5. **TFT & Thyroid Ab:** May indicate associated thyroid disease.

BLOOD PRESSURE REGULATION

Q: What equations describe the relationship between blood pressure & cardiac output?

$$\text{Blood Pressure} = \text{Cardiac Output} \times \text{Systemic Vascular Resistance}$$

$$\text{Cardiac Output} = \text{Heart Rate} \times \text{Stroke Volume}$$

Q: Can you discuss the neurohumoral mechanisms that maintain blood pressure?

Mechanism	Explanation
Baroreceptors	Baroreceptors at e.g. aortic arch & carotid sinus, are stimulated by stretch such that if circulating blood volume falls, less stimulation occurs. **ADH** is also released from the posterior pituitary in response to this, hence preventing diuresis.
Chemoreceptors	Chemoreceptors e.g. aortic & carotid bodies, are stimulated by hypercapnoea, acidosis & hypoxia. If these states ensue during e.g. exercise, cardiac failure or hypovolaemic shock, more stimulation occurs.
Medulla	Baroreceptor & chemoreceptor responses are transmitted to the **cardioinhibitory** (ventral) & **vasomotor** (ventrolateral) centres of the medulla. The response is such that in e.g. exercise, cardiac failure or hypovolaemic shock, SNS activation, PSNS inhibition & catecholamine release occur. Under these circumstances there will be an increase in HR, SV & SVR.
Kidney	Underperfusion activates the renin-angiotensin-aldosterone system, such that sodium & water are retained. This results in raised JVP, peripheral & pulmonary oedema. **Angiotensin II** is an arterial vasoconstrictor (increasing SVR), dipsogen (increasing thirst) & may stimulate **ADH** release from the posterior pituitary.
Heart (Hormonal)	ANP is released by atrial myocytes in response to stretch in e.g. cardiac failure & hypervolaemia. The responses include vasodilation & increased glomerular filtration with diuresis & natriuresis. These responses reduce both afterload & preload.

Mechanism	Explanation
Heart (Intrinsic)	Intrinsic autoregulatory mechanisms include: **Anrep Effect:** An increase in afterload results in an increase in ventricular contractility. **Bowditch Effect:** An increase in HR stimulates inotropy.

Q: Can you discuss the renin-angiotensin-aldosterone system in more detail?

The specialised cells required for this system to function are located in the kidney. **Juxtaglomerular** cells are located in afferent arterioles as they enter their respective glomeruli. They secrete renin in response to decreased afferent arteriole pressure e.g. hypotension & low cardiac output (Fig 3.3). A decrease in blood sodium concentration also results in renin secretion, however this is detected by **macula densa** cells at specialised areas of distal tubules. These cells therefore influence renin in response to certain conditions as follows:

Cells	Detection		Renin Response
Juxtaglomerular	Afferent Arteriole Pressure:	Decrease:	↑
		Increase:	↓
Macula Densa	Blood Sodium Concentration:	Decrease:	↑
		Increase:	↓

↓ Na (macula densa)
↓ Afferent Arteriole Pressure

- ADH Secretion
- Aldosterone Release
- SNS Activity
- Thirst
- Vasoconstriction

RENIN
(juxtaglomerular apparatus)

Angiotensinogen ⟶ Angiotensin I —ACE⟶ Angiotensin II

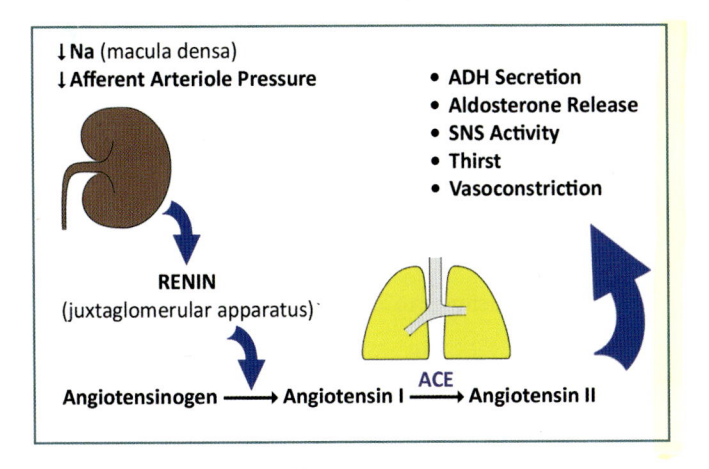

Fig 3.3: Renin-angiotensin-aldosterone system.

Released renin cleaves the circulating peptide angiotensinogen (synthesised by the liver), to angiotensin I. This is converted to angiotensin II by circulating angiotensin converting enzyme (ACE), released by lung endothelial cells. The resulting responses maintain blood pressure & include an increase in:

- ADH Secretion
- Aldosterone Release
- SNS Activity
- Thirst
- Vasoconstriction.

ARTERIAL WAVEFORM & CARDIAC CYCLE

Study the following diagram (Fig 3.4) & answer the questions below:

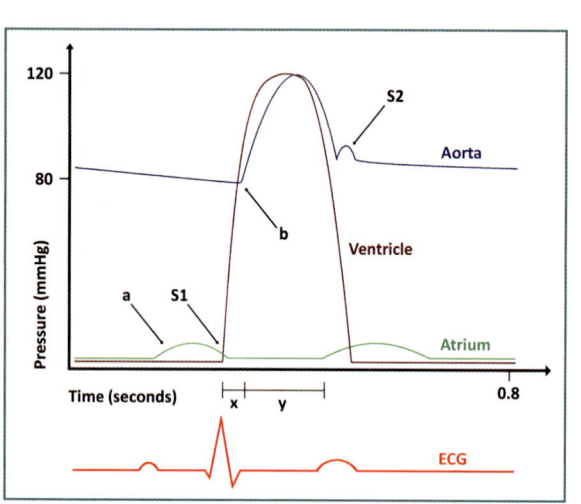

Fig 3.4: Diagram showing pressure changes in the left side of the heart during the cardiac cycle. The ECG waveform has been superimposed.

Q: How long is the cardiac cycle? Can you define stroke volume & ejection fraction?

- The cardiac cycle lasts 0.8 seconds.
- Stroke volume represents the volume of blood ejected by the ventricles during systole = 70mls.
- Ejection fraction is the stroke volume represented as a fraction of the end diastolic volume = 0.60.

Q: What is the significance of points a, b, x, y, S1 & S2?

Point	Significance	Notes
a	Atrial 'Kick'	Active atrial contraction produces 20% of ventricular filling. The remainder of ventricular filling is passive.
b	Aortic Valve Opening	Occurs at the onset of rapid ventricular ejection.
x	Isovolumetric Ventricular Contraction	Both arterial & atrioventricular valves are closed, such that ventricular contraction results in a rapid rise in pressure, without any change in volume.
y	Rapid Ventricular Ejection	The arterial valves are forced open as ventricular pressure exceeds aortic root & pulmonary trunk pressures. This results in rapid ejection of blood volume from the ventricles.
S1	1st Heart Sound	Due to mitral valve closure.
S2	2nd Heart Sound	Due to atrioventricular valve closure. This produces a 'dicrotic notch' in the aortic waveform.

Q: How is mean arterial pressure calculated from the arterial pressure curve?

MAP may be calculated by dividing the area under the arterial pressure curve, by the width of the base of the arterial pressure curve (the time it takes to complete the cardiac cycle). MAP may also be calculated using the following equation:

$$MAP = \text{Diastolic Pressure} + \tfrac{1}{3}(\text{Systolic} - \text{Diastolic Pressure})$$

Q: What effect does exercise have on the cardiac cycle?

There is a shortening of all cardiac cycle phases, with ventricular diastole becoming disproportionately shorter. This is compensated for by an increased contribution to ventricular filling by atrial 'kick'.

Exercise: ↓ systole ↓↓ diastole ↑ atrial kick

Q: What effect does aortic valve disease have on the arterial waveform?

Disease	Effect
Aortic Stenosis	Slow rising waveform with prolonged plateau.
Aortic Regurgitation	Wide pulse pressure, with low diastolic pressure.

CARDIAC ACTION POTENTIALS

Q: Can you draw a diagram & explain the important features of the pacemaker action potential?

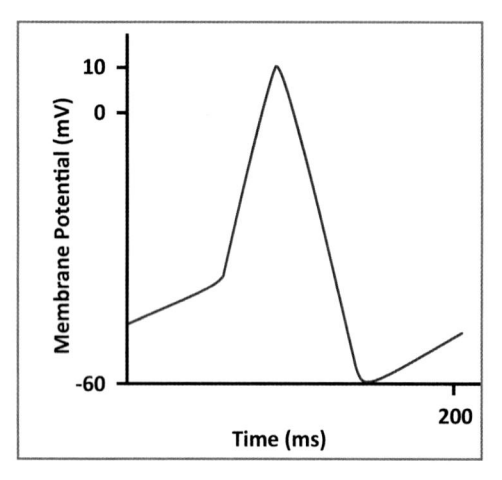

Fig 3.5: Pacemaker potential.

Spontaneous depolarisation is an important feature of the pacemaker potential which begins immediately after repolarisation.

This occurs due to changes in cell membrane permeability & movement of the following ions:

- Na^+ (inward movement)
- Ca^{2+} (inward movement)
- K^+ (decreased outward movement).

Once spontaneous depolarisation has reached the threshold potential (-40mV), depolarisation occurs due to opening of ion channels that allow influx of Ca^{2+} (-60mV). Repolarisation occurs due to opening of ion channels that allow efflux of K^+. Hyperpolarisation occurs as Ca^{2+} channels begin to close.

Q: What are the phases of the ventricular action potential & how do they occur?

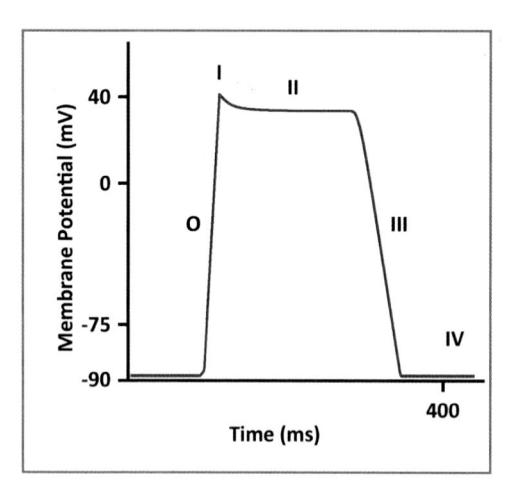

Fig 3.6: Ventricular action potential.

The resting membrane potential of ventricular muscle cells = -90mV.

The action potential commences when the membrane of the ventricular muscle is brought to the threshold potential due to excitation from adjacent cells (-75mV).

Once the threshold has been reached, the action potential proceeds in phases as follows:

Phase	Notes
0	Rapid depolarisation occurs as fast Na⁺ channels open, resulting in rapid influx into the cell.
I	Partial repolarisation occurs as fast Na⁺ channels close & K⁺ channels open, allowing efflux of K⁺ from the cell.
II	A plateau phase occurs due to opening of specialised channels that allow a slow sustained influx of Ca²⁺. **Note: This is important as it provides an absolute refractory period for ventricular muscle, thereby preventing tetany & fatigue.**
III	Repolarisation occurs as K⁺ efflux from the cell continues, coupled with closing of specialised Ca²⁺ channels.
IV	The resting membrane potential of ventricular muscle cells = -90mV. This phase is associated with diastole.

Q: What is the Vaughan-Williams classification system?

This system classifies antiarrhythmic drugs according to their action on cardiac action potentials as follows:

Classification	Action	Examples
I	Inhibit Na⁺ Channels	Procainamide (Ia), Lidocaine (Ib), Flecainide (Ic)
II	β-Blockers	Atenolol, Propanolol
III	K⁺ Channel Blocker	Amiodarone, Ibutilide
IV	Ca²⁺ Channel Blocker	Verapamil, Diltiazem
V	Direct Nodal Inhibition	Adenosine, Digoxin

Handwritten mnemonic:
I — Local, II — Boys, III — kick, IV — Cats, V — & Dogs
Ia — Procainamide, Ib — Lidocaine, Ic — Flecainide

CARDIAC OUTPUT

Q: What is a normal resting value for cardiac output?

5–6 L/min.

Q: What is Frank-Starling's Law of the Heart?

The contractile force generated by the heart is proportional to initial myocardial fibre length due to stretch. This implies that stroke volume is proportional to end diastolic volume, such that increased venous return to the heart results in increased myocardial fibre stretch & subsequent greater force of contractility. This relationship is outlined by the Frank-Starling curve (Fig 3.7). However, there is a point of myocardial fibre stretch, **beyond** which results in a rapid decline in contractile force. This normal relationship may be **shifted up (positive inotropic effect)** or **down (negative inotropic effect)** (Fig 3.7).

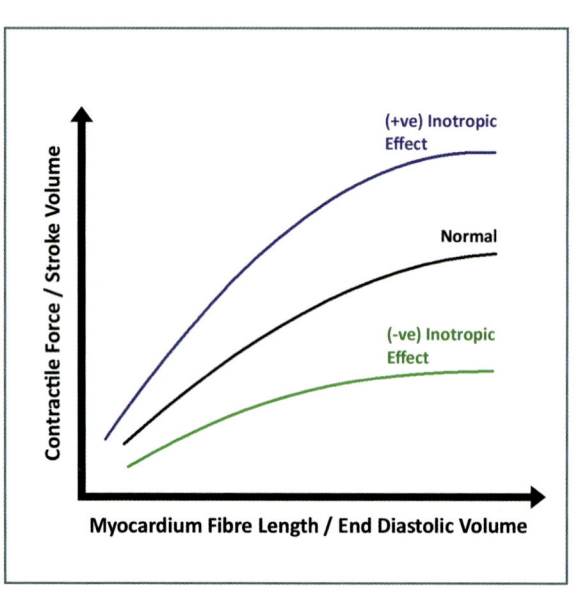

Fig 3.7: Frank-Starling curve.

Shift Up / (+ve) Inotropic Effect:
- Exercise
- Noradrenaline

Shift Down / (-ve) Inotropic Effect:
- β-Blockers
- Cardiac Failure

Q: How is cardiac output measured?

There are numerous methods, some invasive, others non-invasive as follows:

MEASUREMENT OF CO

Methodology	Notes
Fick Principle (invasive)	This is based on the observation that total uptake of a substance by peripheral tissues, is equal to the product of blood flow to those tissues & the concentration gradient of the substance: Cardiac Output = (O_2 Consumption / Arterial-Venous O_2 Gradient) x 100 Thus, the following are required to calculate cardiac output: • **PAC Insertion:** O_2 concentration in mixed venous blood. • **Peripheral Arterial Cannulation:** O_2 concentration in arterial blood. • **Spirometry:** O_2 consumption (closed re-breathing circuit with CO_2 detector).
Dye Dilution / Thermodilution Methods (invasive)	Both methods involve PAC insertion & balloon inflation to float the catheter through the right ventricle. Once lodged in the pulmonary artery, the catheter balloon is deflated. A small volume of dye / known temperature fluid is then injected via the catheter. With both methods, calculating cardiac output first involves testing the concentration of dye / temperature change at a downstream site of known distance. In the case of the dye dilution method, the downstream site is a peripheral artery. In the case of the thermodilution method, the downstream site is 6–10cm further down the pulmonary artery & the temperature is detected using the same PAC. If the cardiac output is high, more dilution / temperature change will occur, however if low, less will occur. A dilution curve is therefore generated that allows for cardiac output calculation.
Doppler USS	Calculations are based on the principle that returning ultrasound waves undergo Doppler shift on return from the heart. This shift is dependent on the velocity of blood through the heart, hence allowing for calculation of cardiac output.
Echocardiogram	Calculations are based on measuring the cross-sectional area of the aorta & utilising the Doppler shift effect to calculate blood velocity. This allows for a more accurate calculation of cardiac output than Doppler USS alone, however requires greater operator skill & training.

SHOCK

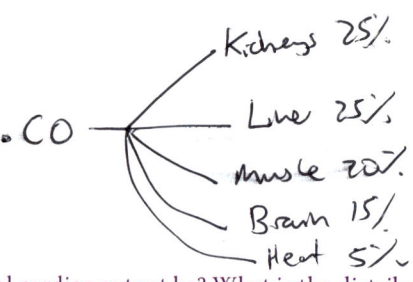

Q: What should normal cardiac output be? What is the distribution to organs / tissues?

Average cardiac output is 5–6L/min. The kidneys & liver each receive approximately 25% of cardiac output. Muscle receives approximately 20%, brain 15%, heart 5% & the remainder of organs & tissues receive approximately 10% of cardiac output.

Q: What is physiological shock?

Acute circulatory failure leading to a generalised state of inadequate organ / tissue perfusion & hypoxia. Cellular dysfunction / damage or major organ failure may ensue.

Q: What types of shock do you know of & what are the hallmark features?

Type	Features
Addisonian	Due to a stress factor in patients with Addison's Disease (e.g. diarrhoea & vomiting, infection, surgery, trauma), or due to non-compliance / abrupt withdrawal of steroids (e.g. not transferring steroids to the drug chart of a patient with IBD). Features may include those of chronic Addison's Disease (e.g. skin & mucus membrane hyperpigmentation) or of a stress factor (e.g. pyrexia, recent scar). When Addisonian crisis occurs & the patient enters shock, features include abdominal pain, nausea & vomiting, cardiovascular collapse, cyanosis, confusion, coma.
Anaphylactic	This is a type I hypersensitivity reaction occurring in previously sensitised individuals *(see pathology chapter)*. Features may occur instantly & include bronchospasm, increased mucus secretion, tachycardia, urticaria, vasodilation & circulatory collapse.
Cardiogenic	Due to pump failure. Initially, the neurohumoral response helps to maintain the falling blood pressure by increasing the SVR (see below). This however makes it harder for the heart to pump blood, resulting in a vicious cycle that may exacerbate pump failure. Furthermore, the neurohumoral response results in a hypervolaemic state, such that a raised JVP, peripheral & pulmonary oedema may be seen.
Hypovolaemic	Due to decreased intravascular volume e.g. diarrhoea, haemorrhage, inadequate fluid resuscitation, 3rd space losses & vomiting. Features are compatible with the percentage of blood loss, memorable by scores in a tennis match *(see below)*.
Neurogenic	Due to acute neurological injury e.g. spinal cord transection. Peripheral vasomotor tone is lost, bradycardia & complete circulatory collapse ensue.
Septic	Due to infection, endotoxin & exotoxin release. Vasodilation ensues resulting in decreased SVR. Features include pink warm peripheries, pyrexia & raised cardiac output with diminished oxygen extraction.
Spinal	This is unrelated to circulatory collapse. Spinal shock is due to spinal cord 'concussion' after trauma. Features include areflexia, hypotonia & paralysis that should, at least partially, recover within 72h.

Q: You are called to the ward, as an emergency, to see a patient who has just been given an intravenous infusion of penicillin. As you approach, you notice that the patient has developed a rash. He is tachypnoeic, tachycardic & hypotensive. What do you do?

This patient is in anaphylaxis. I would do the following as quickly as possible, adhering to ALS guidelines:

- Stop infusion.
- Call for help.
- Ensure airway is maintained (consider advanced airway management) & administer high flow O_2.
- Ensure patient is breathing & ventilating.
- Ensure patient circulatory parameters are adequate.
- Give 0.5mls (1/1000) adrenaline IM *(or 100–200mcg IV & repeat according to response)*.
- Give 20mg chlorpheniramine IV.
- Give 200mg hydrocortisone IV.

Following the above acute management, I would ensure that the patient is placed under close observation & would consider ordering relevant blood tests. Finally, I would come back at a later stage to review the patient.

Q: What are the causes of cardiogenic shock?

The causes of pump failure may be classified as primary or secondary as follow:

Primary	Secondary
IHD & MI	Tamponade
Arrhythmias	Tension Pneumothorax
Cardiomyopathy	Pulmonary Embolism
Dissection	Sepsis

Q: What do you understand by the neurohumoral response to cardiogenic shock?

When pump failure ensues, baroreceptors in the aortic arch, carotid sinus & great vessels are less stimulated by stretch. Furthermore, decreased oxygen delivery to the aortic & carotic bodies results in less stimulation of chemoreceptors. Consequently, there is decreased sensory input to the cardiovascular centres of the medulla. The resulting SNS activation, PSNS inhibition & catecholamine release, directly increase HR, SV & SVR. As the kidneys are underperfused in cardiogenic shock, the renin-angiotensin-aldosterone system becomes activated so that Na^+ & water are retained. This results in the hypervolaemic clinical features that are associated with cardiogenic shock e.g. raised JVP, peripheral & pulmonary oedema.

Q: Can you tell me more about the clinical features & physiology of hypovolaemic shock?

There are 4 classes of hypovolaemic shock, each categorised according to percentage blood volume loss:

Class	Loss	Description
I	15%	Acute blood loss results in decreased venous return & decreased SV (Starling's Law of the Heart). Additionally, baroreceptors & chemoreceptors are less activated by stretch & oxygen delivery respectively. This results in decreased sensory input to the cardiovascular centres of the medulla. SNS activation & PSNS inhibition ensue. As blood loss is still mild at this stage, symptoms may be absent, however, HR may be slightly elevated (<100 bpm) & the patient may be anxious.
II	30%	Decreased venous return to the heart causes a significant drop in SV. Catecholamine release & compensatory HR elevation, maintain CO. Tachycardia >100bpm, narrow pulse pressure, orthostatic hypotension, mild decrease in urine output, mild increase in respiratory rate & further anxiety may be observed.
III	40%	Heart rate is unable to compensate for the further drop in SV, so CO begins to fall. Further catecholamine release ensues, resulting in an increase in SVR to maintain BP. Tachycardia >120bpm, cold & clamminess, narrow pulse pressure, further decrease in urine output, tachypnoea & confusion may be observed.
IV	>40%	SV drops to end-stage levels. HR is unable to maintain CO which then drops further. SVR increases further, but not enough to maintain BP. BP finally drops as a late sign of hypovolaemia. Profound tachycardia >140, hypotension, cold & clamminess, narrow pulse pressure, oliguria, profound tachypnoea & lethargy / unsciousness may be observed.

Note$_1$: Remember these percentages as the scores in a tennis match.

Note$_2$: HR is a very good marker of hypovolaemia & easy to remember relative to class & % blood loss.

Note$_3$: Hypotension is a late, end-stage sign of hypovolaemia.

Q: How would you treat a patient in shock?

Management strategies are dependent on the cause e.g. anaphylaxis is discussed earlier. A general approach must always adhere to ALS / ATLS principles:

- Ensure airway is maintained & administer high flow O_2.
- Ensure patient is breathing & ventilating. A simple manoeuvre, e.g. needle thoracostomy, may improve the problem e.g. tension pneumothorax.
- Ensure patient circulatory parameters are adequate & achieve haemorrhage control.
- Establish IV access with 2 x wide bore cannulae (1 per antecubital fossa) & commence fluid resuscitation (10–20mls/kg).
- Further patient examination e.g. neck veins, abdomen & cardiac trace.
- Placement of other devices e.g. urinary-catheter or central venous-catheter.

- Check blood biochemistry & consider a group-&-save.
- ABG monitoring.
- Appropriate imaging.
- Identify & treat the cause.
- Regularly reassess the patient & fluid challenge as appropriate.
- Consider vasopressors or inotropes.
- Consider transfer to ICU.

Q: What are vasopressors & inotropes?

When a patient is adequately filled yet still shocked, these drugs may be used to improve the cardiac index. For example in sepsis, fluid resuscitation alone may be inadequate to compensate for the degree of vasodilation, leaking capillaries & myocardial depression.

The cardiovascular system has 2 types of adrenergic receptor (α & β). Positive inotropic & positive chronotropic effects result from β1-adrenoceptor stimulation. Vasoconstriction occurs due to α-adrenoceptor stimulation. Vasodilation occurs due to β2-adrenoceptor stimulation. There may be a degree of cross-stimulation as all the aforementioned receptors are adrenergic.

Q: Do you know of any vasopressors or inotropes?

	Noradrenaline	Dobutamine
Type	Vasopressor (primarily)	Inotrope (primarily)
Central Line Administration?	Essential	Yes, or with large peripheral line.
Example Application	Septic Shock	Cardiogenic Shock
Other Considerations	Reduces peripheral & splanchnic supply, with consequences for e.g. free-flap & bowel surgery.	Tolerance may develop over 48–72hours.

Q: Can adrenaline be given for shock?

Yes e.g. for anaphylactic or cardiac shock. However, adrenaline has generalised action on all adrenoceptors. The consequence of this is that the heart & brain receive a large proportion of blood at the expense of other tissues, which may produce a more unfavourable situation.

LUNG FUNCTION

Q: What are the functions of the lungs?

- Oxygenation of Blood
- Elimination of CO_2
- pH Balance
- ACE Release.

Q: What are labels a–g on the spirometry tracing below?

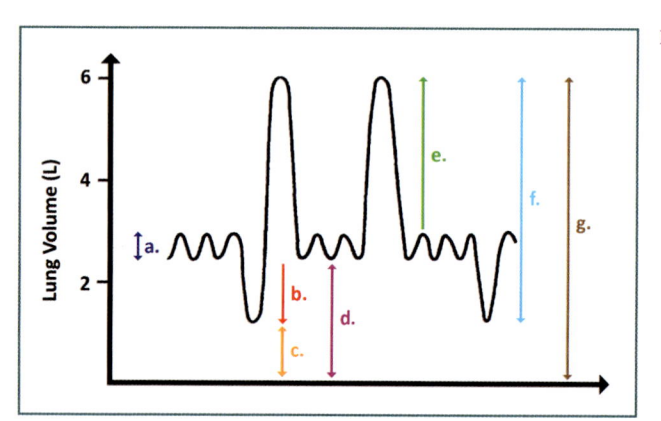

Fig 3.8: Spirometry tracing.

Label	Definition	Notes
a.	Tidal Volume (TV)	Volume of air inspired & expired during normal respiration = 500mls.
b.	Expiratory Reserve Volume (ERV)	Additional volume of air forcibly expired, after a normal tidal breath out = 1250mls.
c.	Residual Volume (RV)	Volume of air remaining in the lungs after a forced breath out = 1250mls.
d.	Functional Residual Capacity (FRC)	Volume of air remaining in the lungs after a tidal breath out = 2500mls. **Note: Calculated as ERV + RV.**
e.	Inspiratory Reserve Volume (IRV)	Additional volume of air forcibly inspired, after a normal tidal breath in = 3000mls. **Note: Calculated as VC – (TV + ERV).**
f.	Forced Vital Capacity (FVC)	Total amount of air forcibly expired, after a forced breath in = 4750mls.
g.	Total Lung Capacity (TLC)	Volume of air within the lungs after a maximum breath in = 6000mls. **Note: Calculated as TV + ERV + IRV.**

Q: Can you briefly outline a technique used to measure residual volume?

RC & TLC cannot be directly measured. However, FRC can be measured using the **helium dilution method**, hence allowing RV & TLC calculation:

- The patient is connected to a closed circuit spirometer containing a known amount & concentration of helium.
- The patient is asked to breathe in & out of the spirometer, after a tidal expiration (hence leaving their FRC in the lungs prior to using the spirometer).
- After 5–10mins, the helium concentration in the lungs & spirometer will equilibrate.
- An in-line CO_2 absorber is in place to prevent CO_2 build up.
- As the helium volume remains constant within this closed system, calculating the final concentration of helium in the spirometer, will contribute to calculating the FRC. The theory behind this statement is that the decrease in helium concentration on the spirometer side is directly due to dilution by the patient's FRC.

Q: A patient comes to clinic with respiratory difficulty. What spirometry test would assist your diagnosis of obstructive vs. restrictive respiratory disease?

FEV_1 / FVC:

- FEV is the expiratory volume recorded during forced expiration from maximum inspiration.
- FEV_1 is the above volume recorded during the 1st second of forced expiration.
    Normal FEV_1 / FVC = 70–75%
    Obstructive Disease   < 70%
    Restrictive Disease   > 75%.

OXYGEN TRANSPORT

Q: How is oxygen transported & what factors affect this?

Method	Amount	Mechanism	Factors
Hb Bound	99%	Up to 4 O_2 molecules may reversibly bind to Hb to form oxyhaemoglobin.	• pH • Temperature • 2,3 DPG • CO & CO_2
In Blood	1%	Dissolved.	• Partial Pressure* • Solubility (affected by temperature)*

*Note: Henry's Law: A Solution's Gas Content = Gas Partial Pressure x Gas Solubility.

Q: What is the oxygen dissociation curve? Can you draw it, labelling its axes?

This sigmoid curve represents Hb's ability to bind O_2 with a differential affinity, depending on the P_aO_2. This means that at the extremes of the curve, large changes in P_aO_2 lead to small changes in % Hb saturation, whereas on the steep part of the curve, small changes in P_aO_2 lead to large changes in % Hb saturation. Patients are able to tolerate a fall in P_aO_2 extremely well, provided it remains above 90%. The P_{50} value = 3.6kPa & this refers to the pressure at which Hb is 50% saturated with O_2.

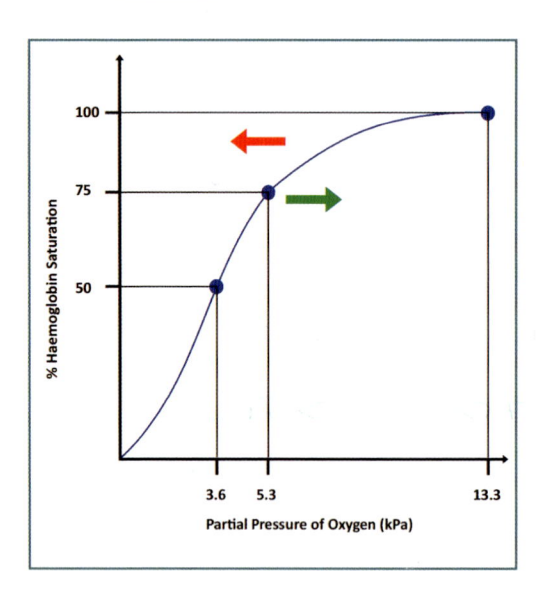

Fig 3.9: O_2 dissociation curve.

Left Shift:
- ↓Temperature
- ↓ H+ (↑pH)
- ↓ 2,3 DPG
- ↓ CO_2
- Foetal Hb

Right Shift:
- ↑ Temperature
- ↑ [H+] (↓pH)
- ↑ 2,3-DPG
- ↑ P_aCO_2

Q: What is cooperative binding & what impact does this have on the O_2 dissociation curve?

Hb binds O_2 with greater affinity, after a subunit has already bound a previous O_2 molecule. This is because the binding of an O_2 molecule facilitates the binding of the next O_2 molecule. This property of Hb is known as cooperative binding & this makes the O_2 dissociation curve sigmoid (Fig 3.9).

Q: What is the Bohr Effect?

An increase in temperature, [H⁺] (↓pH), 2,3-DPG & P_aCO_2 result in a decrease in O_2 affinity of Hb. This means that O_2 is more likely to be transferred from the blood into the tissues. This is known as the Bohr Effect & results in a shift of the O_2 dissociation curve to the right. Other conditions may shift the curve to the left, resulting in a decreased likelihood of transfer of O_2 from the blood into the tissues (Fig 3.9).

Q: What do you know about the O_2 content in blood?

- The solubility of O_2 in blood at 37°C is 0.03ml/L for every 1mmHg rise in partial pressure.
- 200ml O_2 are present in 1L arterial blood.
- 50ml O_2 are taken out per 1L of arterial blood, as it perfuses organs & tissues.
- 150ml O_2 are left per 1L of venous blood.
- 1.34ml O_2 may be bound by 1g Hb.
- The oxygen carrying capacity of blood at 100% saturation is therefore 1.34 x [H⁺].

Total Blood O_2 Content	=	(% Hb Saturation x Blood O_2 Carrying Capacity)	+	O_2 Dissolved in Plasma (Henry's Law)
	=	(S_aO_2 x [Hb] x 1.34) Hb O_2	+	P_aO_2 x 0.03 PLASMA Hb O_2

Q: How would you clinically improve physiological O_2 delivery to tissues?

This is an important principle in critical care medicine & may be achieved by optimising any of the following factors: to support organ-systems whilst optimising the delivery of O_2 to tissues.

Factor	Explanation
S_aO_2	% saturation of Hb may be improved via O_2 therapy.
Cardiac Output	Cardiac output may be optimised by adequately filling the patient, hence optimising Starling's Law of the Heart. Drugs e.g. inotropes may also be indicated.
[Hb]	Hb concentration may be improved via blood transfusion or supplements e.g. Fe^{2+}.

Q: What factors increase the risk of post-operative hypoxaemia in a surgical patient?

Factors	Examples
Comorbidity	• Cardiac e.g. IHD
	• Respiratory e.g. COPD
	• Systemic e.g. Anaemia, DM & Obesity
Physiology	• Hypotension & Hypovolaemia
	• Hyperthermia & Hypothermia
	• Sepsis
Operation	• Major Surgery e.g. Burns, Orthopaedic & Thoracoabdominal

THERMOREGULATION

Q: How are temperature changes detected by the body?

Modality	Location
Core Thermoreceptors	Hypothalamus & Spinal Cord
Peripheral Thermoreceptors	Skin
Higher Processing	Hypothalamus

Q: How does the body respond to hypothermia?

Physiological	Somatic	Behavioural
BMR Upregulation*	Curling Up	Avoid Cold
Piloerection	Shivering (increases BMR)	Central Heating
Sweating (inhibition)		Hot Drinks
Vasoconstriction (peripheral)		Warm Clothes

*Note: Hypothalamic thermoreceptors detect cold, resulting in TRH release = increased thyroid activity.

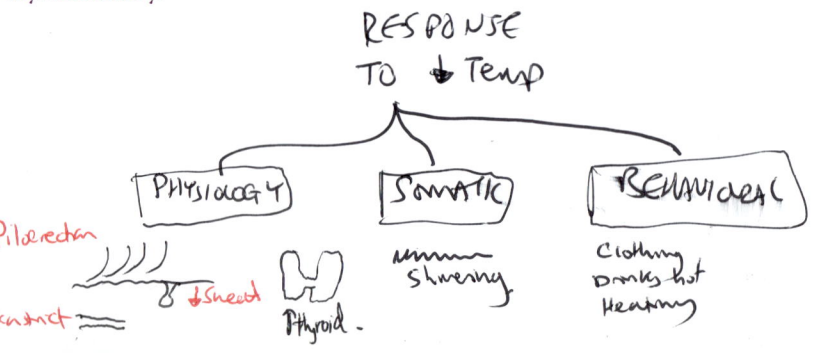

CAUSES OF ↓ TEMP

PATIENT	DISEASE	ENVIRONMENT
- ↑ Age (poor homeostasis)	- AD	- Poverty
- ETOH	- DM	- ETOH/drugs
	- CCF	
	- Infections	
	- Burns/bleeding	

Q: What are the causes of hypothermia?

Classification	Examples
Age Related	Alzheimer's Disease (loss of awareness), Impaired Homeostasis
Disease	Autonomic Neuropathy (DM), Cardiac Failure, MI, Pneumonia
Drugs	Alcohol, Benzodiazepines
Trauma	Burns, Haemorrhage
Social	Poverty

Q: How would you manage a patient with hypothermia?

- ALS / ATLS Approach   (as required)
- Appropriate History & Examination   (within ALS / ATLS framework as required)
- Appropriate Investigations:

Important Blood Tests	Notes
FBC	Rule out anaemia & infection.
U&E	K⁺ abnormalities may precipitate arrhythmias. Blood levels should be repeated during management, as reperfusion injury may result in rhabdomyolysis with hyperkalaemia.
Glucose	Indicator of abnormal glycaemic levels, associated with diabetes. Also important with loss of consciousness, to rule out hypoglycaemia.
TFT	Rule out disease causing decreased thyroid hormone secretion, or inadequate oral replacement therapy.
CK	Rhabdomyolysis is common when patients have been found after a sustained period of immobility. This is due to muscle breakdown & results in an elevated CK.

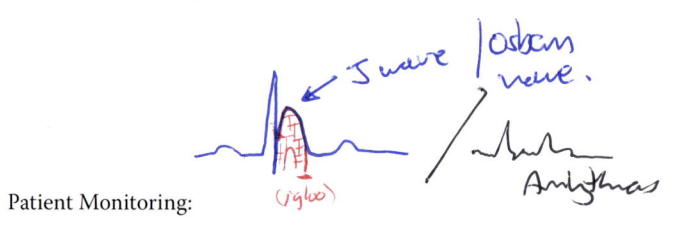

- Patient Monitoring:

Monitoring	Notes
ECG	Arrhythmias, J-Waves
Rectal Thermometer	More Accurate
Urinary Catheter	Fluid Balance, MC+S
ABG	Extreme hypothermia induces peripheral vasoconstriction, such that the receiving tissues are hypoperfused. These tissues then undergo anaerobic metabolism, producing a lactic acidosis (raised lactate). **Note: ABG should be monitored throughout admission.**
Microbiology	Blood Cultures, Sputum, Urine Dipstick, MSU / CSU, Wound Swabs

- **Treatment:** Depends on the clinical scenario. Implementation should be in the context of an ALS / ATLS framework. Investigation & treatment extends beyond the acute setting, so that underlying causes (medical & social) are also addressed. Patient warming methods should be gradual at 1°C/h & include:
    - **Bair Hugger**
    - **Thermal Blanket**
    - **Intravenous Infusion of Warmed Fluids**
    - **Bladder / Intraperitoneal Infusion of Warmed Fluids**
    - **Cardiopulmonary Bypass**
    - **Haemodialysis.**

RENAL FUNCTION

Study this diagram & answer the following questions:

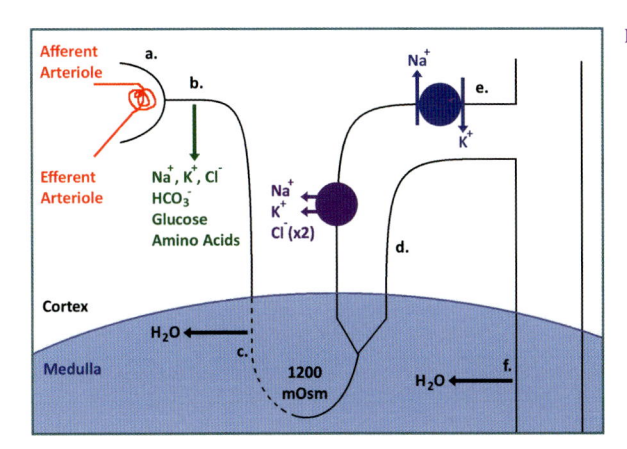

Fig 3.10: Diagram of nephron function.

Q: What are the functions of the kidney?

Function	Examples
Plasma Filtration	Glucose, H_2O, Ions (Na^+, Cl^- & HCO_3^-), Small Amino Acids
Homeostasis	Acid-Base, BP, Electrolytes, Fluid Balance
Hormonal	1,25-Dihydroxycholecalciferol, EPO, Renin
Metabolism	Drugs
Excretion	Urea, Creatinine, H_2O, Drugs & Metabolites

Q: Can you name structures a–f, briefly outlining their function (Fig 3.10)?

Structure	Name	Function
a.	Glomerulus	Ultrafiltration of plasma occurs here. The glomerulus is selectively permeable due to the presence of: • Podocytes (forming slit pores) that allow only small (≤8nm) molecules to be ultrafiltered. • Negatively charged basement membrane that primarily allows ultrafiltration of positive ions.
b.	Proximal Convoluted Tubule	Resorption of Na^+, K^+, Cl^-, HCO_3^-, glucose, amino acids.
c.	Descending Loop of Henle	This is freely permeable to H_2O, which diffuses into the hypertonic renal medulla, resulting in concentration of urine to 1200mOsm.
d.	Ascending Loop of Henle	Active resorption of Na^+, K^+ & Cl^- via K^+-Na^+-$2Cl^-$ cotransporters. The ascending Loop of Henle is impermeable to H_2O, so as the Loop is ascended, ion transfer across the Loop results in a decrease in osmolarity.
e.	Distal Convoluted Tubule	Resorption of Na^+ & excretion of K^+ via Na^+/K^+ ATPase pumps. Stimulation by **aldosterone** increases this process.
f.	Collecting Duct	Resorption of H_2O occurs after stimulation by **ADH**, which increases H_2O permeability. Urine is also delivered to the calyces of the kidney.

Q: Where do diuretics work on the nephron?

Classification	Example	Action
Loop	**Furosemide**	Block K^+-Na^+-$2Cl^-$ cotransporters at the ascending Loop of Henle.
Thiazide	**Bendrofluazide**	Block thiazide sensitive Na^+-Cl^- cotransporters at the distal convoluted tubule.
Potassium-Sparing	**Spironolactone**	Block the action of aldosterone on Na^+/K^+ ATPase pumps at the distal convoluted tubule.

SECTION B: ANATOMY & SURGICAL PATHOLOGY

CHAPTER 4
ANATOMY

BH Miranda
K Asaad
L Clarke
W Birch

CHAPTER CONTENTS

Head & Neck
- Atlanto-Axial Joint & Vertebrae
- Mandible & Temperomandibular Joint
- Tongue
- Parotid Gland & Facial Nerve
- Thyroid Gland
- Triangles of the Neck

Trunk & Thorax
- 1st Rib
- Mediastinum
- Heart
- Lungs
- Diaphragm
- Liver
- Abdominal Aorta & Related Structures
- Penis & Scrotum

Limbs, Spine & Vascular
- Upper Limb Vessels
- Rotator Cuff
- Antecubital Fossa
- Carpal Tunnel
- Dorsum of the Hand
- Femur & Hip Joint
- Lower Limb Vessels
- Femoral Triangle
- Femoral Sheath
- Inguinal Canal
- Adductor Canal
- Knee Joint
- Popliteal Fossa
- Lower Leg Compartments
- Ankle & Foot

Neurosciences
- Skull
- Lateral Cerebral Hemisphere
- Medial Cerebral Hemisphere
- Cerebrospinal Fluid
- Cranial Nerves
- Ascending & Descending Spinal Pathways
- Brachial Plexus
- Carotid Sheath
- Circle of Willis

HEAD & NECK

Atlanto-Axial Joint (Fig 4.1) & Vertebrae

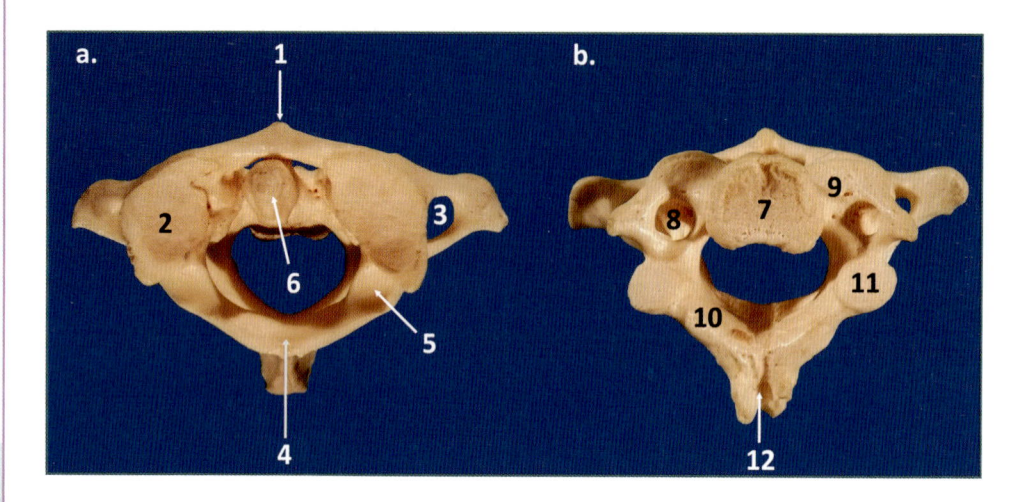

Q: Can you identify images a & b?

a = atlanto-axial joint, superior view onto atlas (C1), b = atlanto-axial joint, inferior view up to axis (C2).

Q: What are structures 1–5?

These are all structures of the atlas: 1 = anterior arch & tubercle, 2 = superior articulating facet of lateral mass, 3 = foramen of transverse process, 4 = posterior arch & tubercle, 5 = groove for vertebral artery.

Q: What are structures 6–12?

These are all structures of the axis: 6 = dens (odontoid process), 7 = body, 8 = foramen of transverse process, 9 = pedicle, 10 = lamina, 11 = inferior articular process, 12 = bifid spinous process.

Q: What type of joint is the atlanto-axial joint & what ligament reinforces it?

Synovial joint, reinforced by the transverse ligament that allows for lateral rotation.

Q: What runs through 8 & what structure does it originate from?

The vertebral arteries run through the vertebral foramina of the C1–C7 vertebrae. They are branches of the subclavian arteries.

Q: What are the features of typical cervical, thoracic & lumbar vertebrae?

Vertebra	Body	Spine	Transverse Process	Plane of Facet Joint	Movements
Cervical	Broad	Small & Bifid	Has Foramen	Oblique	Flexion, Extension, Lateral Flexion
Thoracic	Heart Shape, Has Demifacets	Long & Points Inferiorly	Has Costal Facets	Horizontal-Oblique	Lateral Rotation (primarily)
Lumbar	Kidney Shape	Quadrangular	No Foramen, No Costal Facets	Medial	Flexion, Extension, Lateral Flexion

Mandible & Temperomandibular Joint (Fig 4.2)

Study the skeletal specimen below & answer the following questions:

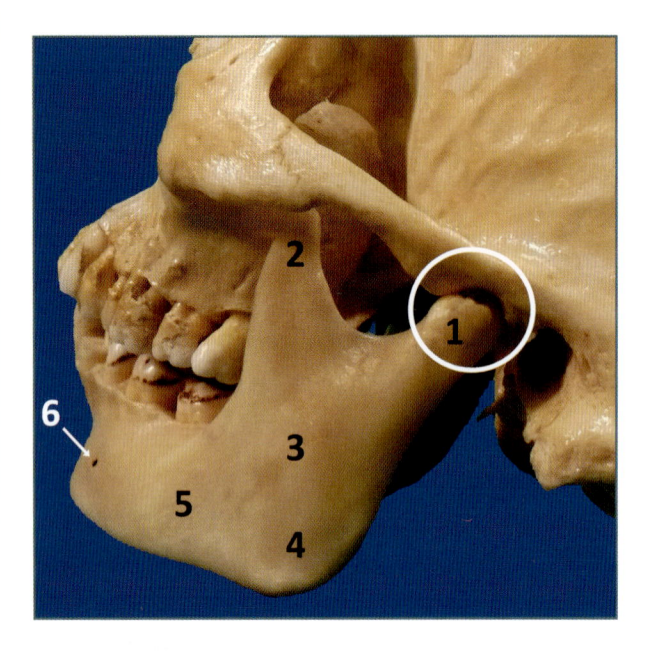

Q: What are the structures labelled 1–6?

This is the left mandible. 1 = condylar head, 2 = coronoid process, 3 = ramus, 4 = angle, 5 = body, 6 = mental foramen.

Q: What runs through 6?

The mental nerve. The inferior alveolar nerve is a branch of the posterior division of V_3 (marginal mandibular nerve). It runs through the mandibular foramen (medial aspect of the mandible) & exits the mental foramen as the mental nerve. The mental nerve supplies sensation to the lower lip & chin.

Q: Can you describe the anatomy of the circled joint?

This is the left temporomandibular joint. It is a synovial joint. The convex mandibular head, articulates with the squamous portion of the temporal bone. The articulating surface of the temporal bone is comprised of a concave articular fossa & convex articular eminence. A saddle shaped meniscus separates the condyle & temporal bone, dividing the joint into superior inferior spaces that contain synovial fluid.

Tongue

Q: What are the muscles of the tongue?

Intrinsic (within the tongue)	Extrinsic (with bony attachment)
Longitudinal	Genioglossus
Transverse	Hyoglossus
Vertical	Palatoglossus
	Styloglossus

Q: What is the innervation of the tongue?

- The motor supply is via the hypoglossal nerve (XII) except palatoglossus which is innervated by the vagus nerve (X) & pharyngeal plexus.
- Somatic sensation from the anterior ⅓ of the tongue is via the lingual nerve, a branch of the mandibular nerve (V3).
- Taste sensation from the anterior ⅔ of the tongue is via the chorda tympani, a branch of the facial nerve (VII).
- Sensation from the posterior ⅓ of the tongue is via the glossopharyngeal nerve (IX).

Q: What taste modalities are detected by the tongue & how is this achieved?

The oral part of the tongue is covered in papillae that are either circumvallate, filiform, foliate or fungiform. All papillae have taste buds except filiform.

- The posterior aspect of the tongue (anterior to the lingual tonsils) senses bitter taste.
- The lateral aspect of the tongue senses sour taste.
- The anterolateral aspect of the tongue senses salty taste.
- The anterior aspect of the tongue senses sweet taste.

Parotid Gland & Facial Nerve (Fig 4.3)

Study the prosection below & answer the following questions.

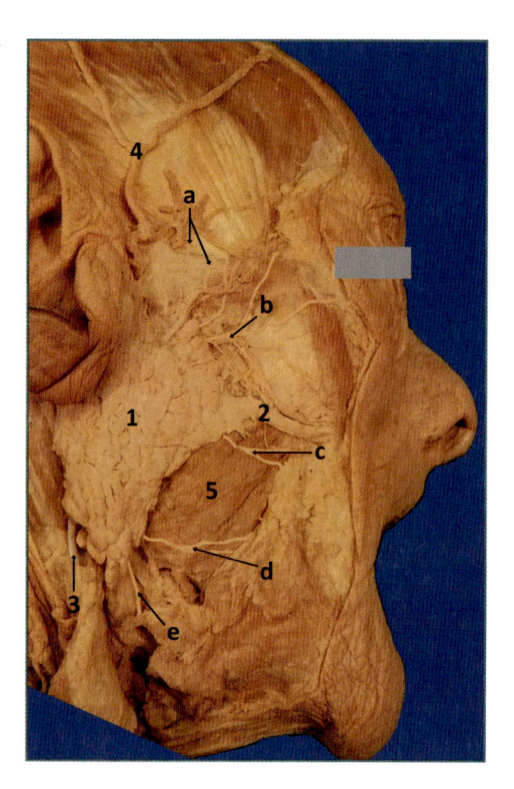

Q: What are structures 1–5?

1 = right parotid gland, 2 = right parotid duct, 3 = right retromandibular vein (drains into the right internal jugular vein), 4 = right superficial temporal artery, 5 = right masseter.

Q: What are structures a–e?

These are the branches of the right facial nerve (VII). a = temporal, b = zygomatic, c = buccal, d = mandibular, e = cervical.

Q: What are the borders of the parotid gland?

Superior = zygomatic arch, inferior = angle of mandible, posterior = sternocleidomastoid, anterior = masseter, deep = styloid apparatus, superficial = investing fascia of neck.

Q: What structures run through the parotid gland?

Facial nerve (VII), external carotid artery (giving off the superficial temporal & maxillary arteries at the level of the mandibular neck), retromandibular vein (formed by the superficial temporal & maxillary veins), lymph nodes.

Q: What is the path / surface anatomy of the parotid duct?

Extends from the anterior border of the parotid gland, over masseter (along a line drawn from the inferior border of the tragus to the midpoint of the filtrum), then pierces buccinator to open in the buccal mucosa at the level of the upper 2nd molar.

Q: Can you describe the path of the facial nerve?

- Originates between pons & medulla.
- Supplies muscles of facial expression.
- Runs with vestibulocochlear nerve (VIII), through the internal auditory meatus of the petrous temporal bone.
- Reaches the middle ear cavity & forms the geniculate ganglion (Fig 4.4).
- Gives off branches including the greater superficial pertrosal nerve, nerve to stapedius & chorda tympani (Fig 4.4).
- Runs posterior along the superior middle ear cavity, then inferiorly along the posterior cavity.
- Exits the petrous temporal bone via the stylomastoid foramen.
- Runs superficial to the mandible.
- Enters the posterior-medial aspect of the parotid gland.
- Passes anteriorly through the parotid gland (dividing the gland into superficial & deep) & gives off 5 branches (Fig 4.3).

Q: What are the branches of the facial nerve?

These may be classified according to function as follows (Fig 4.4):

Function	Branch	Notes
MOTOR	**Stapedius**	Causes hyperacusis if damaged.
	Posterior Belly of Digastric	Elevates hyoid as part of swallowing mechanism.
	Stylohyoid	Elevates hyoid.
	Posterior Auricularis	Moves earlobe.
	5 Divisions Within Parotid Gland	• **Temporal:** Innervates frontalis & orbicularis oculi. • **Zygomatic:** Innervates orbicularis oculi, levator labii superioris & zygomaticus muscles. • **Buccal:** Innervates buccinator, levator anguli oris & nasalis muscles. • **Marginal Mandibular:** Innervates depressor anguli oris, depressor labii inferioris & mentalis. • **Cervical:** Innervates platysma.
SECRETOMOTOR	**Greater Superficial Petrosal Nerve**	Innervates lacrimal, nasal & palatine glands.
	Chorda Tympani	Innervates submandibular & sublingual salivary glands.
TASTE	**Chorda Tympani**	Taste to the anterior ⅔ of the tongue.
OTHER SENSORY	**Multiple Communications**	Communications with trigeminal, glossopharyngeal, vagus, greater auricular & auriculotemporal nerves explain associated mastoid, ear, head & neck pain in herpes zoster & Bell's Palsy.

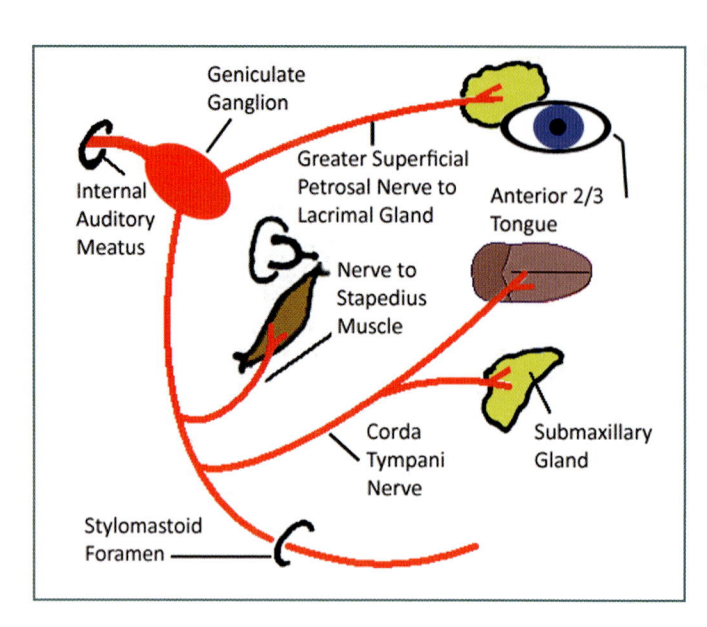

Fig 4.4: Branches of the facial nerve (VII).

Note that after exiting the petrous temporal bone via the stylomastoid foramen, the facial nerve travels superficial to the mandible & towards the parotid gland. It gives off 5 branches within the parotid gland:

1. Temporal
2. Zygomatic
3. Buccal
4. Marginal Mandibular
5. Cervical

Thyroid Gland (Fig 4.5)

Study the prosection below & answer the following questions.

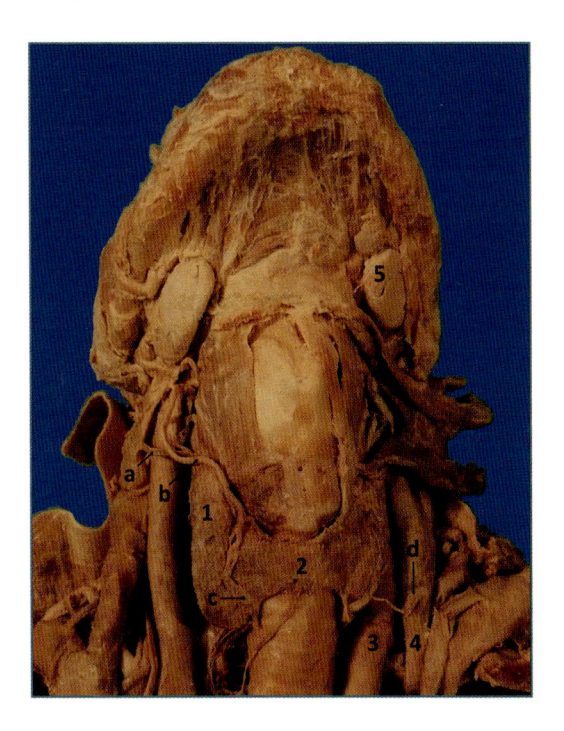

Q: What are structures 1–5?

1 = right thyroid lobe, 2 = thyroid isthmus, 3 = left common carotid artery, 4 = left internal jugular vein, 5 = left submandibular gland.

Q: What are structures a–d?

a = right superior thyroid vein, b = right superior thyroid artery, c = right inferior thyroid vein, d = left middle thyroid vein. **Note: The inferior thyroid artery lies posterior to the thyroid gland.**

Q: What is the blood supply & venous drainage of the thyroid gland?

Arteries	Veins
Superior Thyroid (branch of external carotid)	Superior Thyroid (drains into internal jugular)
Inferior Thyroid (from thyrocervical trunk)	Middle Thyroid (drains into internal jugular)
Thyroid Ima (in 10% of patients – from aortic arch)	Inferior Thyroid (drains into left brachiocephalic)

Q: What is the anatomy of the recurrent laryngeal nerve?

It is a branch of the vagus (X) nerve as it descends into the thorax. The right recurrent laryngeal nerve hooks under the subclavian artery to ascend the right trachea-oesophagus groove. The left recurrent laryngeal nerve ascends the left trachea-oesophagus groove, however it arises, from the vagus (X), within the thorax (so has a longer course) & hooks under the ligamentem arteriosum (under the aorta). The recurrent laryngeal nerve supplies all larynx muscles (except cricothyroid = external laryngeal nerve) & sensation below the vocal folds. Sensation above the vocal folds is supplied by the internal laryngeal nerve.

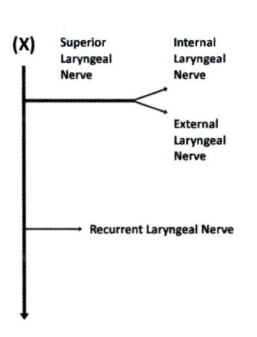

Triangles of the Neck (Fig 4.6)

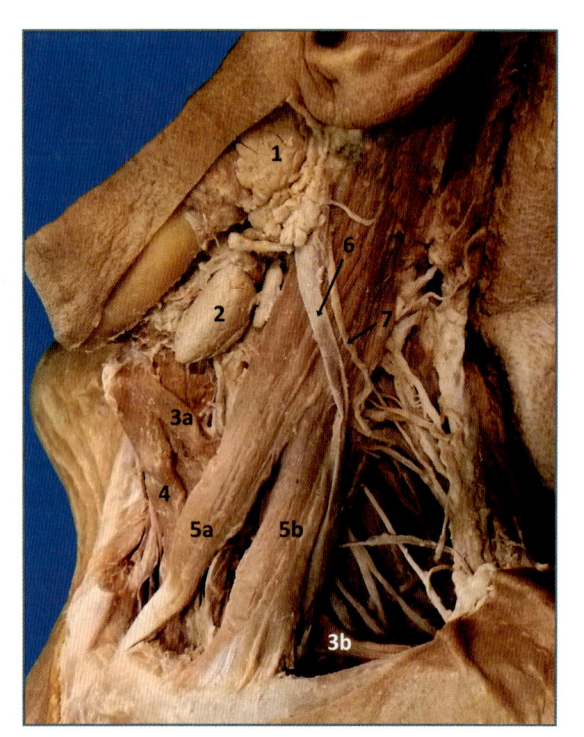

Q: What are structures 1–7?

1 = parotid gland, 2 = submandibular gland, 3a = superior belly of omohyoid, 3b = inferior belly of omohyoid, 4 = sternohyoid, 5a = sternal head of sternocleidomastoid, 5b = clavicular head of sternocleidomastoid, 6 = external jugular vein, 7 = greater auricular nerve.

Q: What is the path / surface anatomy of the spinal accessory nerve?

It traverses the posterior triangle of the neck, from the posterior border of the upper & middle ⅓ of sternocleidomastoid, to the anterior border of the lower & middle ⅓ of trapezius. It supplies both of these muscles.

Q: What are the borders & contents of the anterior & posterior triangles?

Triangle	Border	Notes	Contents
ANTERIOR	Anterior	Neck midline (from chin to jugular notch of manubrium)	• Carotid Sheath • External Carotid Artery • Hyoid Bone • Jugular Veins: Anterior, external & internal • Larynx • Lymph Nodes • Nerves: Ansa cervicalis, vagus (X), hypoglossal (XII) & nerve to myelohyoid • Oesophagus • Parathyroid Glands • Thyroid Gland
	Superior	Inferior border of mandible & line extending from angle of mandible to mastoid process	
	Posterior	Sternocleidomastoid (anterior border)	

Triangle	Border	Notes	Contents
POSTERIOR	Anterior	Sternocleidomastoid (posterior border)	• Arteries: Occipital, superficial cervical & suprascapular • Lymph Nodes (Level 5) • Muscles: Omohyoid • Nerves: Brachial plexus branches & spinal accessory nerve • Veins: External jugular, suprascapular & transverse cervical
	Inferior	Middle ⅓ of clavicle (superior border)	
	Posterior	Trapezius (anterior border)	

Note: The anterior triangle may be further subdivided into carotid, digastric, muscular & submental triangles.

Q: Can you describe the deep cervical fascia & its components?

Fascial Layer	Notes
Investing Deep Cervical	Surrounds the neck, extending from the pectoral girdle (inferior) to base of skull & mandible (superior). It splits to enclose trapezius & sternocleidomastoid muscles.
Pretracheal	Surrounds the larynx, oesophagus, parathyroid glands, pharynx, recurrent laryngeal nerves, thyroid gland & trachea.
Prevertebral	Surrounds the cervical vertebral column, origins of the cervical & brachial plexus, pre- & post-vertebral muscles.
Carotid Sheath	Surrounds the common carotid artery (medial), internal jugular vein (lateral) & vagus (X) nerve (between). **Note: the sympathetic chain lies posterior to the carotid sheath.**

TRUNK & THORAX

1st Rib (Fig 4.7)

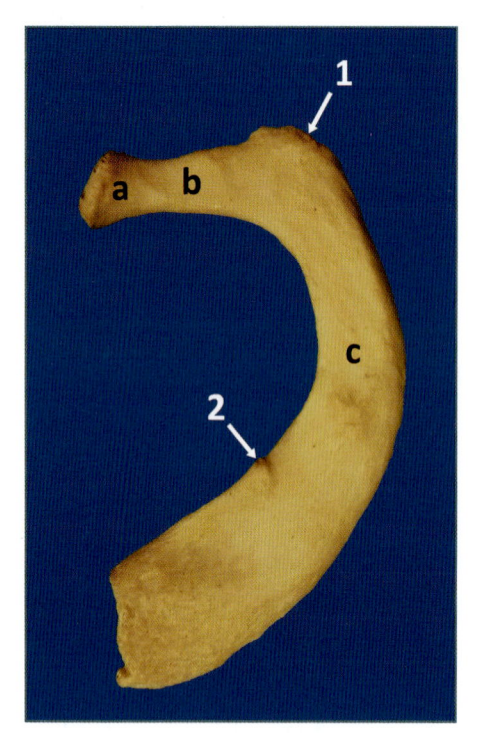

Knowledge of anatomy is clinically important. A patient presents to clinic with tingling that shoots down his arm & into his hand. He has also noticed that his hands turn blue even when it is only slightly cold outside. He is a sales assistant in a supermarket & has noticed that his symptoms are made worse when he is stacking shelves that are above shoulder height. Study this picture & answer the questions below:

Q: Can you identify this bone?

Left 1st rib (superior view).

Q: What are the regions labelled a, b & c?

a = head, b = neck, c = shaft.

Q: What are the protuberances labelled 1 & 2? What inserts here?

1 = tubercle (insertion of lateral costotransverse ligament), 2 = scalene tubercle (insertion of scalenus anterior).

Q: Going from anterior to posterior, what 2 major structures lie in front of & what 2 lie behind the structure that inserts at label 2?

Subclavian vein, phrenic nerve – (scalenus anterior) – subclavian artery, brachial plexus.

Q: What is the likely diagnosis? What are the causes?

Thoracic outlet syndrome which may affect any of the above structures. Causes may be classified as follows:

Anatomical	Traumatic	Neurovascular
Congenital Fibromuscular Bands	Repetitive Postural Movements e.g. Violin Player	Costoclavicular Space Entrapment (between clavicle & 1st rib)
Cervical Rib	Scarring Post RTA	
Scalene Muscle Enlargement	Axillary Vein Thrombosis	

Q: Can you describe Roos' Test?

The patient's arm is placed with 90° of abduction with external rotation at the shoulder & 90° of elbow flexion. The patient is asked to repeatedly open & close their fists. If this reproduces symptoms, thoracic outlet syndrome is likely *(see book 2 Fig 7.1)*.

Q: What treatment options are there for this patient?

After taking a full history, performing a thorough examination & ordering appropriate investigations, treatment options would include:

Conservative	Medical / Invasive	Surgical
Hot / Cold Packs	Muscle Relaxants	Neurolysis
Stretching	Cortisone Injection	Removal of Cervical Rib
Nerve Gliding Exercises	Botulinum Toxin Injection (lasts 3–4 months)	Scalenectomy
Posture Advice & Exercises		Removal of 1st Rib

Note: Approximately 10–15% of patients undergo surgical decompression following trial of conservative therapy.

Mediastinum (Fig 4.8)

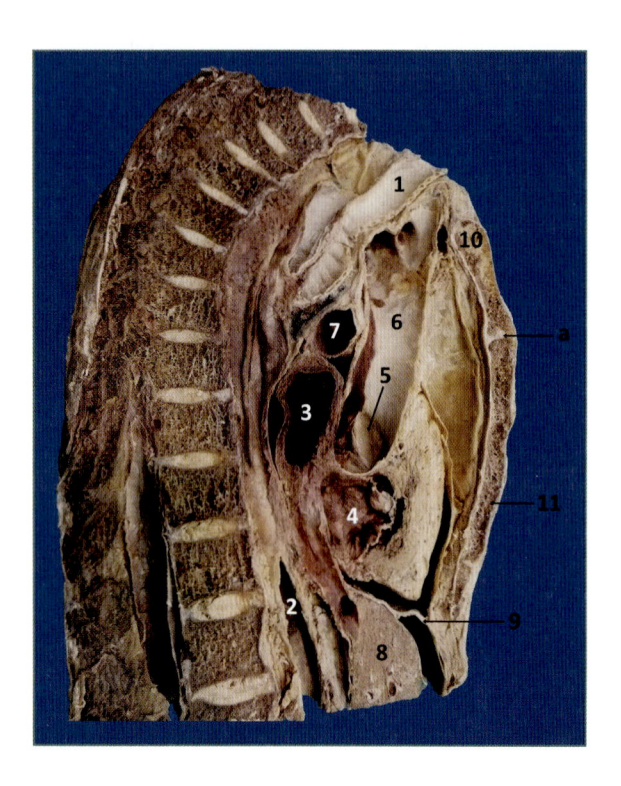

Q: Can you identify this prosection?

Saggital view of the mediastinum, from the right side.

Q: What are structures 1–11?

1 = trachea, 2 = oesophagus, 3 = left atrium, 4 = right ventricle, 5 = aortic valve, 6 = ascending aorta, 7 = right pulmonary artery, 8 = liver, 9 = diaphragm, 10 = manubrium, 11 = body of sternum.

Q: What angle is marked by a?

Angle of Louis (sternal angle).

Q: What are the borders of the mediastinum?

Superior = thoracic inlet, inferior = thoracic outlet, anterior = sternum, posterior = T1-T12 vertebrae, lateral = medial aspects of the lungs.

The mediastinum is further divided into superior & inferior by a line drawn from the Angle of Louis, to the inferior border of T4.

The inferior mediastinum is further divided into anterior (anterior to pericardium), middle (anterior to posterior pericardium) & posterior (posterior to pericardium).

Q: What are the contents of the mediastinum?

(anterior)	Superior Mediastinum		(posterior)
	TVANTODS		
	Thymus, SVC, Aortic Arch, Vagus (X) & Phrenic Nerves, Trachea, s Oesophagus, Thoracic Duct, Sympathetic Chain		
	Inferior Mediastinum		
Anterior	Middle	Posterior	
T	HB	ODDAS	
• Thymus (fat in adults)	• Heart, Pericardium & Phrenic Nerves • Bronchi (primary)	• Oesophagus & Vagus (X) Nerves • Thoracic Duct • Descending Aorta • Azygous Vein • Sympathetic Trunk	

Heart (Fig 4.9)

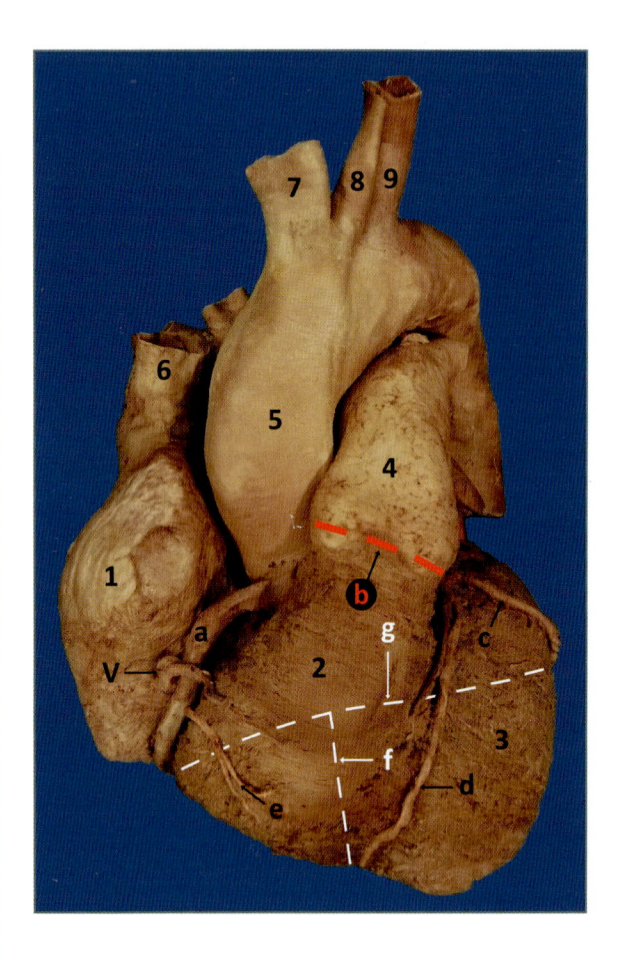

Q: What are structures 1–9?

1 = right atrium, 2 = right ventricle, 3 = left ventricle, 4 = pulmonary trunk, 5 = ascending aorta, 6 = superior vena cava, 7 = brachiocephalic trunk, 8 = left common carotid artery, 9 = left subclavian artery.

Q: What are structures a–f?

The coronary arteries.

a = right coronary artery, b = left coronary artery, c = circumflex artery, d = anterior interventricular artery, e = marginal branch of right coronary artery, f = posterior interventricular artery, g = posterior circumflex artery.

Q: What are the origins of structures a & b?

The right coronary artery (a) originates from the right (anterior) aortic sinus. The left coronary artery (b) originates from the left (posterior) aortic sinus.

Q: What is structure V? What other related structures drain the heart?

V = anterior cardiac vein. The cardiac veins travel (approximately) with the coronary arteries, but incompletely as follows:

- Great cardiac vein with the descending interventricular artery (d).
- Middle cardiac vein with the posterior interventricular artery (f).

The coronary sinus drains the great cardiac & posterior interventricular veins, before draining into the right atrium.

Q: What is the surface anatomy of the heart?

The heart is approximately the size & shape of a closed fist. It sits directly on the diaphragm, without parietal pleura inferiorly. The surface anatomy is as follows:

Border	Surface Anatomy
Superior	Left parasternal at the 2nd rib
Right	Right parasternal from the 3rd to 6th ribs
Cardiac Apex	Left 5th intercostals space, mid-clavicular line
Left	Line drawn from superior border to cardiac apex

Q: What structures cover the heart?

The pericardium covers the heart in 3 layers:

- **Inner Serous Pericardium:** Comprised of inner (**visceral**) & outer (**parietal**) layers, between which pericardial fluid resides to allow free movement of the heart within the pericardial sac.
- **Outer Fibrous Pericardium.**

Lungs (Fig 4.10)

Study the image below & answer the following questions:

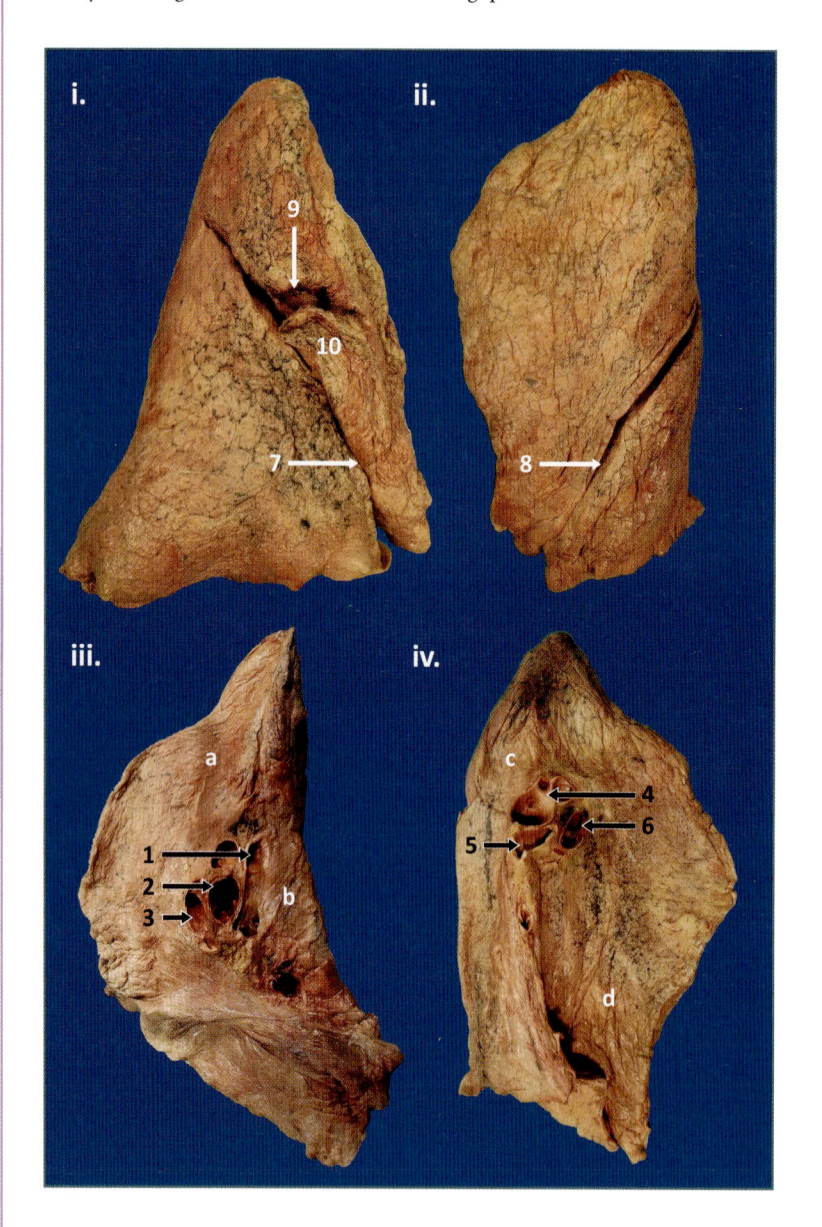

Q: What are the images labelled i–iv?

i = right lung (lateral view), ii = left lung (lateral view), iii = right lung (medial view), iv = left lung (medial view).

Q: What are the structures labelled 1–10?

1.	Right Main Bronchus	6.	Left Pulmonary Vein
2.	Right Pulmonary Artery	7.	Right Oblique Fissure
3.	Right Pulmonary Vein	8.	Left Oblique Fissure
4.	Left Pulmonary Artery	9.	Horizontal Fissure (right only)
5.	Left Main Bronchus	10.	Middle Lobe (right only)

Q: What structures lie in the impressions labelled a–d?

a = superior vena cava, b = azygous vein, c = aortic arch, d = heart.

Q: What is the anatomical position / surface anatomy of the lungs?

Border	Anatomical Position / Surface Anatomy
Apex	Curved line from sternoclavicular joint to 3cm above the junction of the medial ⅓ & intermediate ⅓ of the clavicle.
Anterior	Sternoclavicular joint to xiphisternal joint behind the lateral border of the sternum (note that the left lung deviates laterally from the sternum at the 4th costal cartilage, forming the cardiac notch).
Inferior	6th rib at the mid-clavicular line, 8th rib at the mid-axillary line, 10th rib at the vertebral column.
Posterior	C7 transverse process to T10 transverse process, 4cm from the midline.
Hilum	3rd & 4th costal cartilages, behind the sternal margin at T5, T6, T7.

Q: What structures cover the lung & what is their surface anatomy?

Visceral & parietal pleura. The visceral pleura is adherent to the lung surface & their surface anatomy is identical. The parietal pleura has the following surface anatomy:

Border	Surface Anatomy
Apex	As for lung.
Anterior	As for lung.
Inferior	8th rib at the mid-clavicular line, 10th rib at the mid-axillary line, 12th rib at the vertebral column.
Posterior	C7 transverse process to T12 transverse process, 4cm from midline.

Diaphragm (Fig 4.11)

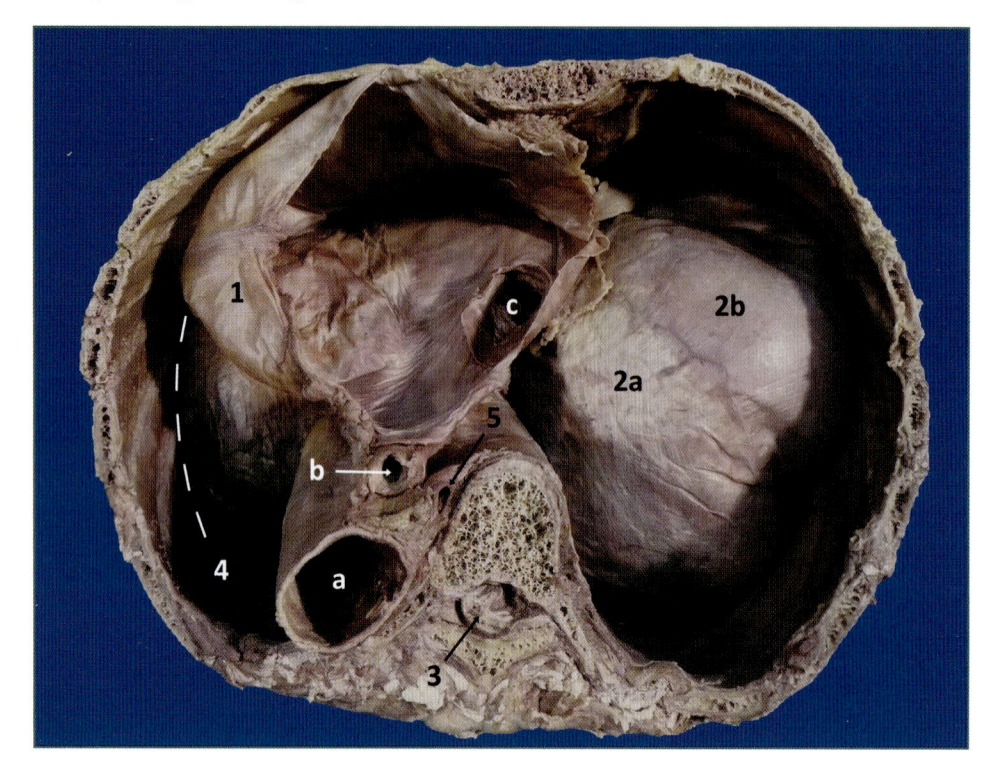

Q: Can you identify this prosection?

Superior view of the diaphragm & associated structures.

Q: What are structures 1–5?

1 = pericardium, 2a = diaphragm tendon (right dome), 2b = diaphragm muscle (right dome), 3 = spinal cord, 4 = left costodiaphragmatic recess, 5 = azygous vein.

Q: What are structures a–c? At what level & with what other structures do they pass from the thorax to the abdomen?

Label	Structure	Thorax to Abdomen Level	Associated Structures
a	Descending Aorta	T12 (passes posterior to diaphragm, through aortic hiatus that is posterior to the median arcuate ligament)	Thoracic Duct & Azygous Vein (to the right), Hemiazygous Vein (to the left)
b	Oesophagus	T10 (pierces diaphragm, through oesophageal opening that is within the right crus)	Right & Left Vagus Nerves (X), Left Gastric Vessels
c	Inferior Vena Cava	T8 (pierces diaphragm, through caval foramen, through central tendon)	Right Phrenic Nerve

Q: What other structure pass from thorax to the abdomen?

- **Left Phrenic Nerve** (pierce left diaphragmatic lobe, muscular portion)
- **Splachnic Nerves** (pierce crura)
- **Superior Epigastric Vessels** (pass between sternal & costal slips of diaphragm)
- **Sympathetic Trunks** (pass posterior to medial arcuate ligament)
- **Neurovascular Bundles** (pass between peripheral muscular slips of diaphragm)

Liver (Fig 4.12 – Inferior View)

Study the image below & answer the following questions:

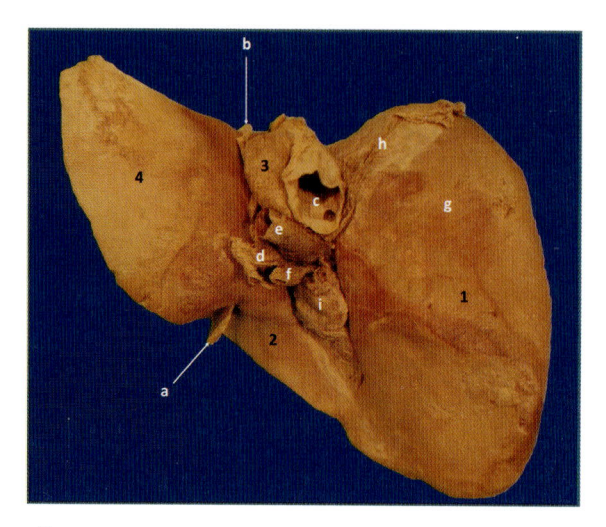

Q: What are structures 1–4?

1 = right lobe, 2 = quadrate lobe, 3 = caudate lobe, 4 = left lobe.

Q: What are structures a–i?

a = ligamentum teres, b = ligamentum venosum, c = inferior vena cava, d = hepatic artery, e = portal vein, f = common hepatic duct, g = indentation for right kidney, h = bare area, i = gallbladder.

Q: What is the porta hepatis?

The porta hepatis is an important region of the liver. Its root (the hilum) contains the hepatic artery, portal vein, common hepatic duct, lymphatics & fibres from the vagus (X) nerve.

Q: What are the falciform ligament, ligamentum teres & ligamentum venosum?

Structure	Notes
Falciform Ligament	A 2-layered fold of peritoneum, connecting the anterior liver surface, to the abdominal wall. It demarcates the right & left liver lobes.
Ligamentum Teres	This is a fibrous remnant of the umbilical vein that runs in the free lower border of the falciform ligament, passing to the visceral surface of the liver.
Ligamentum Venosum	A fibrous remnant of the ductus venosus, which provides a shunt in the foetus, allowing oxygenated placental blood to pass directly from the umbilical vein to the inferior vena cava.

Q: Can you describe the functional anatomy of the liver?

- The liver parenchyma is divided into polyhedral lobules by connective tissue septa.
- Each lobule has a central vein that drains into a tributary of the hepatic vein.
- Each lobule is associated with a number of triads, composed of branches from the hepatic artery, portal vein & bile ducts.
- The portal vein branches drain into the central vein via sinusoids, delivering blood from the small intestine & draining products from hepatocytes.
- The hepatic artery branches feed the hepatocytes, which absorb both nutrients & non-nutrients from sinusoids. Furthermore, hepatocytes store & release carbohydrates, lipids, proteins (including coagulation factors), iron & vitamins (A, D, E, K). They also produce urea & bile, & metabolise drugs, hormones, & toxins.
- The central veins merge to form 3 hepatic veins which in turn drain into the inferior vena cava.

Q: What are the borders of the Winslow's Foramen (epiploic foramen)?

Winslow's Foramen is the communication between the abdominal cavity & omental bursa. The borders are as follows:

Border	Structure
Anterior	Free border of the lesser omentum (within which run the hepatic artery, portal vein & common bile duct).
Posterior	Inferior vena cava (covered by peritoneum).
Superior	Caudate lobe of the liver (covered by peritoneum).
Inferior	Duodenum (1st part)
Left Lateral	Gastrosplenic & splenorenal ligaments.

Q: What is the surgical relevance of Pringle's Manoeuvre?

This technique involves using a haemostat / left hand to control bleeding from the hepatic artery / portal vein intraoperatively. Clamping of these vessels is achieved by passing 1 arm of the haemostat / fingers through Winslow's Foramen, such that the vessels may be compressed between the other arm / thumb. If bleeding continues, it is likely that it originates from the hepatic vein / inferior vena cava.

Abdominal Aorta & Related Structures (Fig 4.13)

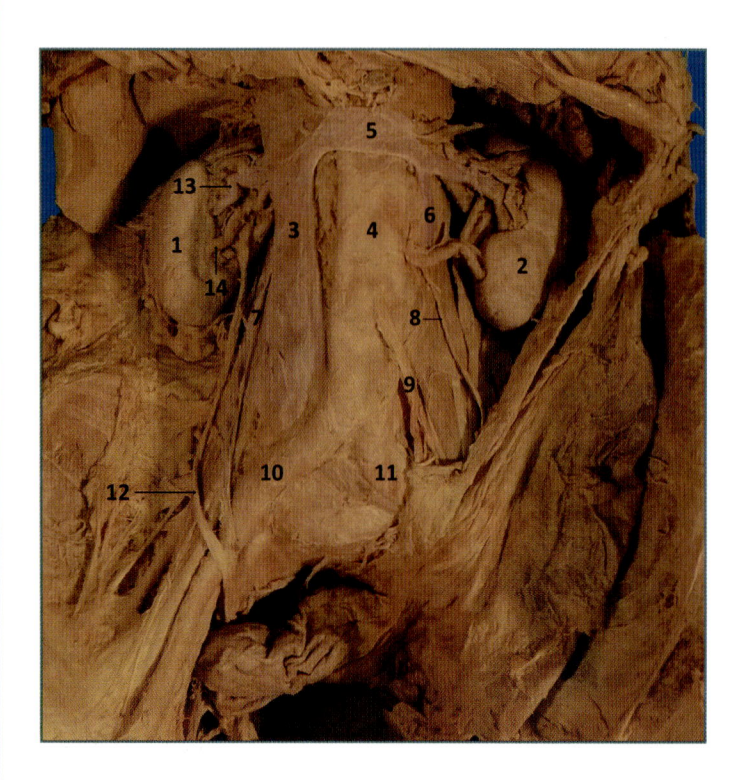

Q: Can you identify this prosection?

This prosection illustrates the retroperitoneal region of the abdomen.

Q: What are structures 1–14?

1 = right kidney, 2 = left kidney, 3 = inferior vena cava, 4 = abdominal aorta, 5 = left renal vein, 6 = left gonadal vein, 7 = right gonadal vein, 8 = left testicular artery, 9 = inferior mesenteric artery, 10 = right common iliac artery, 11 = left common iliac artery, 12 = right ureter, 13 = right renal vein, 14 = right renal artery.

Q: What are the branches of the abdominal aorta?

- **Inferior Phrenic Arteries:**   (T12) level
- **Celiac Trunk:**   (T12) level
- **Superior Mesenteric Artery:**   (L1) level
- **Middle Suprarenal Arteries:**   (L1) level
- **Renal Arteries:**   (L2) level
- **Gonadal Arteries:**   (L2) level
- **Lumbar Arteries:**   (L1–L4) levels
- **Inferior Mesenteric Artery:**   (L3) level
- **Medial Sacral Artery:**   (L4) level
- **Common Iliac Arteries:**   (L4) level

Q: What are the branches of the celiac trunk, superior & inferior mesenteric arteries?

Celiac Trunk (T12)	Superior Mesenteric (L1)	Inferior Mesenteric (L3)

1. Common Hepatic:
 a. Right Hepatic
 b. Left Hepatic
 c. Cystic
 d. Right Gastric
 e. Gastroduodenal
    i) Right Gastroepiploic
    ii) Superior Pancreaticoduodenal
 2. Left Gastric
 3. Splenic
	1. Inferior Pancreaticoduodenal
	 2. Middle Colic
	 3. Right Colic
	 4. Ileo-Colic
	 5. Small Intestine Branches
	
	 Note: The superior mesenteric artery travels within the common mesentery.
		1. Left Colic
		 2. Sigmoid Colon Branches
		 3. Superior Rectal
		
		 Note: The inferior mesenteric artery & branches run mostly in the retroperitoneum, however the vessels to the sigmoid colon run in the sigmoid mesocolon.

Q: What structures lie in the retroperitoneum?

Gastrointestinal	Urological	Vascular
Oesophagus	Adrenal Glands	Aorta
Duodenum (not the 1st part)	Kidneys	Inferior Vena Cava
Pancreas	Ureters	
Colon (ascending & descending only)	Bladder	
Rectum (not lower ⅓)		

Penis & Scrotum (Fig 4.14)

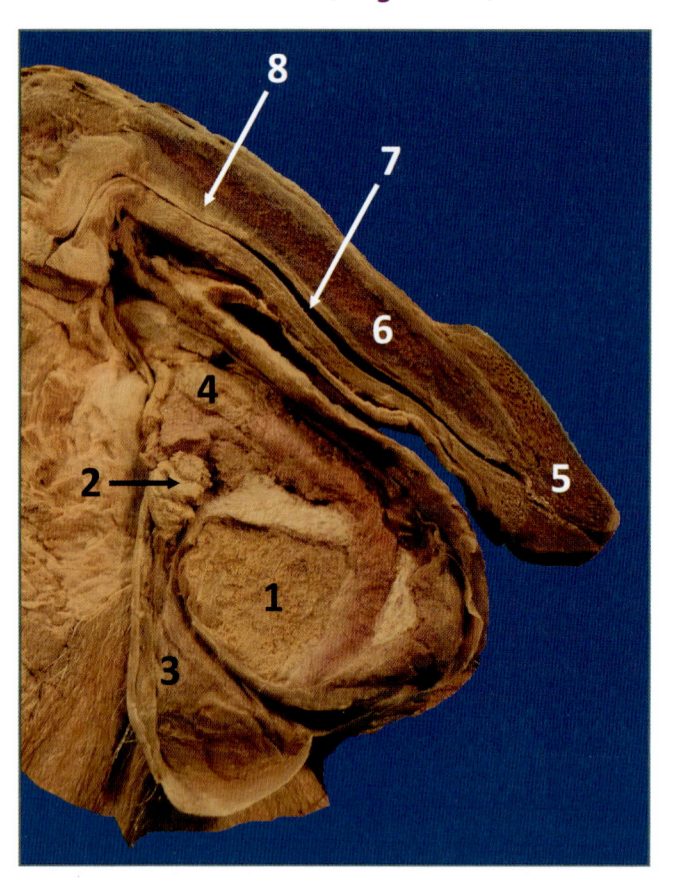

Q: Can you identify this prosection?

Sagittal section of the penis & scrotum.

Q: What are structures 1–8?

1 = testis, 2 = head of epididymis, 3 = tunica vaginalis (parietal), 4 = spermatic cord, 5 = glans penis, 6 = corpus cavernosum, 7 = spongy (penile) urethra, 8 = corpus spongiosum.

Q: What is the lymphatic drainage of the scrotum & testes? What is the clinical & operative significance of this?

The scrotum drains to the inguinal lymph nodes. The testes drain to the para-aortic lymph nodes. Carcinomas confined to the testes thus never result in inguinal lymphadenopathy & are surgically removed via an inguinal incision *(see operative surgery)*.

Q: What is the anatomy of the male urethra?

The male urethra is a 20cm long, fibromuscular tube. It begins at the internal urethral meatus of the bladder & ends at the external urethral meatus of the glans of the penis. The male urethra is described in 3 parts:

Urethra	Notes
Prostatic	3cm long, through the prostate.
Membranous	2cm long, through the pelvic floor & perineal membrane. It is encircled by the main muscle of continence, the external urethral sphincter.
Spongy	15cm long, commencing at the bulb of the penis, traversing the corpus spongiosum & expanding within the glans to form the navicular fossa.

Q: What are the fascial layers of the spermatic cord?

Layer	Fascia	Origin
Inner	Internal Spermatic Fascia	Transversalis Fascia
Middle	Cremasteric Fascia	Internal Oblique
Outer	External Spermatic Fascia	External Oblique

Q: What are the contents of the spermatic cord?

Arteries	Veins
Artery to Vas Deferens	Pampiniform Plexus
Cremasteric Artery	Cremasteric Vein
Testicular Artery	Testicular Vein
Nerves	**Structures**
Genital Branch of Genitofemoral Nerve (L2)	Lymphatics
Sympathetic Nerves (T10)	Obliterated Processus Vaginalis
Ilioinguinal Nerve (runs within the inguinal canal, but outside the cord)	Vas Deferens

LIMBS, SPINE & VASCULAR

Upper Limb Vessels (Fig 4.15)

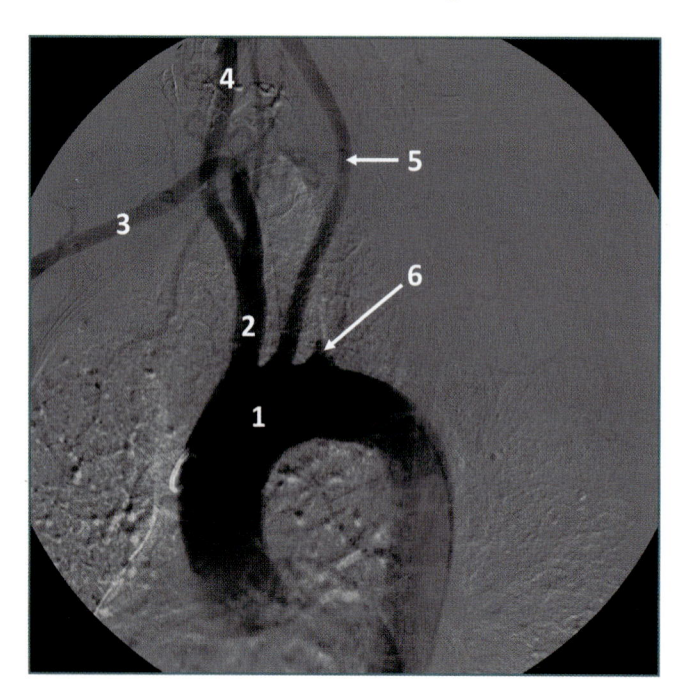

This is an image of a patient who presented with episodic dizziness, vertigo & left arm claudication.

Q: Can you identify this image?

This is a digital subtraction angiogram of the aortic arch & associated arteries.

Q: What are structures 1–6?

1 = aortic arch, 2 = brachiocephalic trunk, 3 = right subclavian artery, 4 = right common carotid artery, 5 = left common carotid artery, 6 = left subclavian artery (root).

Q: What is the diagnosis?

There is occlusion of the left subclavian artery. The associated symptoms indicate subclavian steal syndrome.

Q: Why is the patient experiencing these symptoms?

Occlusion of the left subclavian artery, results in flow reversal in the left vertebral artery. Blood flow is 'stolen' from the contralateral vertebral artery which results in neurological symptoms. The occlusion in the left subclavian artery also decreases perfusion to the limb, resulting in claudication.

Q: What is the major arterial supply & venous drainage to the upper limb?

Arteries	Veins
Subclavian	Subclavian
Axillary	Axillary
Brachial	Brachial
Radial	Cephalic
Ulnar	Basilic
Palmar Arches (superficial & deep)	Medial Cubital
Digital Arteries	Dorsal Digital Veins & Network

Q: What are the branches of the axillary artery?

The axillary artery is divided into 3 parts by pectoralis minor. Each part has its own branches:

1st Part (superior to pectoralis minor)	3rd Part (inferior to pectoralis minor)
• Superior Thoracic Artery	• Subscapular Artery
2nd Part (posterior to pectoralis minor)	• Anterior Humeral Circumflex Artery
• Thoraco-Acromial Artery	• Posterior Humeral Circumflex Artery
• Lateral Thoracic Artery	

Rotator Cuff (Fig 4.16)

Study this prosection carefully & answer the following questions:

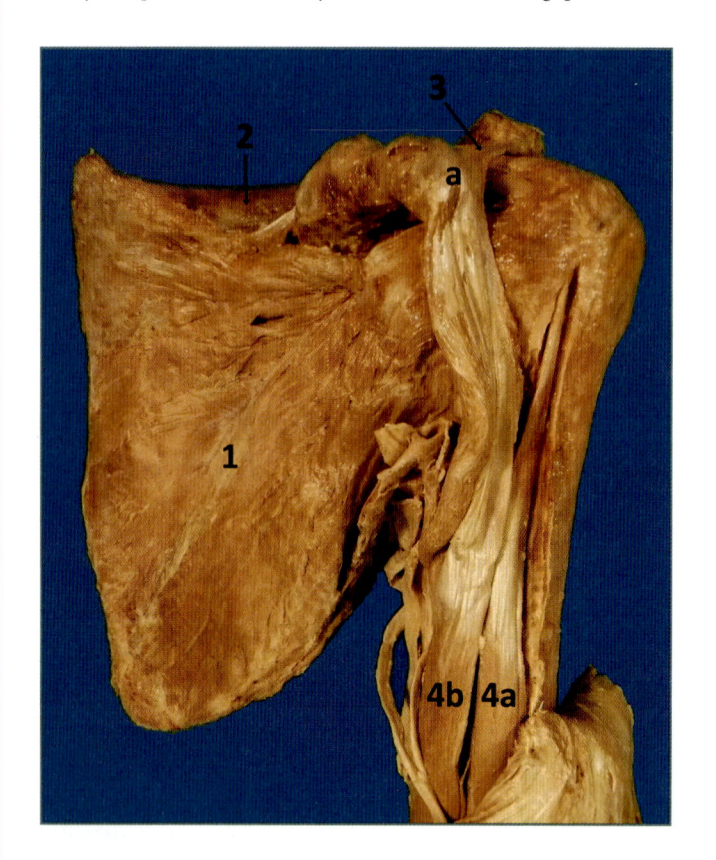

Q: Can you identify this prosection?

Left shoulder, anterior view.

Q: What are structures 1–4?

1. Subscapularis
2. Supraspinatus
3. Coracoacromial Ligament
4. a. Long Head of Biceps Brachii
   b. Short Head of Biceps Brachii

Q: What is structure a? What structures have their origins here?

This is the coracoid process. The following muscles originate here:
- Coracobrachialis
- Pectoralis Minor
- Short Head of Biceps Brachii

Q: What structures ensure stability of the glenohumeral joint?

The following are important with respect to shoulder joint stability, however the rotator cuff muscles are most important:
- Ball & Socket Synovial Joint
- Ligaments – Coracohumeral, Glenohumeral & Transverse
- Joint Capsule
- Rotator Cuff Muscles:

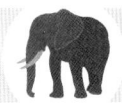

Memory: **'SITS'** for rotator cuff muscles

Muscle	Shoulder Movement	Nerve Innervation & Root
Supraspinatus	0–30° Abduction	Suprascapular (C5–6)
Infraspinatus	External Rotation	Suprascapular (C5–6)
Teres Minor	External Rotation & Adduction	Axillary (C5–6)
Subscapularis	Internal Rotation	Superior & Inferior Scapular (C5–6)

Q: Aside from the rotator cuff, what other muscles are involved in glenuohumeral joint movement?

Joint Movement	Muscles
Abduction	Deltoid (middle fibres)
Adduction	Teres Major, Pectoralis Major, Latissimus Dorsi
Forward Flexion	Biceps Brachii, Coracobrachialis, Deltoid (anterior fibres), Pectoralis Major
Extension	Deltoid (posterior fibres), Latissimus Dorsi, Teres Major
External Rotation	Deltoid (posterior fibres)
Internal Rotation	Deltoid (anterior fibres), Latissimus Dorsi, Teres Major

Antecubital Fossa (Fig 4.17)

Study this prosection carefully & answer the following questions:

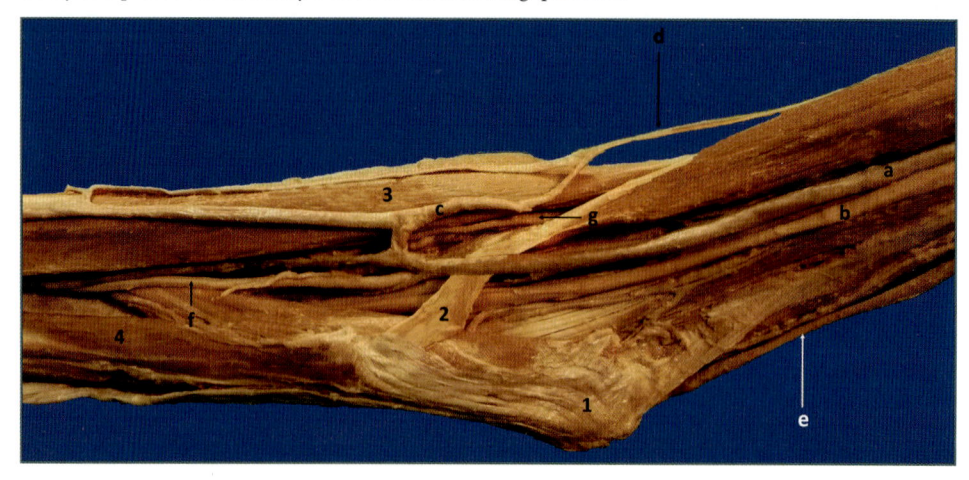

Q: Can you identify this prosection?

Right antecubital fossa.

Q: What are structures 1–4?

1 = common flexor origin at medial epicondyle, 2 = bicipital aponeurosis, 3 = brachioradialis, 4 = flexor carpi ulnaris.

Q: What are structures a–g?

a = basilic vein, b = brachial artery, c = median cubital vein, d = cephalic vein, e = ulnar nerve, f = median nerve, g = radial nerve.

Q: What are the borders of the antecubital fossa?

This is essentially an upside-down triangle with the following borders:

Border	Notes
Superior	Line drawn between the medial & lateral epicondyles of the humerus.
Ulnar	Pronator teres.
Radial	Brachioradialis.
Apex	Meeting point of pronator teres & brachioradialis.
Roof	Superficial fascia.
Floor	Brachialis & supinator.

Q: What are the contents of the antecubital fossa?

The contents are from ulnar to radial:
- Median Nerve
- Brachial Artery
- Biceps Tendon
- Radial Nerve

Note: The radial nerve runs between bracialis & brachioradialis, so it is not always considered part of the antecubital fossa.

Carpal Tunnel (Fig 4.18)

Please study this prosection carefully & answer the following questions:

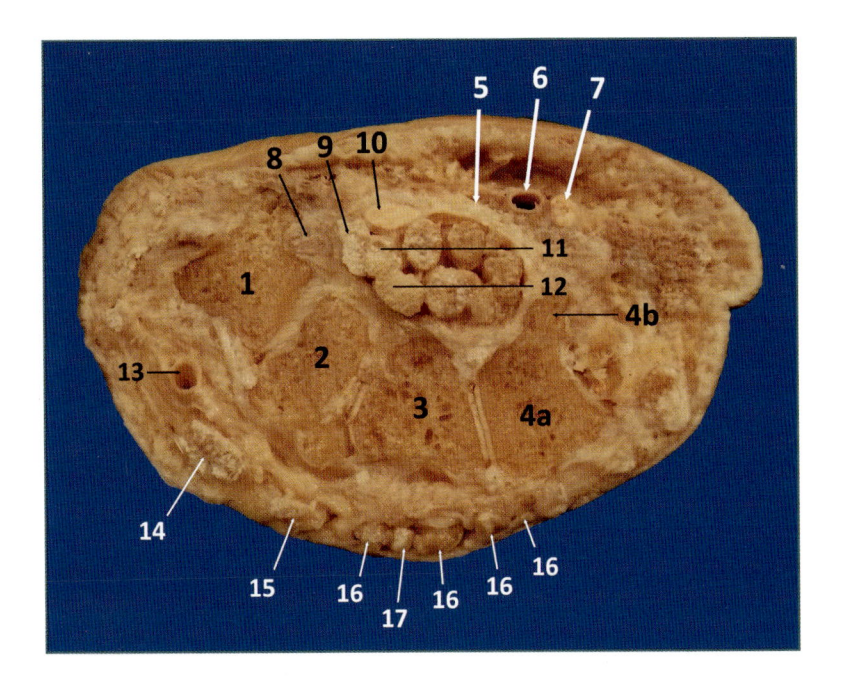

Q: Can you identify this prosection?

A transverse section through the left carpus, showing the carpal tunnel & contents.

Q: What are the structures labelled 1–17?

1.	Trapezium	10.	Median Nerve
2.	Trapezoid	11.	Flexor Digitorum Superficialis Tendons (4)
3.	Capitate	12.	Flexor Digitorum Profundus Tendons (4)
4.	**a.** Hamate **b.** Hook of Hamate	13.	Radial Artery
5.	Flexor Retinaculum	14.	Extensor Carpi Radialis
6.	Ulnar Artery	15.	Extensor Pollicis Longus
7.	Ulnar Nerve	16.	Extensor Digitorum Communis
8.	Flexor Carpi Radialis	17.	Extensor Indicis
9.	Flexor Pollicis Longus		

Q: What is the flexor retinaculum?

A ligament, also known as the transverse carpal ligament, which forms the roof of the carpal tunnel. It has the following attachments:

Radial	Ulnar
Trapezium Tubercle	Hook of Hamate
Scaphoid Tubercle	Pisiform

Q: What is the carpal tunnel?

This is a fibro-osseous passageway, linking the anterior compartment of the forearm with the palm of the hand. It has the following borders:

- **Roof:** Flexor Retinaculum
- **Floor & Walls:** Carpal Bones

Q: What structures pass through the carpal tunnel?

- Medial Nerve
- Flexor Pollicis Longus Tendon
- 4 Flexor Digitorum Profundus Tendons
- 4 Flexor Digitorum Superficialis Tendons

Note: Flexor carpi radialis does not strictly pass through the carpal tunnel, it passes through the flexor retinaculum (Fig 4.18). The ulnar artery & nerve do not pass through the carpal tunnel, they pass through a separate fibro-ossous tunnel called Guyon's Canal.

Dorsum of the Hand (Fig 4.19)

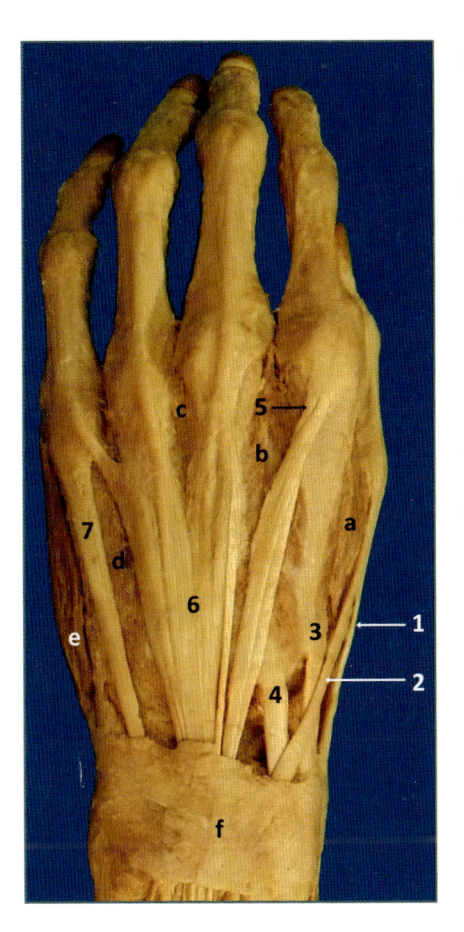

Q: What are structures 1–7?

These are all extensor tendons of the left hand:

1 = extensor pollicis brevis, 2 = extensor pollicis longus, 3 = extensor carpi radialis longus, 4 = extensor carpi radialis brevis, 5 = extensor indicis, 6 = extensor digitorum communis, 7 = extensor digiti minimi.

Q: What are structures a–f?

a = 1st dorsal interosseous, b = 2nd dorsal interosseous, c = 3rd dorsal interosseous, d = 4th dorsal interosseous, e = abductor digiti minimi, f = extensor retinaculum.

Q: What are the borders of the anatomical snuffbox & what is its clinical significance?

Border	Structures
Floor	Radial Styloid, Scaphoid, Trapezium & Base of 1st Metacarpal
Roof	Deep Fascia
Radial	Extensor Pollicis Brevis & Abductor Pollicis Longus Tendons
Ulnar	Extensor Pollicis Longus

Anatomical snuffbox tenderness is associated with a **scaphoid fracture**, one of the most commonly missed traumatic diagnoses. **De Quervain's Tenosynovitis** is a condition where inflammation of the tendons forming the radial border (extensor pollicis brevis & abductor pollicis longus) of the anatomical snuffbox occurs.

Q: What structures run through the extensor compartments?

The extensor compartments house the following tendons:

Compartment	Tendons
I	Abductor Pollicis Longus & Extensor Pollicis Brevis
II	Extensor Carpi Radialis Longus & Extensor Carpi Radialis Brevis
III	Extensor Pollicis Longus
IV	Extensor Digitorum Communis (4 tendons) & Extensor Indicis Proprius
V	Extensor Digiti Minimi
VI	Extensor Carpi Ulnaris

Femur & Hip Joint (Fig 4.20)

Study this bone carefully & answer the following questions:

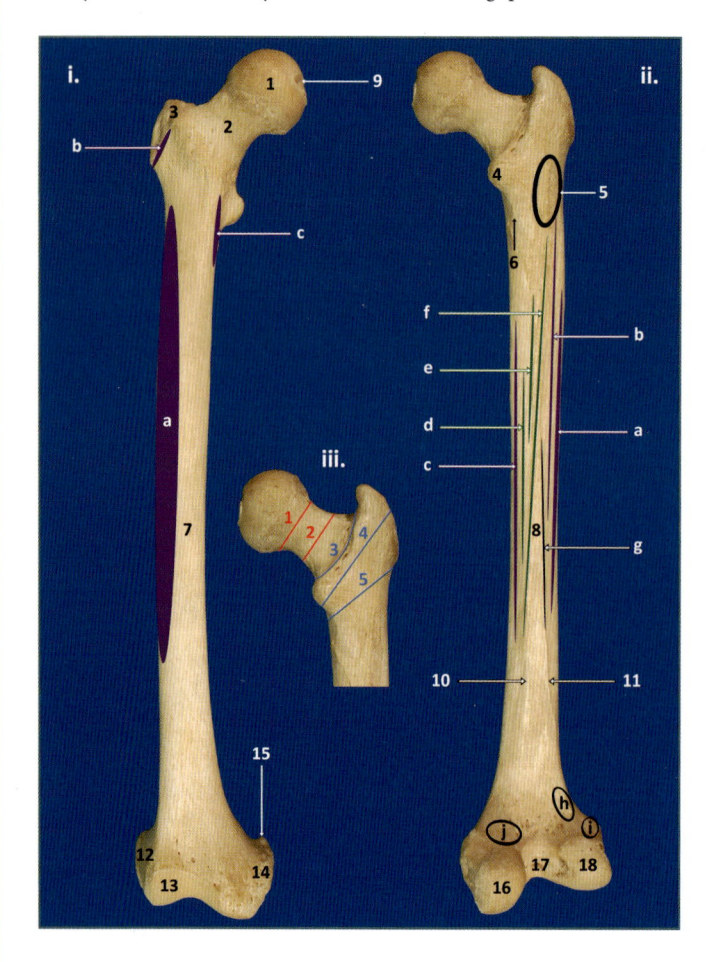

Q: What is the bone shown in (Fig 4.20)?

Right femur:
- i   = anterior view
- ii   = posterior view
- iii   = femoral head posterior view

Q: What are structures 1–18 on i & ii?

1 = head, 2 = neck, 3 = greater trochanter, 4 = lesser trochanter, 5 = gluteal tuberosity, 6 = pectineal line, 7 = shaft, 8 = linea aspera, 9 = fovea capitis, 10 = medial supracondylar line, 11 = lateral supracondylar line, 12 = lateral epicondyle, 13 = patellar surface, 14 = medial epicondyle, 15 = adductor tubercle, 16 = medial condyle, 17 = intercondylar fossa, 18 = lateral condyle.

Q: What are the muscle attachments labelled a–j?

a = vastus intermedius, b = vastus lateralis, c = vastus medialis, d = adductor longus, e = adductor brevis, f = adductor magnus, g = short head of biceps femoris, h = plantaris, i = lateral head of gastrocnemius, j = medial head of gastrocnemius.

Q: What muscles attach to the lateral surface of the greater trochanter?

- Piriformis
- Gluteus minimus
- Gluteus medius

Q: What muscles attach to 4, 5 & 6?

4 = iliopsoas, 5 = gluteus maximus, 6 = pectineus.

Q: What attaches / runs to structure 9?

Ligamentum teres femoris & vessel.

Q: What is the most trauma relevant fracture of this bone? What can happen to structure 1 under these circumstances?

Fractured neck of femur. Avascular necrosis of the femoral head.

Q: What is the blood supply of structure 1?

- Retinacular vessels
- Ligamentum teres vessel
- Interosseous vessels

Q: What are the fracture lines 1–5 shown in Fig 4.20?

1 = subcapital, 2 = transcervical, 3 = basal, 4 = intertrochanteric, 5 = subtrochanteric.

Q: How would you surgically repair the blue fractures 3–5 (Fig 4.20)? What is special about these fractures?

These fractures are **extracapsular**. Repair utilises a **dynamic hip screw** that allows fracture compression during weight bearing for improved healing. Repair of intracapsular fractures is guided by Garden's Classification (Fig 11.6).

Q: How is the hip joint arranged to achieve stability?

- This is a synovial ball & socket joint, surrounded by a joint capsule.
- The femoral head fits snugly inside the acetabulum.
- The acetabulum is further deepened by a ring of cartilage called the labrum, preventing movement of the femoral head within the joint.
- Ligaments further reinforce the joint (iliofemoral, pubofemoral & ischiofemoral).
- Muscles also contribute to joint stabilitiy (quadratus femoris, piriformis, gluteus medius & minimus).

Q: What is the path / surface anatomy of the sciatic nerve?

A line drawn posteriorly, from the midpoint of the ischial tuberosity & greater trochanter, down to the apex of the popliteal fossa.

Lower Limb Vessels (Fig 4.21)

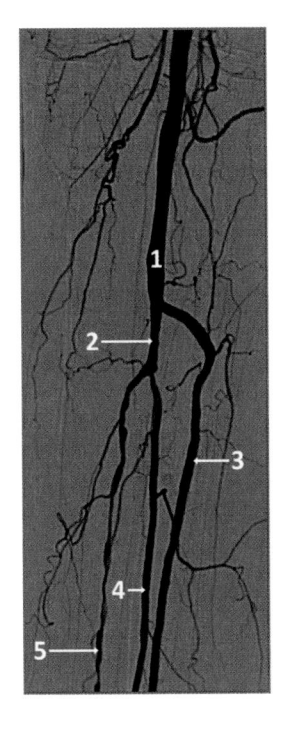

Q: Can you identify this image?

Left-sided digital subtraction femoral angiogram.

Q: What are structures 1–5?

1 = left popliteal artery, 2 = left tibioperoneal trunk, 3 = left anterior tibial artery, 4 = left peroneal artery, 5 = left posterior tibial artery.

Q: How does the arterial supply continue in the foot?

The **anterior tibial** artery continues as the **dorsalis pedis** artery. The **arcuate** artery branches off the dorsalis pedis, providing **metatarsal** & **dorsal digital** arterial branches.

The **posterior tibial** artery branches into **medial** & **lateral plantar** arteries. These are connected by a **plantar arch** which then provides **plantar metatarsal** & **digital** arterial branches.

Q: What veins drain the lower limbs?

- Dorsal & Ventral Digital & Metatarsal Veins
- Dorsal & Plantar Venous Arches
- Great Saphenous Vein   (from dorsal venous arch)
- Small Saphenous Vein   (from dorsal venous arch)
- Anterior Tibial Vein
- Posterior Tibial Vein   (from plantar arch)
- Popliteal Vein
- Femoral Vein
- Profunda Femoris Vein
- Medial & Lateral Circumflex Femoral Veins
- External Iliac Vein

Q: What is the path / surface anatomy of the great (long) saphenous vein?

The great saphenous vein drains the medial margin of the dorsal venous arch. It ascends the lower leg anterior to the medial malleolus, running a hand's breadth posterior to the medial border of the patella. It passes through the saphenous opening of tensor fascia lata and joins the femoral vein at the saphenofemoral junction, approximately 4cm below & lateral to the pubic tubercle.

Q: What is the surface anatomy of the small (short) saphenous vein?

The short saphenous vein drains the lateral margin of the dorsal venous arch & ascends the lower leg posterior to the lateral malleolus. It passes through the subcutaneous fat plane to the midline of the posterior calf, piercing deep fascia to join the popliteal vein at the saphenopopliteal junction.

Femoral Triangle (Fig 4.22)

Study this prosection carefully & answer the following questions:

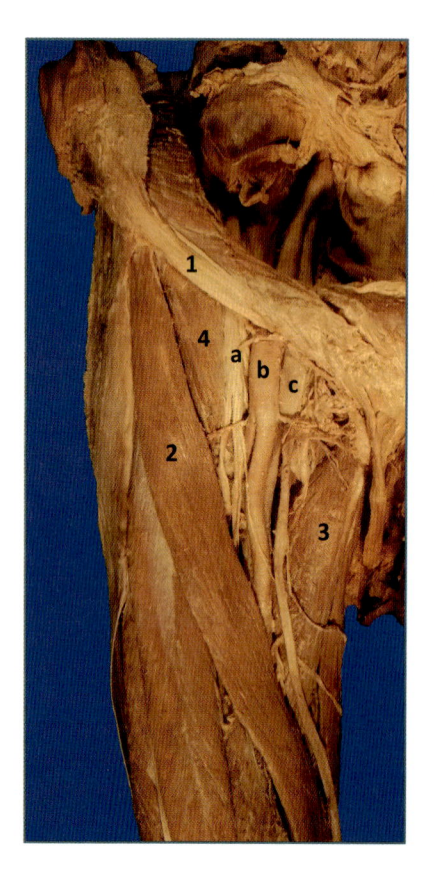

Q: Can you identify this prosection?

Right femoral triangle.

Q: What are structures 1–4?

1 = inguinal ligament, 2 = sartorius, 3 = adductor longus, 4 = iliopsoas.

Q: What are structures a–c?

a = femoral nerve, b = femoral artery, c = femoral vein.

Q: What are the borders of the femoral triangle?

Border	Structure
Superior	Inguinal Ligament
Lateral	Sartorius
Medial	Adductor Longus
Floor	Iliopsoas, Pectineus, Adductor Longus *(from lateral to medial)*
Roof	Fascia Lata

Q: What are the contents of the femoral triangle?

Memory: **'NAVEL'** from lateral to medial.

Nerve   - Femoral
Artery   - Femoral
Vein   - Femoral
Empty Space
Lymph Nodes   - Deep Inguinal

In addition to the above structures, the muscles of the floor border are also contents of the femoral triangle i.e. **Iliopsoas**, **Pectineus** & **Adductor Longus** *(from lateral to medial)*.

Q: What is the origin & attachment of 1?

Anterior superior iliac spine (ASIS) to pubic tubercle.

Q: What is the anatomical position / surface anatomy of the femoral artery?

The mid-inguinal point (½ way from the ASIS to the pubic symphysis).

Femoral Sheath (Fig 4.23)

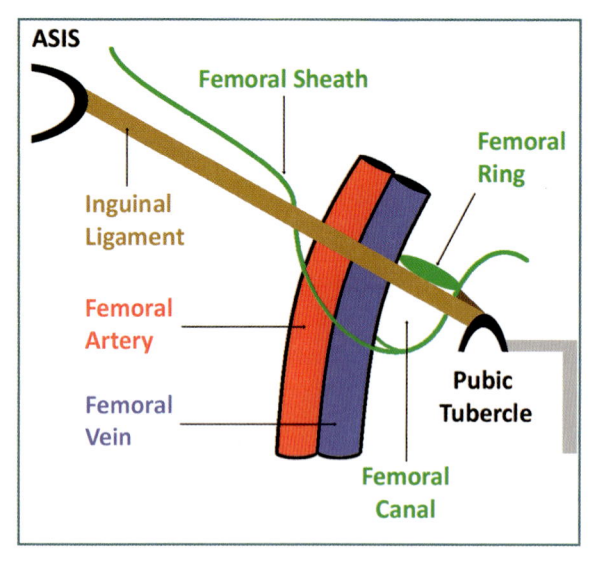

Q: What is the femoral sheath?

This is formed by the thick cribriform fascia of transversalis & iliacus. It 'ensheaths' the femoral artery, femoral vein & femoral canal (Fig 4.23).

Q: What are the borders of the femoral canal?

Border	Structure
Anterior-Superior	Inguinal Ligament
Posterior-Inferior	Pubic Ramus & Pectineus
Lateral	Femoral Vein
Medial	Lacunar Ligament

Q: What are the contents of the femoral canal?

The femoral canal is approximately 2cm long & contains empty space & 1 lymph node (Cloquet's Node).

Q: What are the borders of the femoral ring & what is their relationship?

Anterior border = inguinal ligament, posterior border = pectineal ligament. The inguinal ligament is formed by the inward fold of the external oblique aponeurosis. The lacunar ligament is a continuation of the inguinal ligament that forms the medial border of the femoral canal. A femoral hernia may be 'lacerated' by the lacunar ligament, resulting in perforation. The pectineal ligament runs along the pectineal line & is a continuation of the lacunar ligament as it sweeps posteriorly.

Inguinal Canal (Fig 4.24)

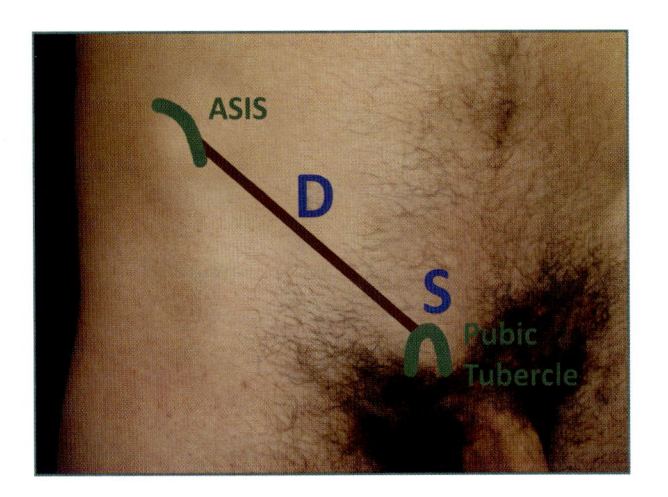

Q: Can you delineate the hernia relevant surface anatomy of the inguinal region?

Anatomy	Notes
ASIS & Pubic Tubercle	The anterior superior iliac spine (ASIS) & pubic tubercles must be identified first.
Inguinal Ligament	Delineate the inguinal ligament which has attachments to both the ASIS & pubic tubercle.
Deep Ring (D)	Point out the location of the deep ring which lies just above the midpoint of the inguinal ligament. It is formed by an aperture through the **transversalis fascia**. Mention that the femoral artery may be palpated below the inguinal ligament at the mid-inguinal point, halfway between the ASIS & pubic symphysis.
Superficial Ring (S)	Point out the location of the superficial ring which lies just above the pubic tubercle. It is formed by an aperture through the **external oblique aponeurosis**.
Inguinal Canal	Finally, explain that the inguinal canal is an oblique communication between the deep & superficial inguinal rings, formed by the arching fibres of the **transversus abdominis** & **internal oblique** muscles.

Q: What are the borders of the inguinal canal?

Border	Anatomy
Posterior Wall	Transversalis Fascia
Anterior Wall	External Oblique Aponeurosis
Floor	Inguinal Ligament
Roof	Arching Fibres of Transversus Abdominis & Internal Oblique

Q: Where would you expect a direct inguinal hernia to be found?

A direct inguinal hernia passes through a weakness in the anterior abdominal wall, commonly within **Hasselbach's Triangle**. This triangle has the following borders; **inferior epigastric artery** (lateral), **linea semilunaris** of rectus abdominis (superior-medial) & **inguinal ligament** (inferior).

Adductor Canal

Q: What are the borders of the adductor canal?

Border	Structures
Proximal	Femoral Triangle Apex
Posterior	Adductor Longus & Adductor Magnus
Lateral	Vastus Medialis
Medial	Adductor Magnus
Anterior	Aponeurosis & Sartorius
Distal	Adductor Hiatus

Q: What is the anatomical position / surface anatomy of the adductor hiatus?

This lies ⅔ the distance along a line drawn from the anterior superior iliac spine (ASIS) to the adductor tubercle of the femur. The most common site of atherosclerosis in the lower limb is within the superficial femoral artery as it passes through the adductor hiatus. Bruits may therefore be auscultated here in such cases.

Q: What are the contents of the adductor canal?

- **Superficial Femoral Artery**
- **Descending Genicular Artery** (superficial femoral artery branch, given off superomedially & just proximal to the adductor hiatus)
- **Femoral Vein**
- **Long Saphenous Nerve**
- **Nerve to Vastus Medialis**

Knee Joint (Fig 4.25)
Study the prosection below & answer the following questions:

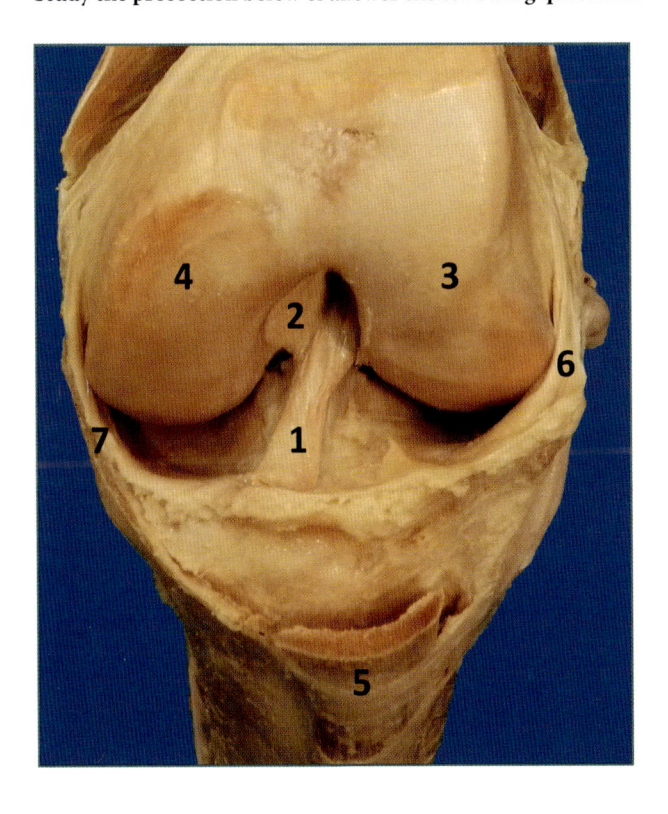

Q: Can you identify this prosection?

Left knee joint, anterior view.

Q: What type of joint is this?

Synovial joint, modified hinge.

Q: What are structures 1–7?

1 = anterior cruciate ligament, 2 = posterior cruciate ligament, 3 = lateral femoral condyle, 4 = medial femoral condyle, 5 = patellar ligament, 6 = lateral collateral ligament, 7 = medial collateral ligament.

Q: What structures provide stability to the knee joint?

Structure	Function
Menisci	Fibrocartilagenous Shock Absorption
Knee Capsule	Posterior & Medial Stability
Cruciate Ligaments	Anteroposterior Stability
Collateral Ligaments	Lateral Stability
Tibial Spine	Lateral Stability
Vasti Muscles	Patella Stability

Popliteal Fossa (Fig 4.26)

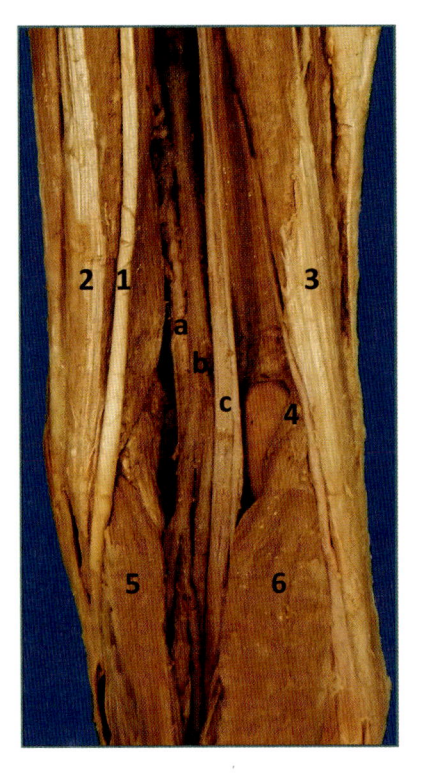

Q: Can you identify this prosection?

Posterior view of right popliteal fossa.

Q: What are structures 1–6 & what do they represent?

These are the borders of the popliteal fossa:

Label	Border	Structure
1	Superior-Medial	Semitendinosus
2	Superior-Medial	Semimembranosus
3	Superior-Lateral	Biceps Femoris
4	Inferior-Medial	Plantaris (deep)
5	Inferior-Lateral	Gastrocnemius (medial head)
6	Inferior-Lateral	Gastrocnemius (lateral head)

Q: What are structures a–c?

These are the contents of the popliteal fossa:

Label	Structure
a	Popliteal Artery
b	Popliteal Vein
c	Tibial Nerve

Lower Leg Compartments (Fig 4.27)

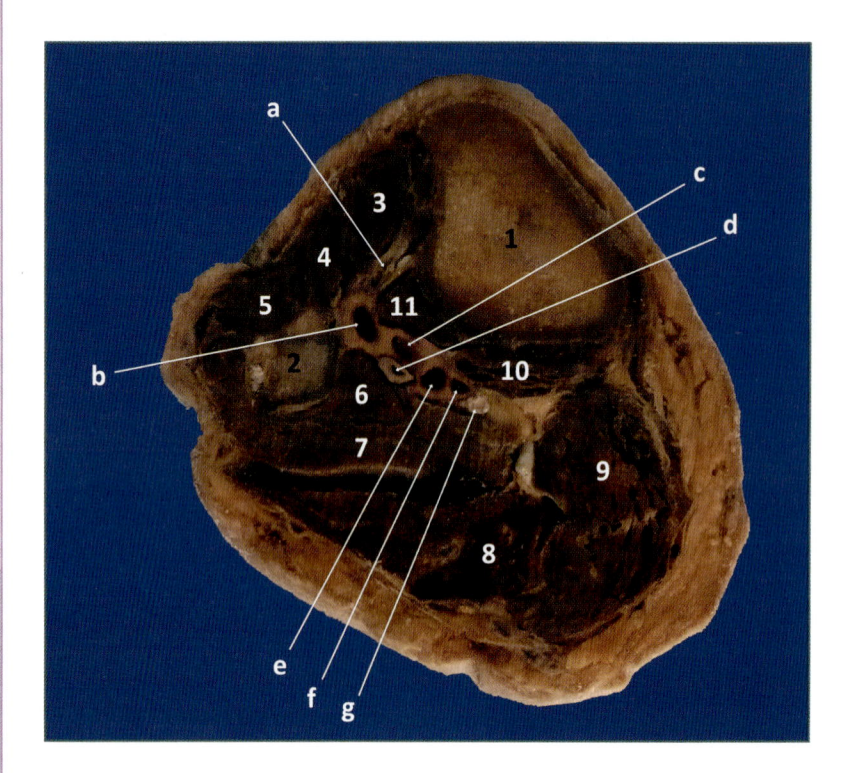

Q: Can you identify this prosection? What are structures 1 & 2?

Cross-section of the right calf (mid-level) inferior view. 1 = right tibia, 2 = right fibula.

Q: What are structures 3–11?

These are all muscles. 3 = tibialis anterior, 4 = extensor digitorum longus, 5 = peroneus longus, 6 = tibialis posterior, 7 = soleus, 8 = lateral head of gastrocnemius, 9 = medial head of gastrocnemius, 10 = popliteus, 11 = flexor digitorum longus.

Q: What are structures a–g?

a = interosseous membrane, b = anterior tibial artery, c = peroneal artery, d = peroneal vein, e = posterior tibial artery, f = posterior tibial vein, g = posterior tibial nerve.

Q: What are the compartments of the lower leg?

Compartment	Muscles	Nerves	Vessels
Anterior (extensor compartment)	• Tibialis Anterior • Extensor Hallucis Longus • Extensor Digitorum Longus • Peroneus Tertius	Deep Peroneal Nerve	Anterior Tibial Vessels
Lateral (peroneal compartment)	• Peroneus Longus • Peroneus Brevis	Superficial Peroneal Nerve	Peroneal Artery & Small Saphenous Vein
Superficial Posterior (flexor compartment)	• Gastrocnemius • Plantaris • Soleus	Tibial Division of Sciatic Nerve	Posterior Tibial Artery & Peroneal Branch
Deep Posterior (flexor compartment)	• Popliteus • Flexor Digitorum Longus • Flexor Hallucis Longus • Tibialis Posterior		

Ankle & Foot (Fig 4.28)

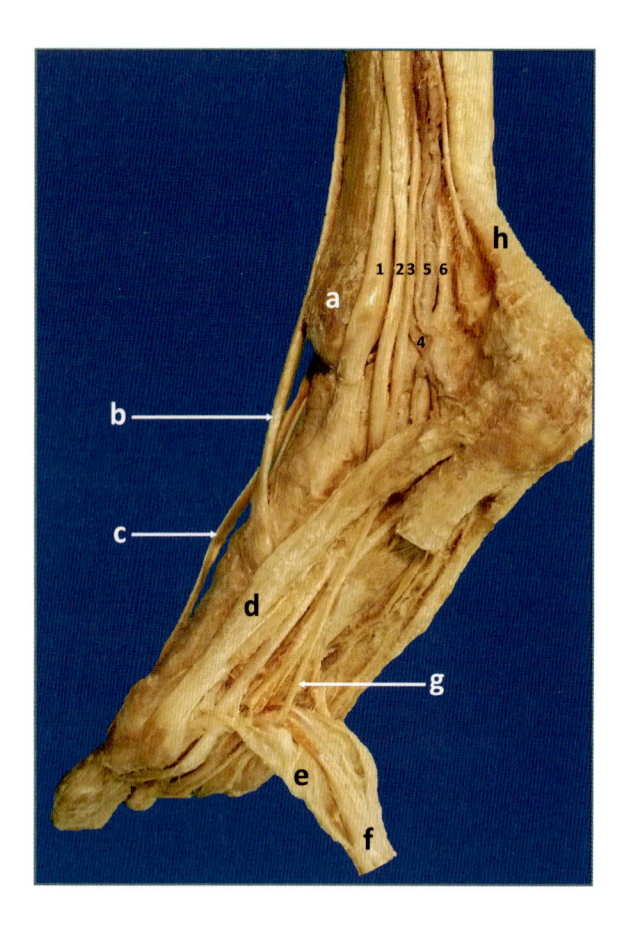

Q: What are structures a–h?

a = medial malleolus, b = tibialis anterior tendon, c = extensor hallucis longus tendon, d = abductor hallucis, e = plantar aponeurosis (cut), f = flexor digitorum brevis (cut), g = medial plantar nerve branches, h = tendo calcaneus (Achilles tendon).

Q: What are structures 1–6?

1 = tibialis posterior, 2 = flexor digitorum longus, 3 = tibial nerve, 4 = posterior tibial artery, 5 = posterior tibial vein, 6 = flexor hallucis longus.

Q: What structure passes under the sustentaculum tali?

Flexor hallucis longus tendon.

Q: What bones contribute to the arches of the foot?

Arch	Bones
Lateral Longitudinal	Calcaneum, Cuboid, 5th Metatarsal
Medial Longitudinal	Calcaneum, Talus, Navicular, 1st Cuneiform, 1st Metatarsal
Transverse	3 Cuneiforms, Cuboid

Q: What are the ligaments of the foot?

Region	Ligaments
Tibia-Fibula	• Anterior & Posterior Tibiofibular • Inferior Transverse
Ankle (Lateral)	• Talofibular • Calcaneofibular • Bifurcate: Calcaneocuboid & calcaneonavicular fibres
Ankle (Medial)	• Deltoid: Superficial fibres pass from the medial malleolus to the navicular (tibionavicular), sustentaculum tali (tibiocalcaneal) & medial talus (posterior tibiotalar). Deep fibres pass from the medial malleolus to medial talus (anterior tibiotalar).
Arches	• Long & Short Plantar: Reinforce the lateral arch. • Spring (plantar calcaneonavicular): Reinforces the medial arch.
Heel	• Anterior & Posterior Tibiofibular

NEUROSCIENCES

Skull (Fig 4.29)

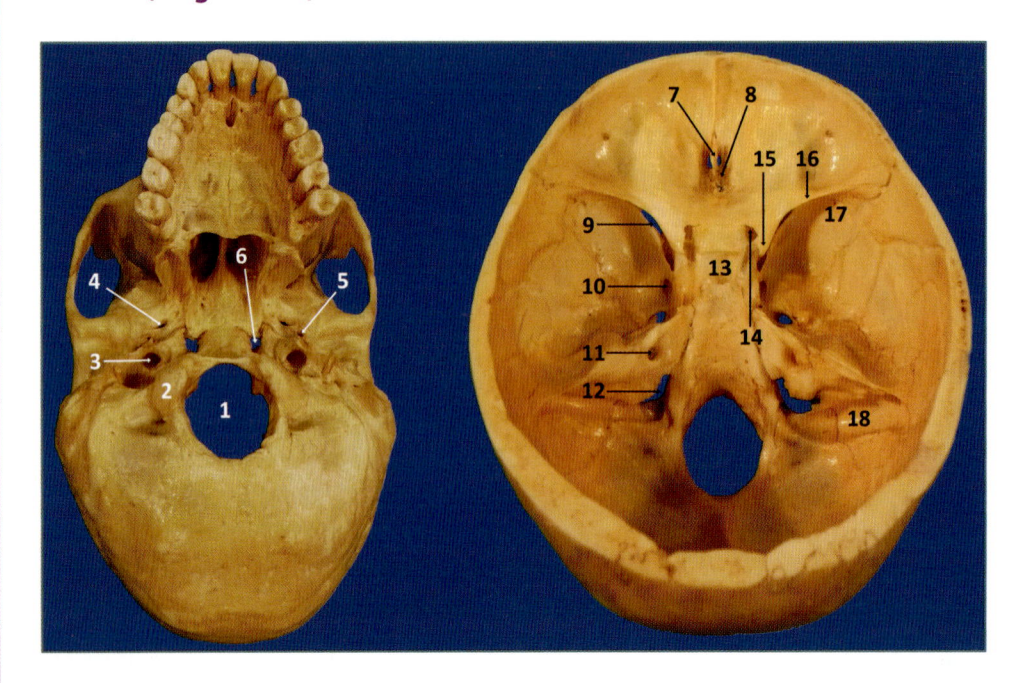

Q: What are structures 1–18?

1 = foramen magnum, 2 = occipital condyle, 3 = carotid canal, 4 = foramen ovale, 5 = foramen spinosum, 6 = foramen lacerum, 7 = crista galli, 8 = cribriform plate, 9 = superior orbital fissure, 10 = foramen rotundum, 11 = internal auditory meatus, 12 = jugular foramen, 13 = sella turcica, 14 = optic canal, 15 = anterior clinoid process, 16 = lesser wing of sphenoid, 17 = greater wing of sphenoid, 18 = groove for sigmoid sinus.

Q: Can you draw & label the bones of the right orbit, anterior view (Fig 4.30)?

a = superior orbital fissure, b = optic canal, c = inferior orbital fissure.

1 = frontal bone (superior border), 2 = maxilla (inferior border), 3 & 4 = ethmoid & lacrimal bones (medial border), 5 = sphenoid (posterior border), 6 = zygoma (lateral border).

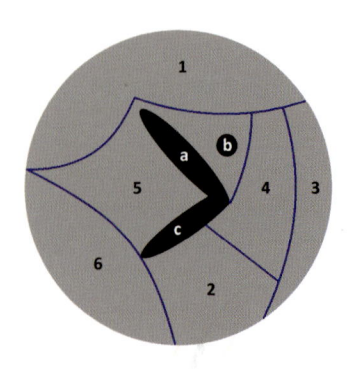

Q: What structures pass through the skull foramina?

Foramen	Structures Passing Through
Cribriform Plate Foramina	Olfactory Nerve Bundles (I).
Optic Canal	Optic Nerve (II), Ophthalmic Artery, Meninges, CSF.
Superior Orbital Fissure	Occulomotor Nerve (III), Trochlear Nerve (IV), Lacrimal Nerve (V1), Frontal Nerve (V1) & Nasociliary Nerve (V1), Abducens Nerve (VI), Superior Ophthalmic Vein, Inferior Ophthalmic Vein.
Supraorbital Foramen	Supraorbital Nerve (a terminal branch of the frontal nerve – V1), Supraorbital Artery, Supraorbital Vein.
Inferior Orbital Fissure	Infraorbital Nerve (V2), Zygomatic Nerve (V2), Infraorbital Artery, Infraorbital Veins, Inferior Ophthalmic Veins.
Infraorbital Foramen	Infraorbital Nerve (a terminal branch of the maxillary nerve - V2), Infraorbital Artery, Infraorbital Vein.
Foramen Ovale	Mandibular Nerve (V3), Accessory Meningeal Artery.
Foramen Spinosum	Middle Meningeal Artery.
Foramen Lacerum	Greater Superficial Petrosal Nerve, Emissary Veins, Cartilage.
Internal Auditory Meatus	Facial Nerve (VII), Vestibulocochlear Nerve (VIII), Labyrinthine Artery
Stylomastoid Foramen	Facial Nerve (VII), Stylomastoid Artery.
Jugular Foramen	Glossopharyngeal Nerve (IX), Vagus Nerve (X), Accessory Nerve (XI), Inferior Petrosal Sinus, Internal Jugular Vein.
Hypoglossal Canal	Hypoglossal Nerve (XII).
Foramen Magnum	Medulla Oblongata, Anterior & Posterior Spinal Arteries, Vertebral Arteries, Meninges, CSF.

Q: What is the clinical significance of the pterion?

This is the junction between the **parietal**, **temporal** (squamous part), **sphenoid** (greater wing) & **frontal** bones. It is situated 3.5cm posterior to & 1cm superior to the frontozygomatic suture. The middle meningeal artery runs beneath the pterion, which is prone to fracture in direct trauma. This may result in arterial rupture causing an extradural haematoma.

Lateral Cerebral Hemisphere (Fig 4.31)

Study the image below & answer the following questions:

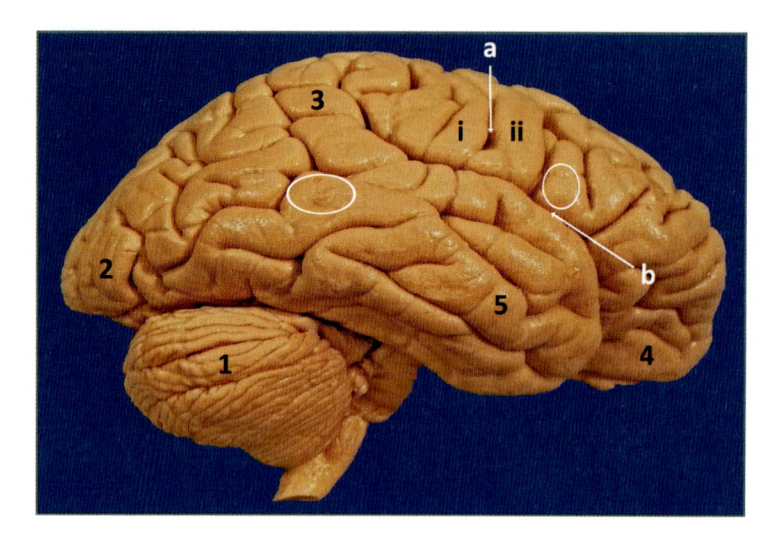

Q: What are the regions labelled 1–5 & what are their functions?

This is the right cerebral hemisphere.

Label	Region	Function
1	Cerebellum	Regulation & Coordination of Movement, Posture & Balance.
2	Occipital Lobe	Visual Processing.
3	Parietal Lobe	Movement, Orientation, Recognition, Perception of Stimuli.
4	Frontal Lobe	Conscious Thought, Reasoning, Planning, Emotions, Problem Solving.
5	Temporal Lobe	Perception & Recognition of Auditory Stimuli, Memory, Speech.

Q: What are the 'spaces' labelled a & b?

a = central sulcus, b = lateral sulcus.

Q: What are functions of the structures labelled i & ii?

Label	Structure	Function
i	Post-Central Gyrus	Sensory Cortex
ii	Pre-Central Gyrus	Motor Cortex

Q: What are the functions of the circled structures?

Circle	Structure	Function
Posterior	Wernicke's Area	Language Comprehension
Anterior	Broca's Area	Speech Production

Medial Cerebral Hemisphere (Fig 4.32)

Study the image below & answer the following questions:

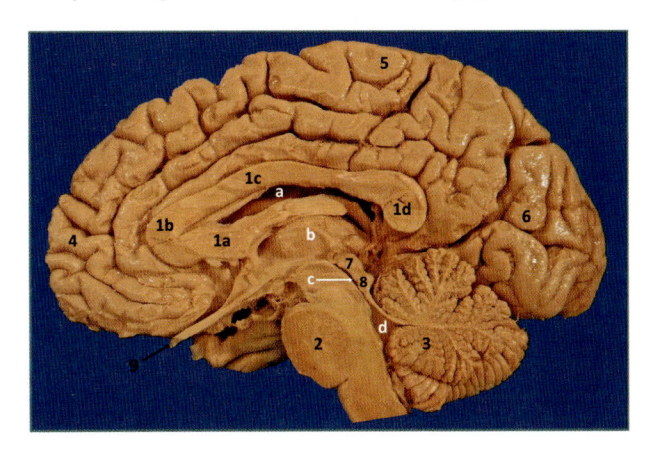

Q: Can you identify this image?

Right cerebral hemisphere (medial view).

Q: What are structures 1a–1d & what is their function?

These are all part of the corpus callosum, the largest white matter structure of the brain. The corpus callosum facilitates communication between the 2 cerebral hemispheres. 1a = rostrum, 1b = genu, 1c = body, 1d = splenium.

Q: What are structures 2–6?

2 = pons, 3 = cerebellum, 4 = frontal lobe, 5 = parietal lobe, 6 = occipital lobe.

Q: What are structures 7–9 what are their functions?

7 = superior colliculus (coordinates eye movement), 8 = inferior colliculus (involved in the auditory pathway), 9 = optic nerve.

Cerebrospinal Fluid

Study (Fig 4.32) & answer the following questions:

Q: What are structures a–d?

a = lateral ventricle, b = thalamus viewed through 3rd ventricle, c = aqueduct of Sylvius, d = 4th ventricle.

Q: Can you describe the flow of cerebrospinal fluid (CSF)?

- 150–200mls of CSF circulates through the cerebral ventricles & subarachnoid space.
- 70% is secreted by the choroid plexuses of the ventricles & the remainder by nearby vessels. A choroid plexus is a vascular invagination of pia mater, lined by ependymal cells.
- Most CSF is produced by the lateral ventricles & this then drains, via the interventricular foramen of Monro, into the 3rd ventricle.
- From here, CSF drains into the 4th ventricle via the aqueduct of Sylvius.
- CSF drains into the subarachnoid space from the 4th ventricle via 2 foramina of **L**uschka (**l**ateral) & 1 foramen of **M**agendie (**m**edial).
- Reabsorption of CSF has been proposed to be via a number of routes including the dural venous sinuses (via arachnoid villi) & lymphatic channels (after draining along cranial nerves & spinal nerve roots).

Cranial Nerves (Fig 4.33)

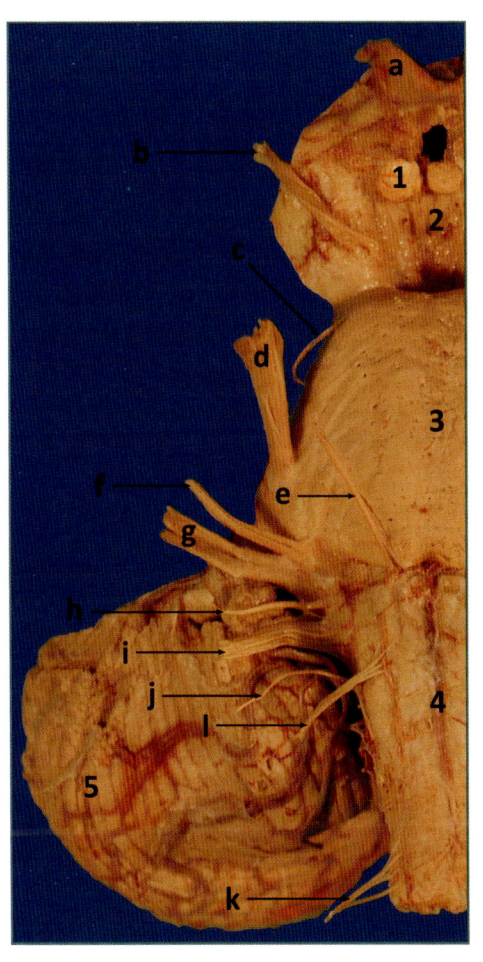

Q: What are structures 1–5?

1 = mamillary body, 2 = mesencephalon, 3 = pons, 4 = medulla, 5 = cerebellum.

Q: What are structures a–l?

These are the cranial nerves.

a = optic (II), b = occulomotor (III), c = trochlear (IV), d = trigeminal (V), e = abducens (VI), f = facial (VII), g = vestibulocochlear (VIII), h = glossopharyngeal (IX), i = vagus (X), j = accessory cranial branch (XI), k = accessory spinal branch (XI), l = hypoglossal (XII).

Q: Where do the cranial nerves originate at the brainstem?

The only cranial nerves that do not originate at the brainstem are (I) & (II).

Origin	Cranial Nerves
Olfactory Epithelium	I (olfactory)
Retinal Epithelium	II (optic)
Mesencephalon	III (occulomotor), IV (abducens), V (trigeminal)
Pons	VI (abducens), VII (facial)
Cerebellopontine Angle	VIII (vestibulocochlear)
Medulla	IX (glossopharyngeal), X (vagus), XI (accessory), XII (hypoglossal)

Ascending & Descending Spinal Pathways

Q: What are the functions of the ascending spinal pathways?

Pathway	Function
Antero-Lateral Spinothalamic Tract	Ascending neurones decussate at the level of the spinal cord & are for **pain & temperature.**
Dorsal Columns	Ascending neurones decussate at the level of the medulla & are for **fine touch, vibration & conscious proprioception.**
Spinocerebellar Tracts	Ascending neurones are for **muscle stretch & unconscious proprioception**. The posterior spinocerebellar tract remains on the ipsilateral side of the spinal column / cerebellum, whereas the anterior spinocerebellar tract decussates at the level of the spinal cord.

Q: What are the functions of the descending spinal pathways?

Pathway	Function
Corticospinal Tracts	Descending neurones decussate at the level of the medulla (pyramidal system) & are for **skilled & discrete movements.**
Extrapyramidal System	This motor pathway receives collective inputs from areas including the cerebral cortex, basal nuclei & cerebellum. They descend the ipsilateral spinal cord to arrive at appropriate motor neurones, resulting in **modulation & regulation of movement**.

Brachial Plexus (Fig 4.34)

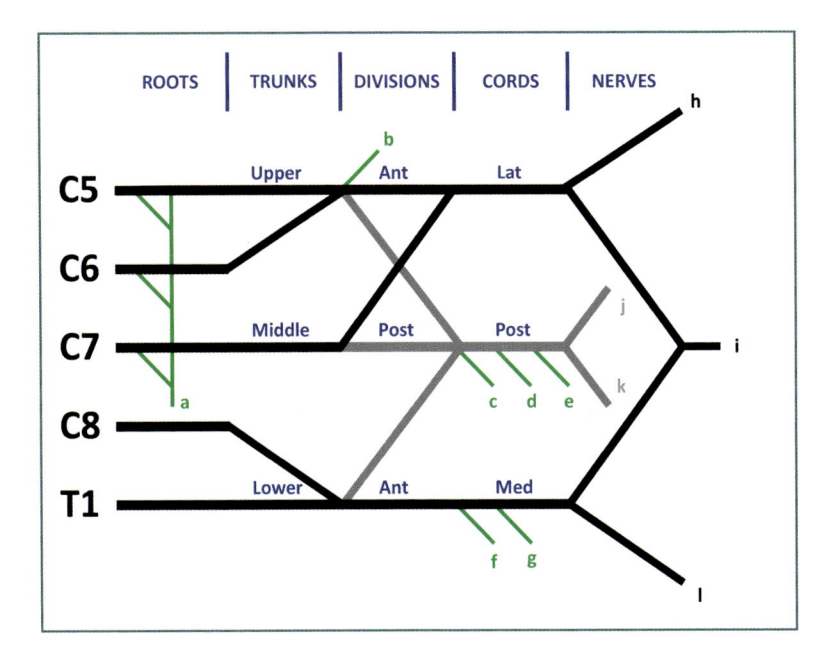

Q: Can you draw & label the brachial plexus?

a = long thoracic nerve of Bell (C5–C7), b = suprascapular nerve (C5–C6), c = upper subscapular nerve (C5–C6), d = thoracodorsal nerve (C5–C6), e = lower subscapular nerve (C5–C6), f = medial pectoral nerve (C8–T1), g = medial cutaneous nerve of the arm (C8–T1), h = musculocutaneous nerve (C5–C7), i = median nerve (C5–T1), j = axillary nerve (C5–C6), k = radial nerve (C5–T1), l = ulnar nerve (C7–T1), m = dorsal scapular nerve.

Q: What clinical features of brachial plexus injuries do you know of?

Feature	Notes
Erb's Palsy	This results from an upper brachial plexus injury, usually arising from shoulder dystocia during birth. Roots C5–C7 are most commonly affected. This results in the affected upper limb lying in an internally rotated, elbow extended & wrist flexed 'waiter's tip' position.
Klumpke's Palsy	This results from a lower brachial plexus injury, arising from a traction injury whilst the shoulder is abducted. Roots C8–T1 are most commonly affected. This results in clawing of the hand of the affected limb due to paralysis of the intrinsic hand muscles. Horner's syndrome may also be present if associated with interrupted sympathetic innervation at that level.

Carotid Sheath

Q: What is the course of the common carotid artery?

There are 2 common carotid arteries. The right originates from the brachiocephalic artery at the level of the sternoclavicular joint, the left originates from the aortic arch directly. The common carotid arteries travel cranially, within the carotid sheaths & divide at the level of C4, giving rise to the internal & external carotid arteries.

Q: What is the carotid sheath & what are the contents?

The carotid sheath is derived from deep cervical fascia. It lies in the lateral border of the retropharyngeal space (deep to sternocleidomastoid) & extends from the level of the 1st rib, to the skull base.

Major Contents	Other Contents
Common Carotid Artery (medial)	Ansa Cervicalis
Internal Jugular Vein (lateral)	Lymph Nodes
Vagus (X) Nerve (between the above)	Glossopharyngeal (IX), Accesory (XI), Hypoglossal (XI) Nerves (pierce the distal sheath fascia)

Q: What are the branches of the external carotid artery?

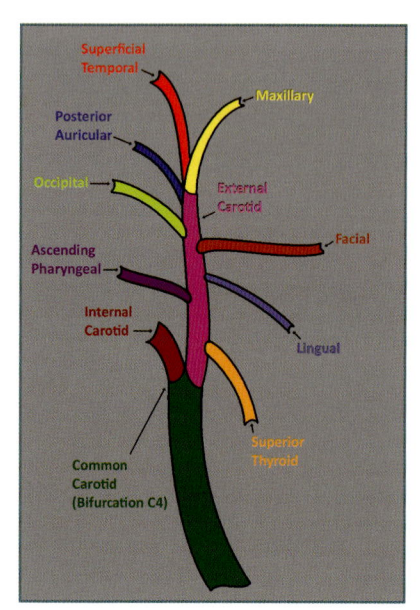

Fig 4.35: Right external carotid artery & branches

There are 4 posterior & 4 anterior arterial branches of the external carotid artery.

Position	Posterior	Anterior
DISTAL	**Superficial Temporal**	**Maxillary**
	Posterior Auricular	**Facial**
	Occipital	**Lingual**
PROXIMAL	**Ascending Pharyngeal**	**Superior Thyroid**

Q: What are the branches of the internal jugular vein?

The internal jugular veins are formed by a confluence of the sigmoid & inferior petrosal sinuses, as they pass through the jugular foramina. They travel down the neck, within the carotid sheath, then drain into the brachiocephalic veins. There are 5 important veins that drain into the anterior portion of the internal jugular vein along its course. From proximal to distal:

1. Pharyngeal Plexus
2. Facial
3. Lingual
4. Superior Thyroid
5. Middle Thyroid

Circle of Willis (Fig 4.36)

Study the image below & answer the following questions:

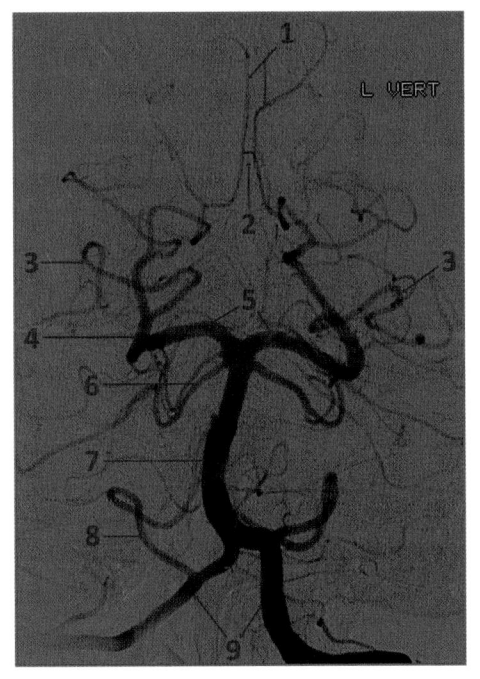

Q: Can you identify this image?

Cerebral angiogram, showing the circle of Willis.

Q: What 'feeds' the structures in this image?

2 x internal carotid arteries feed into the circle of Willis at the level of the middle cerebral arteries.

2 x vertebral arteries feed into the circle of Willis, after joining to become the basilar artery.

Q: What are structures 1–8? What is their function / what do they supply?

These are all arteries of the circle of Willis:

Label	Artery	Function / Supply
1	Anterior Cerebral	Frontal Lobes, Superior-Medial Parietal Lobes
2	Anterior Communicating	Connects Anterior Cerebral Arteries
3	Middle Cerebral	Lateral Cerebral Hemispheres (mostly), Basal Ganglia, Internal Capsule
4	Posterior Communicating	Joins the posterior cerebral artery to the terminal trifurcation of the internal carotid artery. The trifurcation is comprised of the posterior communicating, middle cerebral & anterior cerebral arteries.
5	Posterior Cerebral	Occipital Lobes
6	Right Superior Cerebellar	Right Superior Cerebellum, Parts of Right Midbrain
7	Basilar	Brainstem
8	Right Anterior Inferior Cerebellar	Right Anterior Inferior Cerebellum
9	Vertebral	Deliver Blood to the Circle of Willis

CHAPTER 5
SURGICAL PATHOLOGY

BH Miranda
K Asaad
DJ Tobin

CHAPTER CONTENTS

Biochemistry
- Plasma Proteins
- Calcium
- Hyperuricaemia
- Hepatic Function & Jaundice

Growth, Differentiation & Morphogenesis Disorders
- Atrophy, Hyperplasia & Other Common Phenomena
- Urinary Calculi
- Gallstone Disease
- Amyloid

Haematology
- Anaemias Including Fe^{2+}, B12 & Folate Deficiency
- Sickle Cell Anaemia
- Thalassaemia
- Polycythaemia
- Haemostasis, Platelets & Clotting Cascade
- Disseminated Intravascular Coagulation
- Blood Groups Including ABO & Rhesus Systems
- Blood Transfusion & Blood Products
- Blood Transfusion Reactions & Substitute Blood Products
- Oedema & Lymphoedema

Immunology
- Hypersensitivity, Cytokines & Mediators
- Complement Cascade
- Immunity & Immunoglobulins
- Transplantation

Inflammation
- Acute Inflammation
- Chronic Inflammation
- Cyst, Abscess, Pus & Other Common Phenomena
- Wound Healing

Microbiology
- Surgical Site & Wound Infections
- Pneumonia
- Urinary Tract Infection
- Endotoxin & Exotoxin
- Commensal Bacteria
- Nosocomial Infection
- Immunisation & Vaccination

Neoplasia
- Cell Cycle
- Tumour Markers
- Carcinogenesis
- Malignancy
- Paraneoplastic Syndromes

Vascular
- Clot, Thrombus, Embolus & Virchow's Triad
- Atheroma
- Infarction & Ischaemia
- Aneurysm

BIOCHEMISTRY

Plasma Proteins

Q: What are plasma proteins & where are they made?

These are proteins found in blood serum & represent approximately 7% of total blood volume. They are made in the liver, except for gamma globulins / immunoglobulins that are secreted by plasma cells, also known as B-lymphocytes. Immunoglobulins represent approximately 30% of all plasma proteins.

Q: What are the functions of plasma proteins?

Albumin represents 60% of all plasma proteins. It is a transporter, binding Ca^{2+} & it is also involved in Starling's Law of the Capillaries, maintaining plasma oncotic pressure. Functions of plasma proteins include:

- Complement Cascade Components
- Enzymes & Enzyme Inhibitors
- Clotting Cascade e.g. Factor I / Fibrinogen
- Gene Expression Regulatory Proteins
- Immune System e.g. Gamma Globulins / Immunoglobulins
- Starling's Law of the Capillaries
- Transporter Proteins.

Calcium

Q: What is the normal range for serum calcium & what is corrected calcium?

The normal range is 2.2–2.6mmol/l. Approximately 50% of Ca^{2+} is bound to albumin. Unbound Ca^{2+} is biologically active, so it is important to factor the level of serum albumin into any serum Ca^{2+} measurements. Adjusting for this obtains the corrected Ca^{2+}. A normal serum calcium figure of 40g/l is used in the following equation to calculate corrected Ca^{2+} as follows:

Corrected Ca^{2+} = Total Serum Ca^{2+} + 0.02 (Normal Serum Albumin – Patient's Serum Albumin)

The units for the above calculation are as follows:

Corrected Ca^{2+} & Total Serum Ca^{2+}	= mmol/l
Normal Serum Albumin & Patient's Serum Albumin	= g/l

Q: If a patient has a serum Ca^{2+} of 2.6mmol/l & albumin of 35g/l, what is their corrected Ca^{2+}?

Using the above equation, the patient's corrected Ca^{2+} = 2.7 mmol/l

Corrected Ca^{2+} (mmol/l)	= 2.6 + 0.02 (40 – 35)	
	= 2.6 + 0.02 x 5	
	= 2.6 + 0.1	= 2.7 mmol/l

Hyperuricaemia

Q: What is urate & what is the normal reference range?

Urate, or uric acid, is a product of purine metabolism i.e. adenine & guanine. The normal reference range is 3.5–7 mg/dl.

Q: What are the causes of hyperuricaemia?

These may be classified as primary & secondary as follows:

Primary	Secondary
Idiopathic	Alcohol
Inborn Errors of Metabolism	Diuretics
	Protein Rich Foods

Q: What are the consequences of hyperuricaemia?

These may be classified as acute or chronic as follows:

Acute	Chronic
Gout: classically a hot, painful & swollen MTPJ, although other joints may be affected e.g. ankle, knee, hands, wrist & spine.	Destructive Joint Disease
	Polyarthritis
	Urate Renal Calculi
Low Grade Fever	Renal Failure
Painful Skin Tophi	Skin Tophi Ulceration & Chalky Discharge

Q: What are the pathological features of gout?

10% of patients with hyperuricaemia develop gout. There is rapid uric acid crystal deposition in cartilage, synovium & tendons of the affected joint. Larger deposits, known as **tophi**, may also ulcerate through skin. Joint aspiration reveals negatively birefringent crystals, which appear yellow under polarised light.

Hepatic Function & Jaundice

Q: What are the functions of the liver?

- Bile Production
- Bilirubin Conjugation
- Clotting Factor Synthesis
- Drug Metabolism
- Glycogen Storage
- Plasma Protein Synthesis
- Production of Heat
- Reticuloendothelial System.

Q: What is bilirubin & what is the normal reference range?

90% of RBCs are broken down in the reticuloendothelial system & the remainder are haemolysed within the circulation. Globin & haem are breakdown products of these processes. Bilirubin is a bile pigment. It is produced by the breakdown of haem to biliverdin, followed by conversion, in macrophages, to bilirubin. This occurs within the reticuloendothelial system & the resulting bilirubin is unconjugated & insoluble at this stage. The normal reference range is 3–17μmol/l.

Q: Can you draw the bilirubin metabolism cycle, explaining each step as you go along?

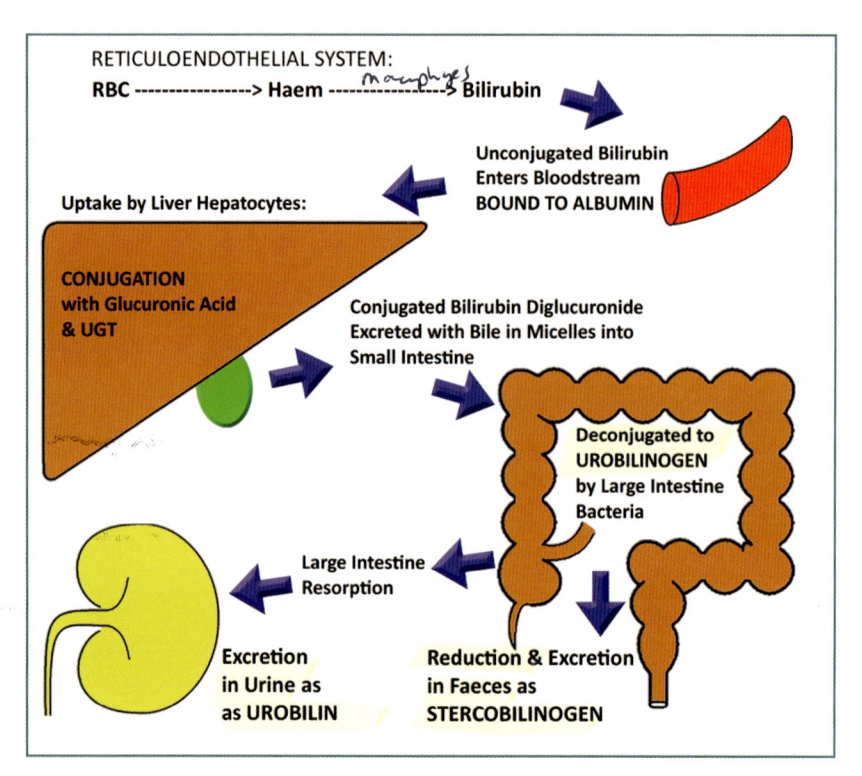

Fig 5.1: Schematic representation of the jaundice cycle.

1. 90% of RBCs are broken down in the reticuloendothelial system & the remainder are haemolysed within the circulation.
2. Unconjugated bilirubin production is the result of haem breakdown (see previous question).
3. Unconjugated bilirubin enters the blood, bound to serum albumin, then transported to the liver.
4. Hepatocytes conjugate bilirubin, with glucuronic acid & the enzyme UGT.
5. Conjugated bilirubin diglucuronide is secreted into the small intestine, with bile, in micelles. It is deconjugated to urobilinogen by large intestine bacteria.
6. Urobilinogen may either be further reduced to stercobilinogen (brown) & excreted in faeces, or reabsorbed & transported to the kidney to be excreted as urobilin (yellow).

GROWTH, DIFFERENTIATION & MORPHOGENESIS DISORDERS

Atrophy, Hyperplasia, Hypertrophy & Other Common Phenomena

Q: What terminology is associated with the failure of growth or growth maintenance?

Terminology	Definition
Agenesis	Abnormal total tissue or organ developmental failure e.g. Corpus Callosum & Renal Agenesis.
Atresia	Failure of normal lumen development within an organ or structure e.g. Biliary & Oesophageal Atresia.
Atrophy	A reduction in size of a tissue or organ that has fully developed. The cells either become decreased in number or size or both. Cells may also have a reduction in organelles, decreased function & display autophagy.
Aplasia	Abnormal, severe tissue or organ developmental failure, with a structure or function that is only partially recognisable e.g. Aplasia Cutis Congenita.
Apoptosis	Programmed cell death. A normal, energy-dependent process that results in the auto-digestion of cells by their own enzymes without damaging the tissue or organism. This process counter regulates normal mitosis.
Hypoplasia	Abnormal, partial tissue or organ developmental failure, with a structure or function that has not reached normal limits, but has developed further than in aplasia e.g. Breast & Optic Nerve Hypoplasia.
Necrosis	Premature death of cells within a living tissue. An abnormal, energy-independent process, associated with inflammation that results in the death of a tissue or organ. This process is caused by influencing factors outside of the affected tissue or organ & is not part of normal counter regulation.

Q: How would you classify the causes of atrophy?

These may be classified as physiological or pathological:

Physiological	Pathological
Late Childhood (Thymus)	Idiopathic (Alzheimer's & Muscular Dystrophy)
Adolescence (Tonsils)	Disuse (Muscle)
Menopause (Breasts, Uterus & Vagina)	Neuropathic (LMN Trauma / Lesion)
	Other (Ischaemia & Osteoporosis)

Q: What is hyperplasia & hypertrophy?

Terminology	Definition
Hyperplasia	An increase in the size of a tissue or organ due to an increase in cell numbers. To increase in number, cells must have the ability to synthesise DNA & divide.
Hypertrophy	An increase in the size of a tissue or organ due to an increase in cell size, with increased synthesis of structural proteins & organelles.

Q: How would you classify the causes of hyperplasia & hypertrophy?

These may be classified as physiological or pathological:

Terminology	Physiological	Pathological
Hyperplasia	Post Hepatectomy (Liver)	Cushing's Disease (Adrenal Glands)
	Pregnancy (Breast, Thyroid & Pituitary)	Graves' Disease (Thyroid)
Hypertrophy	Exercise (Muscle)	Graves' Disease (Thyroid)
	Pregnancy (Uterus)	HOCM (Myocardium)

Q: What is a hamartoma?

This is a benign mass, resulting from abnormal development of tissue native to the organ, arranged in a disorganised manner e.g. CNS Hamartoma (Tuberose Sclerosis), Haemangioma, Juvenile Polyp, Lung, Melanocytic Naevus, Osteochondroma & Peutz-Jeghers Polyp.

Urinary Calculi

Q: What is a calculus & where do calculi form?

An abnormal solid collection that has precipitated within a duct or organ. The commonest sites include Gall Bladder & Biliary Tree, Urinary System, Pancreas, Prostate & Salivary Glands.

Q: What are the different compositions of renal calculi & what is their % occurrence?

Composition	% Occurrence
Calcium Oxalate, Phosphate & Urate	77
Mg^{2+} Ammonium Triple Phosphate (Struvite)	15
Uric Acid*	5
Cysteine	2
Xanthine / Pyruvate	1

*Note: Uric acid calculi are radio-lucent.

Q: How would you classify the causes of urinary calculus precipitation?

Cause	Examples
Anatomy	Horseshoe Kidney, Medullary Sponge Kidney & Vesico-Ureteric Reflux.
Dehydration	Environmental & Poor Fluid Intake.
Infection	*Proteus*, *Klebsiella*, *Serratia* & *Mycoplasma* have the enzyme UREASE. Urease is involved in the hydrolysis of urea, resulting in the production of ammonia & carbon dioxide. The ensuing alkaline conditions are associated with struvite stones that may be florid, causing a STAGHORN CALCULUS.
Stasis	BPH & Urethral Stricture.
Other	Cysteinuria (Cysteine Stones), Crohn's Disease (Oxalate Stones), Hyperoxaluria (Oxalate Stones), Hypercalcaemia (Calcium Stones) & Inborn Errors of Metabolism (Xanthine & Pyruvate Stones).

Q: What are the sequelae of renal calculi?

Sequelae of renal calculi may be classified anatomically as follows:

Kidney	Ureter	Bladder	Urethra
Haematuria	Haematuria	Haematuria	Haematuria
Loin Pain	Renal Colic	Suprapubic Pain	Dysuria
Pyelonephritis	Ureteritis	Cystitis	Urethritis
Hydronephrosis	Hydroureter	Urinary Obstruction	Urinary Obstruction
		Frequency & Urgency	Pain on Passing Stone
		SCC Bladder	

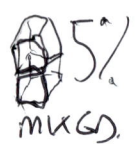

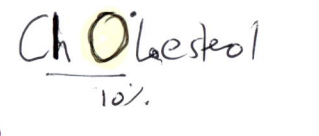

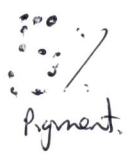

Gallstone Disease

Q: What are the compositions, macroscopic features & % occurrences of gallstones?

Composition	Macroscopic Features	% Occurrence
Mixed	Multiple & Faceted	85%
Cholesterol	Large & Yellow	10%
Pigment	Multiple, Small & Black	5%

Note: 10% of gallstones are radio-opaque due to Ca^{2+} ion precipitation.

Q: What is bile composed of & what is its function?

Up to 1500ml/24h of bile are released into the duodenum. This is mediated by the hormone secretin, which is released by the pancreas. The composition & functions of bile include:

Composition	Function
Bile Pigments	Cholesterol, Drug & Steroid Excretion
Bile Salts	Conjugated Bilirubin Excretion into Small Intestine
Cholesterol	Emulsification of Fat for Digestion
Electrolytes e.g. Bicarbonate	Fat Soluble Vitamin (A, D, E, K) Absorption
Lecithin	Micelle Formation
Phospholipids	Gastric Acid Neutralisation
Water	(due to Bicarbonate Production)

Q: Can you explain the bile production & storage process?

Hepatocytes produce bile that is transported, via bile ducts, for storage in the gallbladder. The gallbladder actively absorbs Na^+ & water. Up to 1500mls/24h may be released, via the common bile duct, Ampulla of Vater & Sphincter of Oddi, into the 2nd part of the duodenum.

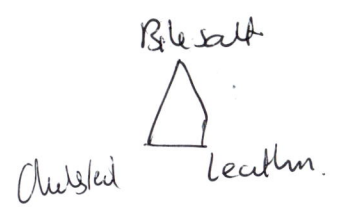

Q: Why do gallstones occur?

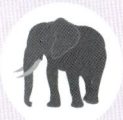

Memory: Imbalanced Heavy Fat Females, Fair & Forty.

Cholesterol stones precipitate due to an **imb**alance between the bile salt : cholesterol : lecithin ratio. Pigment stones are the result of increased **h**aemolysis, with consequent increase in bilirubin production. They are more prevalent in **f**at, **f**emales, with **f**air hair who are **f**orty.

Q: What complications are associated with gallstones?

Within Gallbladder	Within Biliary Tree	Distal to Biliary Tree
Biliary Colic	Obstructive Jaundice	Gallstone Ileus
Carcinoma	Ascending Cholangitis	
Cholecystitis	Pancreatitis	
Empyema		
Mucocoele		

Amyloid

Q: What is amyloid?

Amyloid refers to a group of degradation-resistant proteins, with a characteristic β-pleated sheet structure. Diagnostic biopsy of the affected organ tissue, displays apple-green birefringence with polarised light after staining with Congo red. Clinical features are related to site of deposition.

Q: What types of amyloid do you know of?

Each type may be associated with a particular protein:

Type	Example	Associated Protein
AL / Primary	Myeloma	λ-Immunoglobulin Light Chains
AA / Secondary	Chronic Inflammation	Serum Amyloid Proteins Synthesised by the Liver
AH / Aβ	Alzheimer's Disease	β-Amyloid Protein
PrP	Prion Disease	Prion Protein

Q: What structures are affected by amyloid deposition? What associated conditions do you know?

Most structures in the body may be affected:

Structure	Associated Condition
Heart	Restrictive Cardiomyopathy
Kidney	Nephrotic Syndrome & Renal Failure
Liver	Hepatic Failure (rare in isolated disease)
Nerves	Neuropathy
Pancreas	Diabetes Mellitus
Skin	Visible Dermal Deposition
Spleen	Splenic Function Inhibition (rare in isolated disease)
Thyroid	Medullary Carcinoma

HAEMATOLOGY

Anaemias Including Fe^{2+}, B12 & Folate Deficiency

Q: How would you classify anaemia?

This may be classified as normocytic, microcytic & macrocytic:

Normocytic	Microcytic	Macrocytic
Chronic Disease	Fe^{2+} Deficiency	B12 Deficiency
Renal Failure	Thalassaemia	Folate Deficiency
Sickle Cell Anaemia	Sideroblastic Anaemia	ETOH
Elliptocytosis & Spherocytosis		Hypothyroidism
		Myelodysplasia

Q: What effect does macrocytic anaemia have on bone marrow & circulating blood cells?

Macrocytic anaemia may be sub-categorised into normoblastic & megaloblastic. A normoblast is a nucleated, immature erythrocyte found in the bone marrow e.g. ETOH, Hypothyroidism & Myelodysplasia. A megaloblast is an immature erythrocyte found in the bone marrow, with an abnormally large nucleus e.g. B12 & Folate Deficiency. Normoblasts or megaloblasts are found in the circulation of patients with macrocytic anaemia.

Q: What are the causes of Fe^{2+} deficiency anaemia?

Cause	Example
Blood Loss	Gastrointestinal & Uterine Bleeding.
High Fe^{2+} Demand	Growth & Pregnancy.
Low Fe^{2+} Absorption	Gastric & Small Bowel Disease e.g. Coeliac Disease.
Low Fe^{2+} Intake	Developing Countries.

Q: What would you expect to find in the blood film of a patient with Fe^{2+} deficiency anaemia?

- Hypochromic, Microcytic Cells
- Anisocytosis (variation in the size of erythrocytes)
- Poikilocytosis (variation in the shape of erythrocytes).

Q: What are the causes of B12 deficiency anaemia?

Cause	Example
Autoimmune	Pernicious Anaemia
Diet	B12 present in Eggs, Fish, Meat & Milk
Iatrogenic	Gastrectomy & Ileal Resection
Inflammatory	Crohn's Disease
Malabsorption	Coeliac Disease & Tropical Sprue

Q: What would you expect to find in the blood film of a patient with B12 deficiency anaemia?

- Macrocytic Cells
- Neutrophils with Hypersegmented Nuclei
- Howell-Jolly Bodies (Fig 5.2).

Q: What are the causes of folate deficiency?

Cause	Example
Drugs	Methotrexate, Phenytoin, Sulphasalazine & Trimethoprim
High Folate Demand	*Physiological:* Lactation & Pregnancy
	Pathological: Dialysis & Malignancy
Low Folate Intake	Poor Diet & No Vegetables
Malabsorption	Coeliac Disease & Tropical Sprue

Sickle Cell Anaemia

Q: How would you classify the causes of haemolytic anaemias?

Classification	Subclassification	Example Causes
GENETIC	Enzyme Defects	G6PD & Pyruvate Kinase Deficiency
	Erythrocyte Membrane Abnormalities	Elliptocytosis & Spherocytosis
	Haemoglobinopathies	Sickle Cell & Thalassaemia
		Idiopathic
ACQUIRED	Immunological – Autoimmune	Infectious Mononucleosis
		SLE
	Immunological – Alloimmune	Blood Transfusion Reactions
		Haemolytic Disease of the Newborn
	Immunological – Drug Induced	Methyldopa & Penicillin
		Drugs e.g. Ribavirin
	Non-Immunological	Infection e.g. Malaria & Septicaemia
		Microangiopathic
		Trauma e.g. Cardiac Valve Replacement

Q: What is the pathogenesis of sickle cell anaemia?

- An autosomal recessive, haemolytic anaemia. RBC lifespan is reduced from 120 to 10–20 days.
- It is more prevalent in Afro-Caribbean & Mediterranean individuals.
- Heterozygotes have sickle cell trait & homozygotes have sickle cell disease.
- Normal adult HbA has 2 α- & 2 β- chains; however glutamic acid is replaced by valine at position 6 on the β chain in sickle cell anaemia.
- This results in an abnormal, less soluble HbS tetramer that represents approximately 30% of the total Hb in heterozygotes & >90% of the total Hb in homozygotes.
- Certain 'states' result in HbS polymerisation & the formation of characteristic sickle cells which result in vaso-occlusive disease, causing tissue ischaemia & pain crises.

Q: What 'states' result in vaso-occlusive disease in sickle cell anaemia?

- Dehydration
- Hypoxia
- Infection
- Hypothermia.

Q: What are the clinical features of sickle cell anaemia?

These may be classified as follows:

Haemolytic	Vaso-occlusive
Anaemia	Pain e.g. Bone Crisis
GSD	Priapism
Jaundice	Focal Neurology
Cardiac Failure	Ocular Events
Sequestration Crisis	**Infective**
Hepatomegaly	Acute Chest Syndrome (Chlamydia & Mycoplasma)
Splenomegaly	Aplastic Crisis (Parvovirus B19)
	Osteomyelitis (Salmonella)

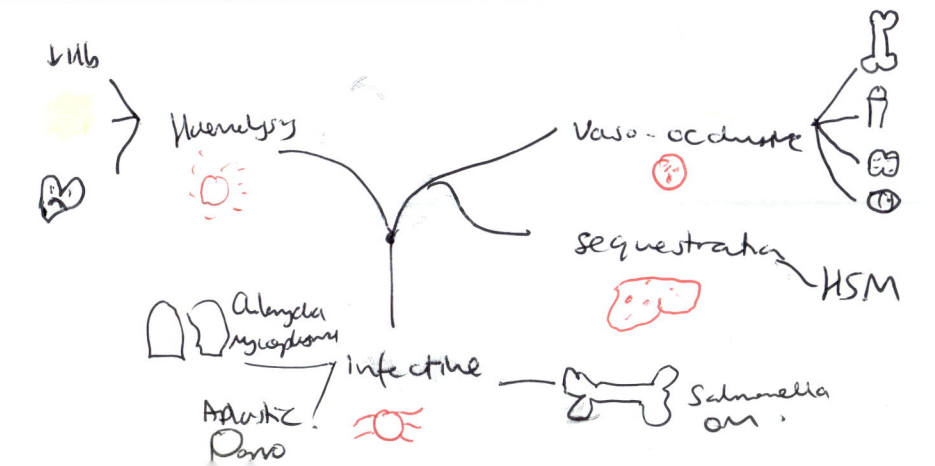

Q: What management strategies should be addressed in a surgical patient with sickle cell anaemia?

Strategy	Explanation
Oxygen	Prevent hypoxia
Temperature	Prevent hypothermia
Fluids	Prevent dehydration
Antibiotics	Prevent infection
Analgesics	Control pain & beware of opioid dependence
Blood Transfusion	Prevent / treat anaemia
Tourniquets	Use with caution, particularly intra-operatively

Q: What would you expect to find in the blood film of a patient with sickle cell anaemia?

- Normochromic Cells
- Fragmented Cells
- Reticulocytes
- Sickle Shaped Cells (Fig 5.2)
- Target Cells (Fig 5.2)
- Howell-Jolly Bodies (Fig 5.2)

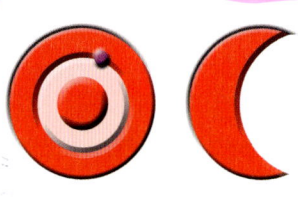

Fig 5.2: Target Cell & Howell-Jolly Body (left); Sickle Shaped Cell (right).

Thalassaemia

Q: What is the genetic basis of thalassaemia?

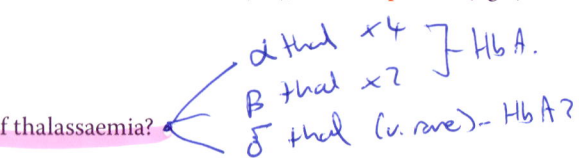

- This is an autosomal recessive haemolytic anaemia.
- There are 3 types of thalassaemia, each is named after the particular defect in globin chain synthesis that occurs in adult Hb. 95% of adult Hb is HbA & this will be affected by both α- & β-thalassaemia. 3% of adult Hb is HbA2 & this will be affected by δ-thalassaemia.
- Only 3% of adult Hb is HbA2, hence δ-thalassaemia is less clinically relevant.
- α-thalassaemia is more prevalent in Afro-Caribbean & Asian individuals; 2 linked genes on chromosome 16 code for α-globin chains.
- β-thalassaemia is more prevalent in Afro-Caribbean & Mediterranean individuals; 1 gene on chromosome 11 codes for β-globin chains.
- Human cells are diploid, hence up to 4 alleles may be involved in α-thalassaemia & 2 alleles that may be involved in β-thalassaemia.
- The severity of thalassaemia is governed by the number of genes affected.

Q: What types of α-thalassaemia do you know of?

These are defined by the number of genes that are affected that code for the α-globin chain:

Type	Explanation
Silent	Only 1 allele is affected. This is clinically silent.
Trait	2 alleles are affected. There is mild, microcytic, hypochromic anaemia only.
HbH Disease	3 alleles are affected. Tetrameric β-chains are produced in this type of α-thalassaemia, resulting in HbH that has a high oxygen affinity, so a microcytic, hypochromic anaemia ensues. The presence of Heinz bodies, target cells (Fig 5.2) & splenomegaly is characteristic.
Hydrops Foetalis	All 4 alleles are affected. Foetal Hb is composed of 2 α- & 2 γ-chains, however only tetrameric γ-chains are produced in this type of α-thalassaemia, resulting in HbBarts that is incompatible with life. Neonates are therefore stillborn.

Q: What types of β-thalassaemia do you know of?

Type	Explanation
Major	Both alleles are affected. Patients are affected by microcytic, hypochromic anaemia that requires frequent transfusion. Splenomegaly may be present & bone marrow transplant may offer a cure. Average life expectancy is approximately 30 years. The commonest cause of death is cardiac siderosis due to Fe^{2+} overload, secondary to chronic transfusion.
Minor	1 allele is affected. A mild microcytic, hypochromic anaemia ensues that may only present, for example in pregnancy. Splenomegaly is uncharacteristic.
Intermedia	Patients present with symptoms that fall in between major & minor forms. Episodic transfusion may be required.

Q: What would you expect to find in the blood film of a patient with β-thalassaemia?

- Hypochromic Cells
- Reticulocytes
- Target Cells (Fig 5.2)
- Howell-Jolly Bodies (Fig 5.2).

Q: What characteristic features may be present in a patient with β-thalassaemia?

Feature	Clinical Sequelae
Marrow Hyperplasia	Frontal bone bossing & hair-on-end appearance of skull on radiography.
Fe²⁺ Overload	Cardiac siderosis, endocrine disease e.g. hypothalamopituitary & thyroid disease, liver cirrhosis, pancreatitis & reduced sexual development.
Hypersplenism	Anaemia, leucopaenia & thrombocytopaenia.

Polycythaemia

Q: What is polycythaemia?

This is a condition reflecting an increase in the concentration of red blood cells. There is usually an accompanying increase in haematocrit & Hb.

Q: How would you classify polycythaemia?

Primary	Secondary	Relative
Polycythaemia Vera	**Appropriate:**	Burns
	Altitude	Dehydration
	Emphysema	Diuretics
	Right to Left Shunt	ETOH
	Inappropriate:	
	HCC	
	Phaeochromocytoma	
	RCC	

Q: What underlying mechanisms allow for conditions, that cause polycythaemia, to be classified?

Classification	Mechanism
Primary	This is a direct result of bone marrow disease.
Secondary	*Appropriate:* This is due to appropriate release of EPO.
	Inappropriate: This is due to inappropriate release of EPO.
Relative	This is an 'apparent' polycythaemia, actually caused by decreased plasma volume.

Haemostasis, Platelets & Clotting Cascade

Q: What occurs during haemostasis?

- Vasoconstriction
- Platelet Activation & Aggregation
- Clotting Cascade.

Q: What are the functions of platelets?

Platelets, also known as thrombocytes, are anucleated cells with an average life span of 10 days. They contain & may release a number of substances that include ADP, ATP, TXA2, actin & myosin. Their roles include involvement in:

- Haemostasis
- Phagocytosis
- Cytokine Signalling.

Q: Describe the role of platelets in haemostasis.

- Endothelial damage results in release of vWF from endothelial cells.
- Platelet activation, adherence & aggregation ensue.
- ADP release results in further platelet aggregation.
- TXA2 release results in further platelet activation.
- Actin & myosin myofilament contraction results in platelet plug reinforcement.

Q: What is the clotting cascade?

A complex series of reactions, involving clotting factors & enzymes, that results in the conversion of soluble plasma proteins into an insoluble fibrin meshwork. It plays a vital role in haemostasis.

Q: Where are clotting factors made & what are they?

All clotting factors are synthesised by the liver except IV, which is Ca^{2+}. Furthermore, VIII is primarily synthesised by the vascular endothelium. Aside from IV (Ca^{2+}), most clotting factors are serine proteases, however V & VIII are glycoproteins & XIII is a transglutaminase.

Intrinsic (APTT): Twelve Eleven Nine Ten
Eight
Extrinsic: 7 (imagine funnel)
(PT)

Ca
Protein C
Xa
Prothrombin → Thrombin → Plasmin
(II)   *Plasmin*
Fibrinogen → Fibrin
Ca
XIII
Platelet

Q: Can you draw the clotting cascade?

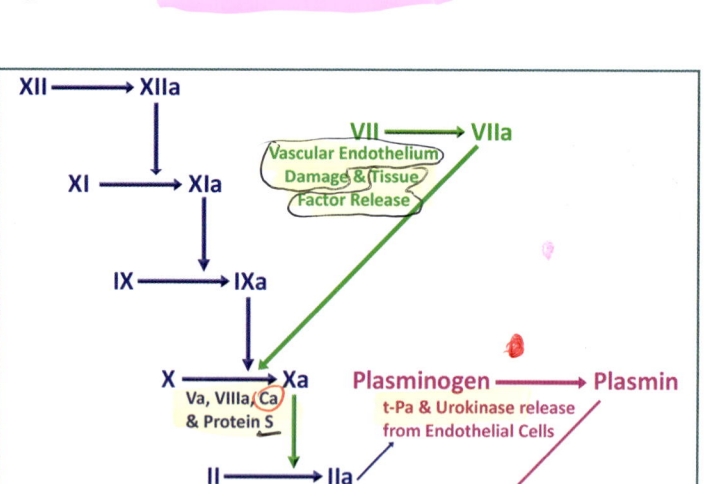

Fig 5.3: Simplified diagram of the clotting cascade.

Extrinsic Pathway

Intrinsic Pathway

Final Common Pathway

Fibrinolytic System

XII → XIIa
XI → XIa
IX → IXa
VII → VIIa (Vascular Endothelium Damage & Tissue Factor Release)
X → Xa (Va, VIIIa, Ca & Protein S)
Plasminogen → Plasmin (t-Pa & Urokinase release from Endothelial Cells)
II → IIa (Prothrombin) (Thrombin) Protein C & Ca
I → Ia (Fibrinogen) (Fibrin) XIIIa, Ca & Platelet PL

Pathway	Notes
Extrinsic	Activated by endothelial damage & tissue factor exposure.
Intrinsic	Comprised of blood components only.
Final Common	Generation of an insoluble fibrin meshwork.
Fibrinolytic System	Thrombin stimulates endothelial cell release of t-Pa & urokinase. These convert plasminogen to plasmin, a fibrinolytic. This system counter-regulates the cascade.

Q: Do you know of any pathways that counter-regulate the clotting cascade?

Antithrombin ⊖ 2, 9, 10, 11, 12

Counter-Regulator	Notes
Antithrombin	This serine protease inhibitor degrades the serine proteases IIa, IXa, Xa, XIa & XIIa.
Cascade Progression	Results in clotting factor depletion.
Fibrinolytic System	See earlier.
Protein C	Binds to the vascular endothelium & is activated. This in turn inactivates Va & VIII.

Protein C ⊖ 5, 8

Disseminated Intravascular Coagulation

Q: What is DIC?

Disseminated **i**ntravascular **c**oagulation is initially characterised by clotting cascade activation. The result is widespread intravascular coagulation. Once clotting factors have been consumed & the fibrinolytic system has become effective, bleeding ensues.

Q: What are the causes of DIC?

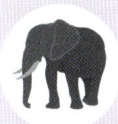

> Memory: 'I Be SAT at Tea'
>
> **I**nfection
> **B**leeding
> **S**hock
> **A**denocarcinoma
> **T**ransfusion
> **T**rauma.

Q: What pathological features & investigations assist diagnosis of DIC?

- APTT & PrT are both prolonged.
- Fibrin degradation products are increased in urine & serum.
- Fibrinogen is decreased in plasma.
- Schistocytosis (RBC fragmentation).
- Thrombocytopaenia.

Q: How would you treat a patient with DIC?

- Fluid resuscitation & careful maintenance.
- Blood products may be required e.g. to replace depleted clotting factors & platelets.
- Search & treat cause.
- Management on ICU.
- Antithrombin infusion.
- In severe cases, antithrombin or activated protein C infusions may be used. Antithrombin is a potent inhibitor of the coagulation cascade. Activated protein C inactivates clotting factors V & VIII, hence terminating coagulation.

Blood Groups Including ABO & Rhesus Systems

Q: What is the ABO blood group system?

This is the most important blood group system in humans & is coded by 3 alleles; A, B & O. These alleles govern the synthesis of enzymes that add carbohydrate to glycoproteins on the RBC surface. The O allele differs from the A allele by 1 guanine nucleotide deletion at position 261. The enzyme required for the addition of carbohydrate to glycoproteins on the RBC surface is therefore not produced. There are 6 genotypes & 4 phenotypes or blood types; O, A, B & AB. Phenotypes are dictated by the antigen that is present on the RBC surface. Serum contains antibodies against the antigen that is not present, according to phenotype as follows:

Phenotype	O	A	B	AB
Genotype	OO	AA / AO	BB / BO	AB
RBC Antigens	O	A	B	AB
Serum Antibodies	Anti-A & Anti-B	Anti-B	Anti-A	Nil

Q: What is the universal donor & recipient? What blood groups can receive & donate to each other?

O is the universal donor due to a lack of A & B antigens on the RBC surface. AB is the universal recipient due to a lack of serum antibodies. Incompatible blood donation results in agglutination & damage of RBCs. Blood group compatibility is as follows:

Phenotype	O	A	B	AB
RBC Antigens	Nil	A	B	AB
Serum Antibodies	Anti-A & Anti-B	Anti-B	Anti-A	Nil
Receives From	O	O & A	O & B	O, A, B & AB
Donates To	O, A, B & AB	A & AB	B & AB	AB

Q: Can you describe the Rhesus system?

This is a blood group system, defined by the presence or absence of the Rh-D antigen on the RBC surface. The 2 alleles involved are D & d. Homozygous dd individuals do not have the Rh-D antigen on their RBC surfaces & they are therefore Rh-D negative. Rh-D positive implies the presence of the Rh-D antigen. This antigen is immunologic, so that Rh-D negative individuals, who come into contact with Rh-D positive blood, are very likely to produce anti-Rh-D antibodies. Sensitisation classically occurs during pregnancy or transfusion. This is particularly important when a sensitised Rh-D negative mother, falls pregnant with a Rh-D positive baby. The sensitised mother's anti-RhD IgG antibodies may cross the placenta, causing haemolytic disease of the newborn. Rh-D negative mothers are always given anti-Rh-D during pregnancy.

① O⁺ 40%
② A⁺ 35%

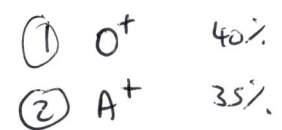

Q: How prevalent are the blood types of the ABO & Rhesus group systems?

% Prevalence	Blood Group System & Blood Group Type			% Prevalence
	ABO	Rh-D	
45	O	+	40
		−	5
40	A	+	35
		−	5
10	B	+	8
		−	2
5	AB	+	3
		−	2

Blood Transfusion & Blood Products

Q: What does group & save mean? What is a cross match?

Terminology	Definition
Group & Save	Prior to a procedure that is unlikely to require blood transfusion, the patient's blood may be tested for common antigens e.g. ABO & Rhesus systems. The sample is stored for approximately 7 days & then discarded. Storage allows rapid emergency cross-matching & generation of allogenic blood units for transfusion, if requested.
Cross Match	Cross matching minimises transfusion reactions due to patient-donor blood type incompatibility. Prior to receiving transfusion, the patient's blood is ABO & Rhesus system typed. Additional antigens are also typed e.g. Duffy, Kell & Kidd. Group compatible erythrocytes from donor blood are mixed with recipient serum. Agglutination will occur if the donor blood is incompatible. A procedure-specific number of allogenic blood units may be requested to be on standby for the patient by 'cross-matching' e.g. elective AAA repair may require 6 units to be cross-matched.

Q: What is autologous blood transfusion?

This is the principle of using the patient's own blood when required for transfusion. This is usually performed in elective procedures where blood loss is predicted. The patient may begin donating blood from 35 days prior to the procedure, until approximately 3 days before surgery. No more than 2 donations per week is advisable & the blood is stored until the patient's surgery. A cell saver may also be used, if appropriate, to achieve autologous blood transfusion intraoperatively *(see later)*.

Q: What are the advantages & disadvantages of autologous blood transfusion?

Advantages	Disadvantages
Conservation of Allogenic Blood Supplies	Unnecessary Blood Transfusion due to Existence of Autologous Supply
Exact Blood Type Minimises Transfusion Reactions	Mislabelling / Accidental Use of Allogenic Blood
Less Risk of Infection Transmission	Infection Contamination Possible when Transfusing
Patient Reassurance by Using Their Own Blood	Processing for Storage is Expensive
Supply is Renewable by Patient's Bone Marrow	Disposal of Unused Units is Common

Q: What is a cell saver & why is it important in surgery?

Also known as an intraoperative cell salvage machine, this collects, washes, filters & transfuses autologous blood intraoperatively. This is advantageous as it reduces the risk of requiring intra- or post-operative allogenic transfusion by improving the tendency towards bloodless surgery. Furthermore, as the blood is continuously processed, the possible volume of transfusion is not limited by the availability of allogenic blood. Use of such a machine may be vital when operating on patients e.g. Jehovah's Witnesses, whose beliefs disallow the transfusion of blood products from another individual. Cell saver use is contraindicated in malignancy & infection.

Q: In transfusion, how is whole blood 'processed' & what products are commonly used?

Commonly transfused whole blood products include RBCs, platelets, FFP & cryoprecipitate. Donor blood may be treated as follows:

Process	Explanation
Screening	Reduces the risk of CMV, HBV, HCV, HIV & syphilis transmission.
Centrifugation	Separates blood into constituent components.
Leucofiltration	Removes lymphocytes, reducing the risk of CMV transmission & non-haemolytic febrile transfusion reactions.
Irradiation	Inactivates donor T-lymphocytes, reducing the risk of graft versus host disease, which is of particular importance in immunodeficient patients.

Q: What factors are important with respect to blood storage?

Temperature & time are vital. These vary, according to the particular product in question, as follows:

Product	Storage Temperature	Storage Time
RBCs	1–6 °C	35 days
Platelets	20-24 °C (constant agitation)	5 days
FFP	-30 °C	1 year
Cryoprecipitate	-30 °C	1 year

Q: What is the relationship between FFP & cryoprecipitate?

FFP is the top layer produced by the centrifugation of whole blood. It may be administered to patients at a dose of 15ml/kg & contains albumin, all clotting factors, complement components, fibrinogen & vWF. Cryoprecipitate may be thought of as a sub-component of FFP as it contains factor VIII, factor XIII, fibrinogen & vWF. FFP & cryoprecipitate are both devoid of RBCs, leucocytes & platelets.

Blood Transfusion Reactions & Substitute Blood Products

Q: How would you classify transfusion reactions?

These may be classified as immune, due to massive transfusion & general reactions as follows:

Classification	Example
IMMUNE	**Acute Haemolytic Reaction:** ABO incompatibility may result in severe haemolysis, loin pain, pyrexia, renal failure & shock over 1–10 minutes. This is most commonly caused by clerical error.
	Non-Haemolytic Febrile Transfusion Reaction: Donor leucocytes release pyrogens that may result in a slow developing & mild pyrexia over 1–6 hours.
	Delayed Haemolytic Reaction: Previous recipient sensitisation to certain RBC antigens may result in a delayed immune response & haemolysis over 1–4 weeks.
	Graft Versus Host Disease: Donor immune competent T-cells attack recipient tissues that may result in abdominal pain, fever, profuse diarrhoea, rash & vomiting over 4–30 days. It is fatal in approximately 80–90% of cases.
	Transfusion Related Acute Lung Injury: Donor plasma anti-HLA & anti-HNA antibodies, cause granulocytes to release cytokines & vasoactive substances. This may result in non-cardiac pulmonary oedema over 10 minutes to several hours.
	Anaphylaxis: Donor plasma protein allergens, particularly in patients with IgA deficiency, may precipitate a type 1 hypersensitivity reaction with dizziness, urticaria, oedema, bronchospasm, tachycardia & shock over 1–10 minutes.
MASSIVE TRANSFUSION	Citrate Toxicity
	Coagulopathy
	Hyperkalaemia, Hypocalcaemia (from citrate binding) & Fe^{2+} Overload
	Thrombocytopaenia
	Metabolic Acidosis
	Fluid Overload & Congestive Cardiac Failure
GENERAL	DIC
	Infection
	Thrombophlebitis

Q: Do you know of any blood transfusion substitutes?

These may be classified as fluids or oxygen-carrying products as follows:

Fluids	Oxygen-Carrying Products
Colloid:	Hemopure™
Gelofusin	Oxygent™
Crystalloid:	Perftec™
Hartman's Solution	Perftoran™
Normal Saline	PolyHeme™

Oedema & Lymphoedema

Q: What is oedema, lymphoedema, exudate & transudate?

Terminology	Definition
Oedema	Generalised or localised collection of extracellular fluid. This may be an exudate or transudate.
Exudate	This occurs across an intact capillary endothelium & is defined by a protein content >30g/l.
Transudate	This occurs across an intact capillary endothelium & is defined by a protein content <30g/l.
Lymphoedema	Oedema due to obstruction of lymphatic drainage. This may be primary or secondary.

Q: What forces govern the net filtration across a capillary?

Starling's Law of the Capillaries describes net fluid filtration across a capillary & is as follows:

Net Filtration = (Capillary – Interstitial Hydrostatic Pressure) – (Capillary – Interstitial Oncotic Pressure) & Lymph Drainage

It is dependent on a balance between the capillary & interstitial, hydrostatic & oncotic pressures. Lymphatic drainage is also involved, draining excess fluid filtered from the capillary (Fig 5.4).

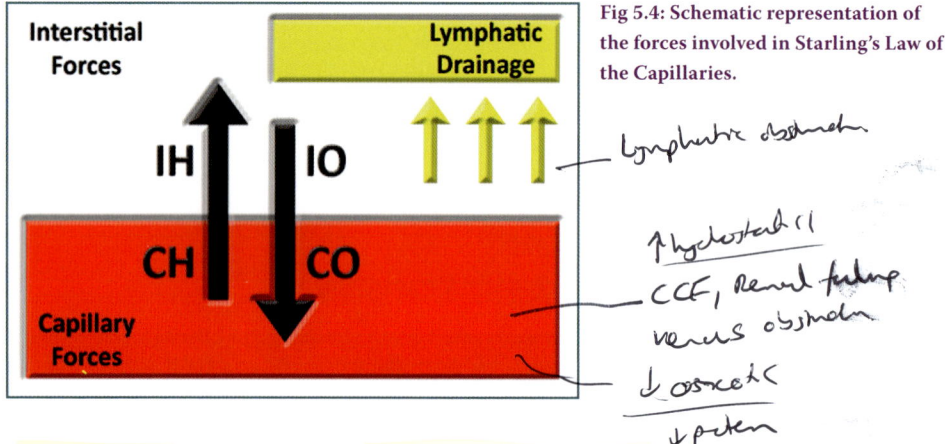

Fig 5.4: Schematic representation of the forces involved in Starling's Law of the Capillaries.

- Lymphatic obstruction
- ↑ Hydrostatic
  - CCF, Renal failure
  - venous obstruction
- ↓ oncotic
  - ↓ protein

Fluid is pushed out of the capillaries by the higher capillary hydrostatic pressure (CH), relative to the lower interstitial hydrostatic pressure (IH).

Fluid is retained in the capillaries by the higher capillary oncotic pressure (CO), relative to the lower interstitial oncotic pressure (IO).

Lymphatics drain excess interstitial fluid.

Q: What are the causes of oedema?

These may be classified by their relationship to Starling's Law of the capillaries *(see previous question)* & other causes as follow:

Classification	Example
Increased Capillary Hydrostatic Pressure	Congestive Cardiac Failure, Intravascular Fluid Retention e.g. Renal Failure & Venous Obstruction e.g. Venous Thrombosis
Decreased Capillary Oncotic Pressure	Hypoproteinaemia e.g. Malnutrition, Liver Failure & Nephrotic Syndrome
Capillary Leakage	Allergy & Inflammation
Lymphatic Drainage Obstruction*	PRIMARY: Congenital e.g. Milroy's Disease SECONDARY: Infection e.g. Filiariasis, Radiotherapy, Surgery & Tumour
Other	**Drugs** e.g. Nifedipine, NSAIDs & Steroids **Gravitational** e.g. Standing Long Periods **Physiological** e.g. Menstrual Cycle

*Note: This is Lymphoedema

Q: What are the treatment options for lymphoedema?

Treatment modalities may be classified as conservative, medical & surgical as follows:

Treatment	Examples
Conservative	Compression Stockings, Leg Elevation, Massage & Manual Lymphatic Drainage
Medical	Antibiotics (as required)
Surgical	EXCISIONAL: Charles Procedure: *circumferential excision & SSG.* Homan's Procedure: *raise skin flaps, debulk subcutaneous tissue & close flaps.* Liposuction. PHYSIOLOGICAL: Lymphovenous Anastomosis

IMMUNOLOGY

Hypersensitivity, Cytokines & Mediators

Q: What is a hypersensitivity reaction?

This is a negative event, produced by a competent immune system, usually requiring pre-sensitisation. Reactions may be classified according to type as follows:

Type	Example	Mediators
I (Allergic)	Anaphylaxis Asthma	IgE
II (Cytotoxic)	Autoimmune Haemolytic Anaemia Goodpasture's Syndrome	IgG, IgM Complement
III (Immune Complex)	Serum Sickness SLE	IgG Complement
IV (Cell Mediated)	Chronic Transplant Rejection Crohn's Disease TB	T-Cells

Q: What pathophysiological processes occur in type I hypersensitivity conditions such as asthma?

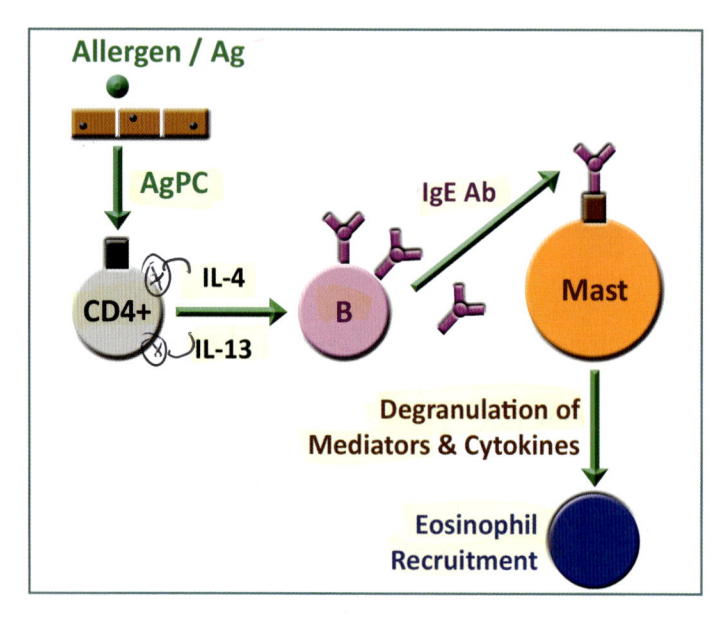

Fig 5.5: Schematic representation outlining the events in type I hypersensitivity reactions.

Allergen / Ag & AgPC

CD4+ Helper T-Lymphocytes release IL-4 & IL-13

B Cells release IgE Ab

Mast Cells Degranulate Mediators & Cytokines after Binding IgE Ab

Eosinophil Recruitment Occurs

- Allergens (Ag) are inhaled (or ingested).
- These allergens / antigens are recognised by dendritic antigen presenting cells.
- CD4+ T-helper cells are targeted by antigen presenting cells.
- T-helper cells release IL-4 & IL-13.
- B-cells produce IgE antibodies (Ab) that are antigen-specific, in response to IL-4 & IL-13 release.
- IgE antibodies bind to mast cells & basophils which degranulate & release mediators & cytokines.
- Mediators & cytokines result in symptoms & recruitment of cells e.g. IL-5 & eosinophils.

Q: What mediators & cytokines do you know of & what are their actions?

	Examples	Effects
MEDIATORS	Bradykinin	Hypotension, Increased Vascular Permeability, Pain, Smooth Muscle Spasm & Vasodilation. **Note:** Kininogenase, released by mast cells, acts on plasma kinins & bradykinin is produced.
	Histamine	Gastric Acid Secretion, Increased Vascular Permeability, Mucus Production, Pruritis, Smooth Muscle Spasm & Vasodilation.
	Leukotrienes	**B4:** Activation & Chemotaxis of Neutrophils. **C4, D4 & E4:** Bronchoconstriction & Increased Vascular Permeability. **Note:** These are products of the lipoxygenase pathway.
	Prostaglandins	**D2:** Bronchoconstriction, Neutrophil Chemotaxis, Platelet Aggregation Inhibition & Peripheral Vasodilation. **F2:** Bronchoconstriction & Coronary Vasoconstriction. **Note:** These are products of the cyclo-oxygenase pathway.
	TXA2	Bronchoconstriction, Platelet Aggregation & Vasoconstriction. **Note:** This is a product of the cyclo-oxygenase pathway.
	PAF	Bronchoconstriction, Chemotaxis & Degranulation of Eosinophils & Neutrophils, & Increased Vascular Permeability. **Note:** This is synthesised by membrane phospholipids.
CYTOKINES	IL-4	CD4+ T-helper Cell Proliferation & B-cell IgE Synthesis.
	IL-5	Basophil Histamine & Leukotriene Release. B-cell proliferation & Ig production. Eosinophil Activation & Chemotaxis.
	IL-6	Mucus Production.
	IL-13	CD4+ T-helper Cell Proliferation.
	TNFα	Neutrophil Activation.

Complement Cascade

Q: What is the complement cascade?

This is part of the innate immune system & is not adaptable, although it may be activated by elements of the adaptive immune system. It is primarily involved in the clearance of pathogens & is comprised of a complex network of cytokines, proteases & proteins. There are 3 pathways that converge on a final common pathway, at the stage of C3 involvement, primarily involved in the clearance of pathogens. The end point of the final common pathway produces the MAC. This inserts into & creates a channel within the target cell membrane. This channel allows for osmotic lysis of the target cell.

membrane attack complex.

Q: Can you draw & discuss the 4 pathways involved in the complement cascade?

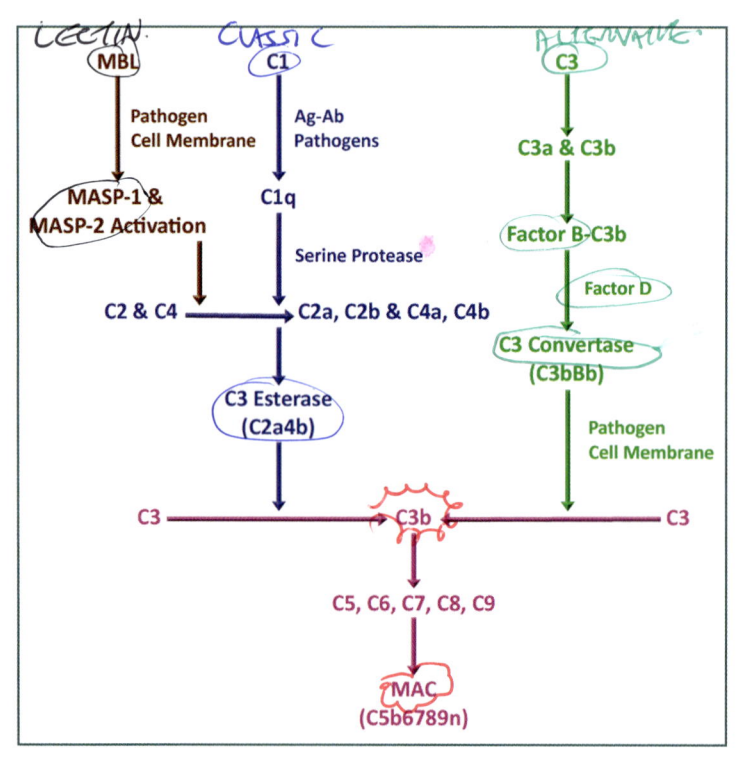

Fig 5.6: Simplified diagram of the complement cascade.

Lectin Pathway
Classic Pathway
Alternative Pathway
Final Common Pathway

LECTIN
- MBL
- Pathogen Cell Membrane
- MASP-1 & MASP-2 Activation
- C2 & C4 → C2a, C2b & C4a, C4b
- C3 Esterase (C2a4b)
- C3 → C3b
- C5, C6, C7, C8, C9
- MAC (C5b6789n)

CLASSIC
- C1
- Ag-Ab Pathogens
- C1q
- Serine Protease

ALTERNATIVE
- C3
- C3a & C3b
- Factor B C3b
- Factor D
- C3 Convertase (C3bBb)
- Pathogen Cell Membrane
- C3

Pathway	Notes
Classic	C1 complex is activated due to binding of C1q with antigen-antibody complexes or directly with bacteria. C1q then undergoes conformational change & activates serine protease enzymes. A set of cleavage reactions ensue, resulting in the production of C2a & C4b fragments, due to cleavage of C2 & C4. C2a & C4b form the C2aC4b complex, also known as C3 esterase, that cleaves C3.
Alternative	Hydrolysis of C3, produces C3a & C3b. Factor B binds C3b. In the presence of Factor D, further cleavage reactions ensue, resulting in C3bBb complex, also known as C3 convertase, formation. This complex cleaves C3 after attaching to pathogen cell membranes. This pathway is therefore independent of antigen-antibody (Ag-Ab) complex formation.
Lectin	Mannose-binding lectin is a serum protein & opsonin that binds to the pathogen cell membrane. This activates mannose-binding lectin associated serine proteases MASP-1 & MASP-2 which cleave C2 & C4, feeding into the classic pathway. This pathway is therefore independent of antigen-antibody complex formation.
Final Common Pathway	This is the point of convergence of the above 3 pathways at the point of C3 cleavage. Further cleavage reactions ensue which involve C5, C6, C7, C8 & C9, resulting in production of C5b6789n, also termed the MAC. MAC formation is crucial, as it inserts as a channel into the pathogen cell membrane, resulting in osmotic lysis. In addition, chemotaxis & inflammation occur.

Q: Why is the complement cascade important?

The complement cascade is part of the innate immune system. It is important for the following reasons:

- Lysis of cells & pathogens.
- Opsonisation of pathogens.
- Promotion of the inflammatory response.
- Deficiency increases infection & sepsis risk.
- Deficiency is associated with autoimmune disorders e.g. SLE.
- Overactivation e.g. C1q esterase deficiency is associated with angioedema.

Immunity & Immunoglobulins

Q: What are immunoglobulins & what structure do they adopt?

Immunoglobulins are gamma globulin proteins that are present in serum & body secretions. They are secreted by plasma cells, also known as B-lymphocytes, as part of the immune system response to pathogens. Their structure is outlined below (Fig 5.7):

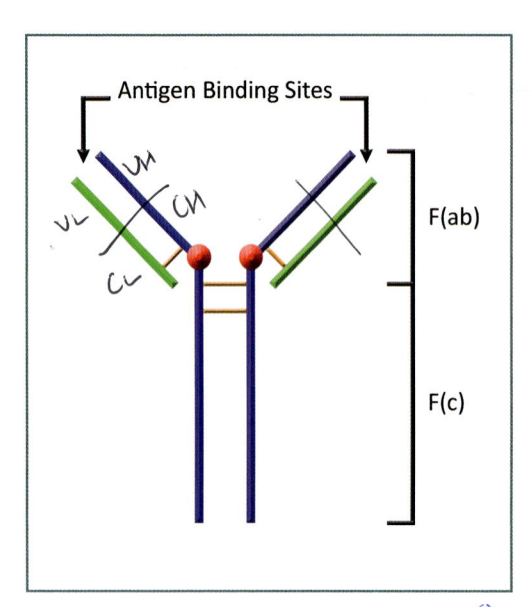

Fig 5.7: Simplified diagram of immunoglobulin structure.

Light Chain

Heavy Chain

Hinge Region

Disulphide Bonds

F(ab): The fragment antigen binding region is composed of 1 constant & 1 variable domain from both heavy & light chains. Ag-binding sites are located here.

F(c): The fragment crystallisable region interacts with cell surface Fc receptors & various complement cascade proteins, thus allowing immune system activation.

Q: What is immunodeficiency?

This refers to the body's inability to fight disease, either partially or completely, due to a problem with the immune system. Conditions that suppress the immune system may be classified as primary or secondary as follows:

Primary (rare)	Secondary
Complement Deficiency	Chemotherapy, Immunosuppressants & Steroids
DiGeorge Syndrome	DM
G6PD Deficiency	DMARDS, Penicillamine & Phenytoin
Hypogammaglobulinaemia	HIV & AIDS
Severe Combined Immunodeficiency	Malignancy e.g. Leukaemia, Lymphoma & Myeloma

Q: What do you understand by the term immunity?

Immunity implies resistance of an individual, to infection by pathogens. It may be classified as cell-mediated or humoral as follows:

Classification	Notes
Cell-Mediated	This does not involve antibodies or the complement cascade. It is protective by activating cytotoxic (CD8) T-lymphocytes, macrophages & natural killer cells. It also stimulates cells that release cytokines & mediators, hence it is involved in the adaptive & innate immune response.
Humoral	This is defined by antibody release & associated events such as complement cascade activation, cytokine production, opsonisation & phagocytosis.

Q: What classes of antibodies do you know of?

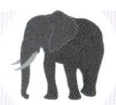

Memory: **My Good Antibodies Eat Disease.**

Ab Class	Notes
IgM	The 1st Ab released by the humoral response to pathogenic insult. It binds & agglutinates micro-organisms whilst sufficient quantities of IgG are being synthesised.
IgG	This provides the majority of humoral immunity after pathogenic insult & is released after IgM. It is the only Ab capable of crossing the placenta & it may also enter into extravascular spaces. The F(c) portion binds to C1q & phagocytic cell receptors.
IgA	The primary Ab present in body secretions e.g. breast milk, saliva, sweat, tears & urine. It is protective against colonisation by pathogens.
IgE	Binds to mast cells & basophils to promote degranulation of cytokines & mediators e.g. Type I hypersensitivity reactions.
IgD	This is present on the surface of B-lymphocytes & binds Ag. This results in B-lymphocyte activation for participation in the humoral response.

Transplantation

Q: What types of transplant do you know of?

Transplant Type	Definition
Autograft	An organ or tissue transplanted from one area of the body to another, on the same individual e.g. skin grafting or long saphenous vein harvesting for CABG.
Allograft	An organ or tissue transplanted between genetically non-identical individuals.
Isograft	An organ or tissue transplanted between genetically identical individuals.
Xenograft	An organ or tissue transplanted from a different species e.g. porcine heart valves.

Note: Generally, autografts & isografts are more likely to take successfully than allografts & xenografts.

Q: What drugs may be used in transplantation & rejection?

These may be classified as steroids, immunosuppressants & antibody preparations as follows:

Steroids	Immunosuppressants	Antibody Preparations
Hydrocortisone	Azathioprine	Anti-Lymphocyte Globulin
Prednisolone	Cyclosporin	Basiliximab
	Mycophenolate Mofetil	
	Tacrolimus	

Q: What side effects are associated with non-steroidal immunosuppressant use in transplantation?

Side effects may vary considerably between drugs & patients. Many symptoms e.g. rash, headache, diarrhoea, nausea & vomiting may be common. Certain key side effects are associated with more commonly used drugs:

Drug	Side-Effects
Azathioprine	Alopecia, cholestasis, hepatitis & myelosuppression.
Cyclosporin	Gingival hyperplasia, hyperkalaemia & hypomagnesaemia & nephrotoxicity*.
Tacrolimus	Alopecia, hirsutism, nephrotoxicity* & neurotoxicity.

*Note: Mycophenolate mofetil is used, often in triple therapy combination with steroids & azathioprine, to reduce the risk of nephrotoxicity in renal transplant patients.

Q: What is transplant rejection?

This refers to when a donor organ or tissue is not accepted by the recipient's body. Rejection may be classified as hyperacute, acute & chronic as follows:

Classification	Time Frame	Notes
Hyperacute	Minutes–Hours	Due to circulating preformed Ab in the recipient, against the donor organ or tissue. It is a complement system mediated process which results in small vessel microthrombosis & subsequent rejection of the organ or tissue. Lymphocytotoxic cross matching minimises the risk of occurrence.
Acute	Weeks	Recipient T-cell mediated destruction of the donor organ or tissue occurs. The donor organ or tissue may be tender & swollen & biopsy may reveal a mononuclear cell infiltrate. There may be accompanying organ-specific signs e.g. hypertension & decreasing urine output in the case of renal transplantation. HLA typing minimises the risk of occurrence.
Chronic	Months–Years	May be of unknown aetiology, or may occur after recurrent acute rejection episodes. Biopsy of the affected organ or tissue may reveal arteriosclerosis, collagen deposition or scarring. Treatment often has limited effect.

INFLAMMATION

Acute Inflammation

Q: What are the 5 features of acute inflammation?

Traditional Terminology (original description by Celsus)	Signs & Symptoms
Rubor	Red
Calor	Hot
Dolor	Painful
Tumor	Swollen
Functio Laesa (added by Virchow)	Loss of Function

Q: What are the processes of acute inflammation?

- Vasoconstriction
- Vasodilation & increased vascular permeability
- Leucocyte margination & emigration
- Phagocytosis.

Q: What is leucocyte margination & emigration?

Leucocytes flow in the axial (central) zone of the blood stream. Margination refers to their movement into the outer (plasmatic) zone. Emigration refers to their adherence (pavementing), then active amoeboid migration across the endothelium of veins & venules. Neutrophils respond prior to monocytes.

Q: What might the final result of an acute inflammatory episode be?

- Resolution
- Suppuration
- Repair & Organisation
- Fibrosis
- Chronic Inflammation (progression from acute inflammation)
- Location & disease specific e.g. IBD & RA.

Chronic Inflammation

Q: What are the causes of chronic inflammation?

Cause	Example / Description
Acute Inflammation	Osteomyelitis. May progress from acute to chronic.
Chronic Infection	TB, Leprosy & Syphilis. Mycobacteria are low toxicity intracellular microbes that evoke an immunological response & result in granulomatous inflammation.
Toxic Materials	Asbestos & Silica. Due to prolonged exposure.
Autoimmune	RA.

Q: What is a granuloma?

A collection of modified macrophages, resembling epithelial cells, with or without a surrounding rim of lymphocytes. The following diseases may be characterised by the presence of granuloma; Histoplasmosis, Leprosy, Sarcoid & TB.

Q: What cellular processes occur during chronic inflammation?

- Immune system activation of T-lymphocytes produces lymphokines.
- Lymphokines e.g. IFNγ, activate Macrophages.
- Activated macrophages release growth factors e.g. IL-1, IL-6 & TNFα, & monokines to stimulate B-cells & CD4 T-helper cells.
- Fibroblast proliferation occurs.
- Neovascularisation occurs.
- Tissue destruction occurs due to protease & oxygen FR release.

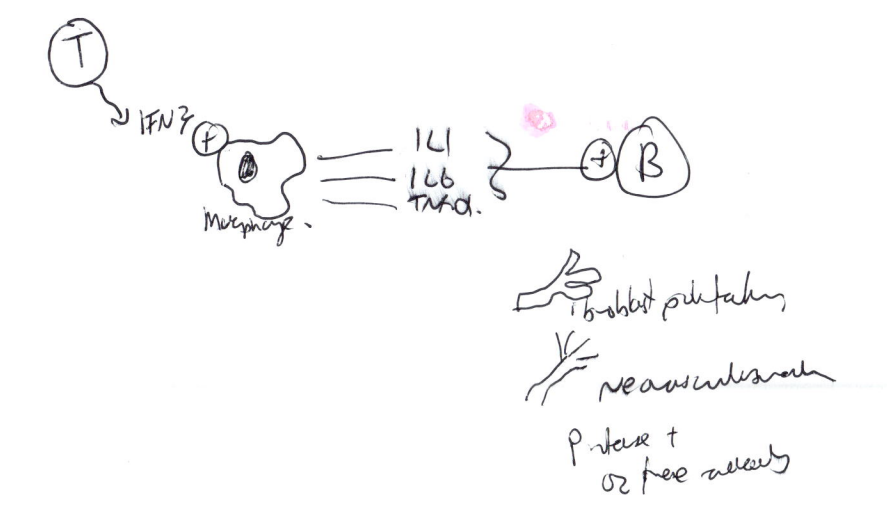

Cyst, Abscess, Pus & Other Common Phenomena

Q: What is a cyst, pseudocyst, abscess, sinus & fistula?

Definition	Explanation
Cyst	An abnormal, membrane-lined sac composed of epithelial cells, containing fluid.
Pseudocyst	An abnormal collection of fluid, surrounded by granulation or fibrous tissue & without a true membrane composed of epithelial cells e.g. Pancreatic Pseudocyst & Amoebic Liver Cyst.
Abscess	A localised or loculated collection of pus, surrounded by granulation tissue. Polymorphs (neutrophils & macrophages), release enzymes which split large molecules into small molecules. The result is an increase in osmotic pressure & subsequent fluid collection within the abscess. This collection will therefore either discharge via the path of least resistance or resolve spontaneously.
Sinus	A blind ending tract in communication with an epithelial surface. May be normal e.g. Cardiac Sinus, or abnormal e.g. Osteomyelitis & Pilonidal Sinus.
Fistula	An abnormal communication between 2 epithelial surfaces. Anal fistula is the most common presenting fistula, however an ear piercing is the most prevalent overall!

Q: How would you classify cysts?

Classification	Example
Idiopathic	Simple Cyst
Congenital	Branchial Cyst, Cystic Hygroma, Dermoid Cyst & Thyroglossal Cyst
Degenerative	Bone Cyst (in OA), Cerebral Cyst (post infarction)
Hyperplastic	Breast Cyst & Endometrium Cyst
Implantational	Epidermal Cyst & Dermal Cyst
Infective	Amoebic Cyst (*Entamoeba histolytica*) & Hydatid Cyst (*Echinococcus granulosus*)
Neoplastic	Ovarian Cyst & Pancreatic Cyst
Obstructive	Epididymal Cyst & Meibomian Cyst

Q: What is a dermoid cyst?

This is a cystic teratoma, containing mature skin, hair follicles & sebaceous glands that become trapped during embryological development; further contained structures may include bone & teeth. Dermoid cysts are consequently present at birth, however they are often noticed during childhood, or in young adults, due to their slow growing nature. Anatomical sites include Forehead, Neck, Midline, Ovary, Spinal Cord, Brain & Nasal Sinus.

Q: What is a sebaceous cyst?

This is a closed cyst below the skin surface, filled with sebum & with a central punctum. Sebum is produced by the sebaceous glands of hair follicles. The cyst contents may become semi-solid, caseous & foul smelling. Causes may be hereditary e.g. Gardner's Syndrome, or associated with Blocked Sebaceous Glands & High Testosterone levels.

Q: What is pus composed of?

Pus has fluid & solid components:

Fluid	Solid
An Exudate of:	*Live & Dead:*
• Clotting Factors	• Bacteria
• Complement Components	• Polymorphs (Neutrophils & Macrophages)
• Cytokines	*With:*
• H_2O	• Dead Human Cells
• Immunoglobulins	• Fibrin Meshwork

Wound Healing

Q: What are the stages of wound healing?

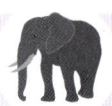

Memory: **C**utting (1) **I**s (2) **P**leasingly (3) **R**epetitive (4).

COAGULATIVE → INFLAMMATORY → PROLIFERATIVE → REMODELLING

Stage:	1. Coagulative	2. Inflammatory	3. Proliferative / Fibroblastic	4. Remodelling / Maturation
Timing:	Immediate	Immediate – 3 days	3 days – 3 weeks	3 weeks – 2 years
Characteristics:	**Vasoconstriction** (Platelets secrete ADP, Serotonin & TXA2)	**Vasodilation**	**Granulation** (Fibroblasts secrete GAGS, Collagen & Elastin Fibres. New Capillaries are Formed)	**Reorganisation** (Haphazardly laid collagen is restructured)
	↓	↓	↓	↓
	Platelet Adhesion & Activation (Damaged endothelial cells release vWF. Platelets adhere & become activated)	**Exudation** (Polymorphonuclear & Mononuclear Lymphocytes. Cytokines e.g. VEGF, PDGF & TGFβ)	**Contraction** (Wound edges pull together)	**Regression** (Initially laid capillaries involute)
	↓	↓	↓	↓
	Fibrin Clot (Clotting Cascade)	**Phagocytosis** (Macrophages)	**Epithelialisation** (Epithelial cell migration)	**Scar Tissue** (80% of original tissue strength)

Q: What are the roles of macrophages in wound healing?

Macrophages are essential to wound healing as they carry out the following:
- Tissue debridement
- Phagocytosis & destruction of micro-organisms
- Release of growth factors e.g. IL-1, PDGF, TGFβ.

MICROBIOLOGY

Surgical Site & Wound Infections

Q: What are surgical site infections?

Surgical site infections are those that affect the surgical scar or anatomical structures encountered during surgery. They occur in approximately 5% of surgical procedures & may be classified as follows:

Classification	Areas Affected
Superficial Incisional	Skin & Subcutaneous Tissues
Deep Incisional	Deeper Tissues e.g. Fascia & Muscle
Organ / Space	Organs & Spaces (manipulated during the operation outside of the initial incision)

Q: What organisms are involved in wound colonisation & surgical site infections?

Most wounds are colonised by micro-organisms. Colonised wounds may be associated with exudate, malodour & surrounding skin erythema. If the pathogen is able to overcome immune defence mechanisms, infection may ensue. In addition to the signs of colonisation, infected wounds may be associated with cellulitis & purulent exudate. Common micro-organisms involved in surgical site infections include:

Memory: Surgical Events Ended Prematurely And the Bar Ended Kevin's Symptoms.

Staphylococcus

Enterococcus

Escherichia coli

Pseudomonas

Acinetobacter

Bacillus

Enterobacter

Klebsiella

Streptococcus.

Q: What factors increase the risk of wound infection?

Risks may be classified as operative, patient & wound factors:

Operative Factors	Patient Factors	Wound Factors
Contamination	Age	Foreign Material
Inappropriate Antibiotic Prophylaxis	Comorbidity e.g. Carcinoma & Cardiac Failure	Haematoma
Operative Time	Steroids & Immunosuppressants (immunosuppression e.g. DM, HIV)	Inadequate Debridement of Dead Tissue
Poor Surgical Technique		Poor Skin Preparation
Poor Ventilation	Malnutrition	Pre-Existing Infection
Suboptimal Thermoregulation	Obesity	

Pneumonia

Q: What are the risk factors for the development of pneumonia?

Risk Factor	Notes
Age	Very Young & Very Old Patients
Drugs	Intravenous Drug Use (*Staphylococcus aureus*)
Immunosuppression	DM, HIV Immunosuppressants & Steroids
Lifestyle	Alcohol & Smoking
Neurological	CVA & PD
Respiratory Disease	Asthma, Bronchiectasis, COPD & Cystic Fibrosis
Other	Immobility & Surgery e.g. Cardiothoracic & Gastrointestinal

Q: How does neurological disease increase the risk of developing pneumonia?

Increased risk of pneumonia in neurological disease occurs either due to a lack of innervation to the respiratory musculature or due to impaired consciousness & control of swallowing. In the case of decreased innervation, respiration is insufficient to clear pathogens. In the case of impaired consciousness & control of swallowing, aspiration pneumonia is more likely.

Q: What bacterial micro-organisms cause pneumonia?

Bacterial pneumonia may be classified as community acquired, hospital acquired & atypical. Atypical pneumonia implies a less severe & gradual onset respiratory presentation, often consisting of a dry cough only. Extrapulmonary symptoms may be more troublesome to the patient e.g. diarrhoea, fatigue, headache, myalgia, nausea, sore throat & vomiting.

Community Acquired	Hospital Acquired	Atypical
Streptococcus pneumoniae (70%)	Pseudomonas	Mycoplasma
Haemophilus influenzae*	Klebsiella	Legionella
Chlamydia	Staphylococcus	Chlamydia
Legionella	Escherichia coli	
Mycoplasma		

*Note: *Haemophilus* is traditionally more common in children, however, HiB vaccination is resulting in a decreasing prevalence.

Q: Aside from bacteria, what other micro-organisms cause pneumonia?

Parasites, fungi & viruses may all cause pneumonia. HSV affects newborns & CMV classically affects immunosuppressed patients.

Parasites	Fungi	Viruses
Toxoplasma	Histoplasma	Adenovirus
Strongyloides	Cryptococcus	Influenza
	Pneumocystis	RSV
		HSV (newborns)
		CMV (immunosuppressed)

Q: What are the complications of pneumonia?

These may be classified as pulmonary or extra-pulmonary as follows:

Pulmonary	Extrapulmonary
Empyema	*General:*
Lung Abscess	DVT (dehydration & immobility)
Pleural Effusion	Post-Streptococcus GN
Pneumothorax	*Due to Septicaemia:*
Post-Infective Bronchiectasis	Cerebral Abscess
	Endocarditis
	Meningitis
	Septic Arthritis

Urinary Tract Infection

Q: What are the risk factors for developing a UTI?

Risk Factor	Notes
Catheters	Provide an entry point for micro-organisms from the outside world into the urinary tract. Indwelling catheters classically increase the risk of nosocomial infections.
Constituents	Abnormal urine constituents may provide better bacterial growth media e.g. glucose in DM.
Congenital	Anatomical abnormality e.g. Posterior Urethral Valves & Vesico-Ureteric Reflux.
Female Sex	Due to close anatomical relationship between anus & urethra.
Immunosuppression	DM, HIV Immunosuppressants & Steroids.
Pregnancy	Due to urinary tract dilation & flow stagnation.
Urinary Stasis	Due to e.g. BPH, Calculus, Tumour & Neurogenic Causes.

Q: What micro-organisms cause UTI?

90% of UTIs in the developed world are due to *Escherichia coli*, a normal constituent of gut bacterial flora. Bacterial STIs, parasites, fungi & rarely viruses, may also cause UTI. These micro-organisms may be classified as follows:

Bacteria – General	Bacteria – STI	Parasites	Fungi
Escherichia coli (90%)	Chlamydia	Wuchereria bancrofti (Filariasis)	Candida
Proteus	Gonorrhoea		**Viruses**
Staphylococcus		Schistosoma mansoni (Schistosomiasis)	Adenovirus
Klebsiella			HSV
Pseudomonas		Trichomonas vaginalis. (Trichomoniasis)	
TB			

Q: What is the pathogenesis of UTI? What are the clinical features & how are they classified?

Escherichia coli possesses adhesins, cytolysins, P-fimbriae & toxins that help it adhere to the urothelium & cause ascending infection. The UTI may therefore spread from the urethra, to the bladder, ureters & to the kidneys. Direct spread, such as via a vesico-colic fistula, haematogenous & lymphatic spread is also possible. Clinical features may be classified according to the site of involvement as follows:

Site of UTI	Clinical Features
Urethra	Cloudy Urine, Dysuria (like passing razorblades), Frequency, Malodour & Urgency.
Bladder	Sensation of Incomplete Emptying & Suprapubic Pain.
Kidney / Pyelonephritis	Fever, Loin Pain, Rigors & Vomiting. Children with congenital anatomical abnormalities e.g. Vesico-Ureteric Reflux, may suffer with recurrent acute attacks. These recurrent attacks may lead to chronic pyelonephritis & subsequent chronic renal failure in later life. As children often only present with e.g. Failure to Thrive, Fever, Lethargy or Diarrhoea & Vomiting, full investigation of the urinary tract is essential when faced with any of these presentations.

Q: What are the key points in relation to MSU collection & processing?

MSU collection occurs in the middle of urination to collect micro-organisms that truly reside within the bladder. For example, urine collected at the start of the stream may contain perineum or urethral micro-organisms. The specimen is labelled & sent for microscopy, micro-organism culture & antibiotic sensitivity. The following results are useful to know with respect to MSU microscopy & culture:

MSU Analysis Modality	Result	Interpretation
Microscopy	>10 WBCs / ml	Pyuria
Culture	>10^5 c.f.u. / ml	Pyuria has an Infective Cause

Q: What are the complications of UTI?

- Ascending Infection
- Septicaemia
- Calculi Formation e.g. Proteus & Staghorn Calculi
- Recurrence
- Chronicity
- Renal Scarring.

Endotoxin & Exotoxin

Q: Bacteria may secrete endotoxins or exotoxins. What are the differences between these?

Endotoxins & exotoxins may have specific or general effects on the body. They differ (generally) as follows:

Property	Endotoxin	Exotoxin
Released by	Gram Negative Organisms	Gram Positive Organisms
Constitution	Lipopolysaccharide from Outer Cell Membrane	Secreted Protein
Immunogenic	No	Yes
Thermo-Stability	Heat Stable	Heat Labile
Effects on Body	Generalised	Specific
Pyrogenic	Yes	Occasionally

Q: How may endotoxins result in generalised body effects?

Endotoxin effects may be classified as those that result in activation, degradation & formation of the following:

Activation	Degradation	Formation
Clotting Cascade	Fibrin	Cytokines
Complement Cascade		Leukotrienes
		NO
		PAF
		Prostaglandins

Q: How may exotoxins result in specific effects on the body?

Exotoxin effects may be classified as those with cell surface action, intracellular action & those that result in membrane damage as follows:

Action	Exotoxins	Example Bacteria
Cell Surface	Superantigen	Staphylococcus aureus & Streptococcus pyogenes
	Enterotoxin	Escherichia coli
Intracellular	AB	Bordatella pertussis, Shigella dysenteriae & Vibrio cholerae
	Injected	Yersinia enterolitica
Membrane Damage	Channel-Forming	Staphylococcus aureus
	Enzymatic	Clostridium perfringens exotoxin has phospholipase activity.

Q: What diseases or effects on the body are due to endotoxin & exotoxin release?

Endotoxin	Exotoxin
DIC	Botulism
Hypotension	Cholera
Pyrexia	Diphtheria
Septic Shock	Food Poisoning
Multiple Organ Failure	Gas Gangrene
	Tetanus
	Toxic Shock Syndrome

Commensal Bacteria

Q: What are commensal bacteria? Can you give some examples?

Commensal bacteria are those that live on, or in a host to their own benefit, but without detriment to the host itself. Examples can be given according to their expected location within or on the body as follows:

Location	Examples
Skin	Staphylococcus epidermidis, Corynebacteria, Mycobacteria & Propionibacteria
Oral Cavity	Staphylococcus, Streptococcus, Lactobacillus & Neisseria
Upper Respiratory	Staphylococcus epidermidis, Streptococcus pneumonia, & Neisseria
Gastrointestinal	Bacteroides, Enterococcus & Lactobacillus
Urethra	Staphylococcus, Streptococcus & Diphtheroids
Vagina	Lactobacillus

Nosocomial Infection

Q: What is a nosocomial infection? What increases the risk of contracting a nosocomial infection?

This is a hospital acquired infection that has been contracted after admission. Factors that increase the risk of contraction may be classified as iatrogenic, institutional & patient factors as follows:

Iatrogenic	Institutional	Patient
Antibiotic Misuse	Air-Conditioning Contamination	Co-morbidity
Contaminated Equipment	Close Proximity Beds	Immobility
Indwelling Urinary Catheters	ICU Admission	Immunocompromise
Intravascular Catheters	Lack of Isolation Bays	Length of Stay
Intubation & Ventilation	Large Open Wards	Nutrition
Poor Hand Washing by Staff	Low Staff to Patient Ratio	Unkempt

Immunisation & Vaccination

Q: What is your understanding of the concept of immunisation?

The term 'immunisation' is commonly reserved for the process by which individuals are made resistant to particular infections. This is achieved either actively by vaccination, or passively by Ig administration. This results in immunity, without the need for exposure to natural infection. The concept behind immunisation is disease containment, disease eradication e.g. smallpox, or occupationally-protective e.g. HBV & healthcare workers.

Q: What types of vaccine do you know of?

Vaccines may be derived from bacteria, viruses or their components. They are either antigenic, inactivated or live-attenuated. Antigenic & inactivated vaccines have no ability to replicate & therefore are usually safe in immunocompromised or pregnant individuals. Live-attenuated vaccines have low pathogenicity & therefore should be avoided in immunocompromised or pregnant individuals. See below:

Immunisation	Type	Examples
ACTIVE	Antigenic Vaccine	Streptococcus pneumoniae
	Inactivated Vaccine	Bordetella pertussis
	Live-Attenuated Vaccine	Measles, Mumps, Rubella & Polio Viruses MMR/POLIO
	Toxoid Vaccine	Corynebacteriam diphtheriae & Clostridium tetani
PASSIVE	Immunoglobulin	HBV, VZV & Tick-Borne Encephalitis Ig

NEOPLASIA

Cell Cycle

Q: Can you draw & label the cell cycle, describing each phase?

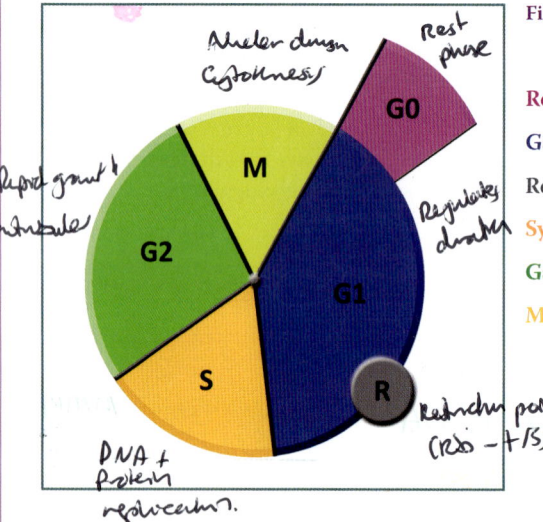

Fig 5.8: Schematic representation of the cell cycle.

- Resting Phase
- Gap 1 Phase
- Restriction Point
- Synthesis Phase
- Gap 2 Phase
- Mitosis Phase

Key	Description
G0	Resting phase, prior to re-entering the cell cycle.
G1	Gap 1 phase. The most important phase for regulating the duration of the cell cycle.
R	Restriction point. The Rb gene is a tumour suppressor gene, the product of which acts as a rate limiting checkpoint for the G1 phase.
S	Synthesis phase. DNA replicated & proteins synthesised.
G2	Gap 2 phase. Period of rapid growth, with microtubules forming spindles in preparation for mitosis. A second checkpoint allows for progression to mitosis.
M	Mitosis phase. Nucleus genetic material is separated equally, giving rise to two equal daughter nuclei. **Cytokinesis** is the process of cell division, giving rise to daughter cells with equally distributed chromosomes & other cellular structures.

Q: What factors control progression of the cell cycle?

Stimulation of Progression	Inhibition of Progression
Cyclins (Cyclin D & E)	Cyclin Dependent Kinase Inhibitors (p53, p21, p27)
Cyclin Dependent Kinase (CDK 4 & 2)	Rb Gene

Q: What factors control cellular growth during inflammation & wound healing?

Stimulation of Growth	Inhibition of Growth
Cytokines (IGF-1, TNFα)	Heparin
EGF	IFNα
PDGF	Prostaglandin E2
VEGF	

Q: What is dysplasia, metaplasia & neoplasia?

Terminology	Definition
Dysplasia	Abnormal cell development, resulting in atypical cells with differentiation abnormalities that display aneuploidy & pleomorphism. Cells are PREMALIGNANT & changes may resolve after removal of stimulus e.g. Cervical Carcinoma.
Metaplasia	Replacement of one fully differentiated cell type with another fully differentiated cell type e.g. Barrett's Oesophagus.
Neoplasia	An abnormal mass of tissue due to uncontrolled & progressive cell division. This may be BENIGN or MALIGNANT. Malignancy may be PRIMARY or SECONDARY.

Tumour Markers

Q: What is a tumour marker?

A molecule or substance found in the blood, urine or tissues that is detectable in the presence of a particular neoplasm. The marker will disappear after successful treatment & will become detectable again with recurrence. Tumour markers are not pathognomonic, however they are very useful when monitoring the patient's response to treatment.

Q: Do you know of any tumour markers?

Classification	Tumour Marker	Associated Tumour (carcinoma unless otherwise stated)
CANCER ANTIGENS	CA 15-3	Breast
	CA 19-9	Colorectal & Pancreas
	CA-125	Ovary
ENZYMES	Acid Phosphatase	Prostate (now replaced by PSA)
	Alkaline Phosphatase	Testicular Seminoma
		Colorectal, Lung & Pancreas
	PSA	Prostate
HORMONES	β-HCG	Testicular Teratoma & Choriocarcinoma
	Calcitonin	Medullary Thyroid
	ACTH	Small Cell Lung
ONCOFETAL ANTIGENS	α-FP	HCC & Testicular Teratoma
	CEA	Colorectal

Carcinogenesis

Q: What is carcinogenesis?

Definition	Explanation
Carcinogenesis	Process where normal cells are converted to abnormal cells capable of becoming neoplasms. May involve a carcinogen, initiator & promoter.
Carcinogen	A substance or agent that causes carcinogenesis.
Initiator	Alters cellular DNA resulting in an abnormal progeny of cells.
Promoter	Alters normal or initiated cells, resulting in altered gene expression.

Q: What cancers & corresponding carcinogens do you know of?

Cancer	Corresponding Carcinogen
Bladder	β-Naphthylamine (dyes)
	Nitrosamines (bacon, cured meats, metal industry, pesticides & rubber industry)
Burkitt's Lymphoma	EBV
Cervix	HPV
Cholangiocarcinoma	Liver Fluke Parasite (*Clonorchis sinensis, Fasciola hepatica* & *Opisthorchis* species)
Hepatocellular	Aflatoxin, HBV & HCV
Kaposi's Sarcoma	HHV8
Leukaemia (T-cell)	HTLV
Lymphoma	Cyclophosphamide
Lung	Asbestos & Tobacco
Nose	Sawdust
Skin	Irradiation & UV-light

Q: How would you classify carcinogens?

Classification	Example
Chemical	Dyes, Nitrosamines & Tobacco
Environmental	UV-light
Fungal	Aflatoxin (toxin produced by *Aspergillus flavus*)
Immunosuppressant	Cyclophosphamide
Occupational	Asbestos, Sawdust
Viral	EBV, HBV, HCV, HHV8, HPV & HTLV

Malignancy

Q: What are the pathological features of malignancy?

These may be classified as macroscopic & microscopic:

Macroscopic	Microscopic
Growth	More frequent mitosis
Haemorrhage	Pleomorphism (variation in cell size & shape)
Infiltration	High nucleus : low cytoplasm ratio in cells
Necrosis	Hyperchromatism (dark staining nucleus)
Metastasis	

Q: Do benign or non-neoplastic masses have the potential to cause morbidity & mortality?

Yes. This is usually due to a local effect, however one should also consider general effects:

Local	General
Haemorrhage	Malignant Transformation
Infarction	Psychological Effect of Visible Mass
Infection	Sequela of Mistaken Malignant Diagnosis & Subsequent Treatment
Obstruction	
Pressure Effect on Surrounding Structures	

Q: What malignant tumours do you know of?

Classification	Definition
Carcinoma	Malignant tumour of epithelial cells. e.g. Adenocarcinoma, Squamous Cell, Transitional Cell & Anaplastic.
Sarcoma	Malignant tumour of connective tissue cells. Accounts for 1% of all cancers. e.g. Chondrosarcoma, Leiomyosarcoma & Osteosarcoma.
Blastoma	Rare, locally aggressive tumour of embryonic cells, with risk of metastasis. CHILD variety most common e.g. Medulloblastoma, Nephroblastoma (Wilm's Tumour), Neuroblastoma, Pleuropulmonary & Retinoblastoma. ADULT variety less common e.g. Chondroblastoma, Glioblastoma multiforme & Osteoblastoma.
Teratoma	Tumour composed of cells that may give rise to all 3 germ layers. May contain normal tissue from other sites e.g. bone, hair & teeth. May be malignant or benign. e.g. Gonads (1% of testicular teratomas are benign, 1% of ovarian teratomas are malignant) & Midline Structures (hypothalamus, neck & mediastinum).

Q: What types of carcinoma are there?

Classification	Definition
Adenocarcinoma	Arising from glandular cells with secretory properties. e.g. Breast, Cervix, Colorectal, Gastric, Lung, Oesophagus, Pancreas & Prostate.
Squamous Cell	Arising from squamous cells. e.g. Bladder, Cervix, Lung, Oesophagus, Penis, Rectum & Skin.
Transitional Cell	Arising from transitional cells of the urothelium. e.g. Renal Pelvis, Ureters & Bladder.
Anaplastic	Highly aggressive & poorly differentiated, with a high propensity for metastasis. e.g. Thyroid, Anaplastic Large Cell Lymphoma.

Q: In what organs is carcinoma most prevalent?

Overall	Males	Females
Skin (non-melanomatous)	Skin (non-melanomatous)	Skin (non-melanomatous)
Lung	Prostate	Breast
Prostate	Lung	Lung
Breast	Colorectal	Colorectal
Colorectal	Bladder	Uterus & Ovary

Q: What carcinomas are associated with the highest mortality rates?

Overall	Males	Females
Lung	Lung	Lung
Colorectal	Prostate	Breast
Breast	Colorectal	Colorectal
Prostate	Oesophagus	Ovary
Oesophagus	Bladder	Pancreas

Paraneoplastic Syndromes

Q: What are paraneoplastic syndromes?

Symptoms or diseases caused by a tumour, not due to the local presence of the tumour itself. It is due to the release of substances or factors, such as hormone or cytokines, by tumour cells. Breast, Lung, Ovarian, Pancreatic & Renal Carcinoma & Lymphoma often result in paraneoplastic syndromes. Early symptom detection is important in recognising malignancy early.

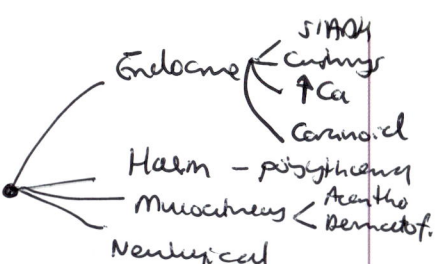

Q: How would you classify paraneoplastic syndromes?

Classification	Syndrome	Associated Tumour (carcinoma unless stated)	Causal Factor
ENDOCRINE	Cushing's	Small Cell Lung Pancreatic	ACTH or related polypeptide
	SIADH	Small Cell Lung	ADH or related polypeptide
	Hypercalcaemia	Squamous Cell Lung Breast Ovarian RCC	PTHRP
	Carcinoid	Lymphoma Carcinoid Lung Tumour Gastric Pancreatic	Serotonin, Somatostatin & Bradykinin
HAEMATOLOGICAL	Aplastic Anaemia	Thymus	Possible Immunological
	Polycythaemia	HCC RCC	EPO
MUCOCUTANEOUS	Acanthosis Nigricans	Gastric Lung	EGF & Immunological
	Dermatomyositis	Breast Lung	Immunological
NEUROLOGICAL	Cerebellar Degeneration	Lung Ovarian Breast	Immunological
	Lambert-Eaton Myasthenic Syndrome	Lung Prostate Cervix	Immunological

VASCULAR

Clot, Thrombus, Embolus & Virchow's Triad

Q: What is a clot, thrombus & embolus?

Terminology	Definition
Clot	A collection of solid material formed in stationary blood, involving the intrinsic & extrinsic clotting cascade.
Thrombus	A collection of solid material formed in flowing blood, involving platelets & the components that contribute to Virchow's Triad.
Embolus	An abnormal mass of undissolved material that has detached from an initial site & travelled via the bloodstream to a distant site. This may be composed of e.g. air, clot, fat, foreign body material, micro-organisms, thrombus & tumour cells.

Q: What is Virchow's Triad?

This describes 3 broad categories that contribute to thrombosis:

Endothelial Damage	Hypercoagulable States	Stasis / Turbulent Blood Flow
Atheroma	Antiphospholipid Antibodies	Aneurysm
Radiotherapy	Antithrombin Deficiency	Cardiac Valves
Trauma e.g. Cannulation	Dehydration	DVT History
	Factor V Leiden	Immobility
	Malignancy	Obesity
	OCP & HRT	Pelvic & Lower Limb Surgery
	Protein C & S Deficiency	Stents

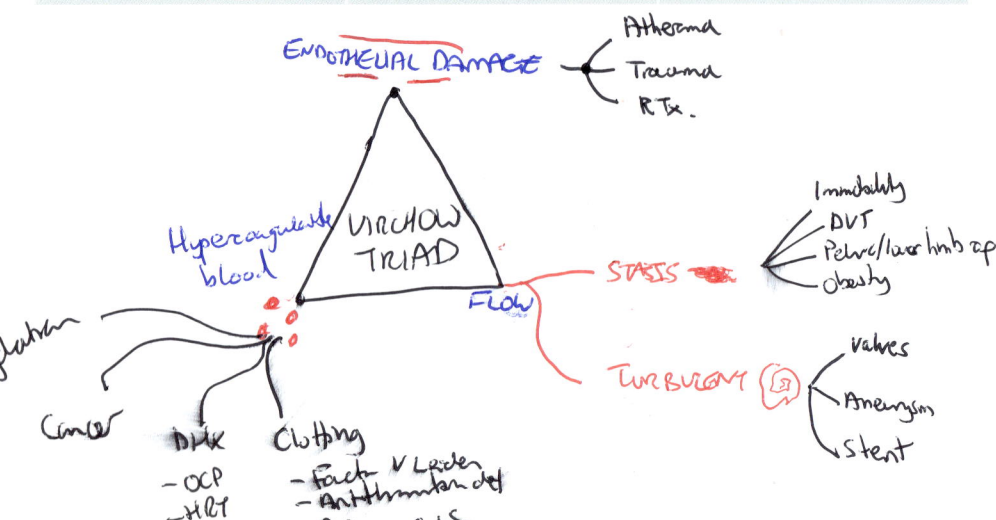

Atheroma

Q: What is an atheroma?

This is an abnormal lipid collection within the tunica intima of medium & large sized arteries. This lipid collection may either be free or within macrophages that are then termed foam cells. The lipid collection is associated with calcification, smooth muscle hyperplasia & fibrosis.

Q: What are the risk factors for atheroma formation?

Risk factors may be classified as follows: MODIFIABLE v. NON MODIFIABLE

Modifiable	Non-Modifiable
Diabetes	Family History
Hyperlipidaemia	Familial Hyperlipidaemia
Hypertension	Male Gender
Smoking	

Q: What are the theories that contribute to atheroma formation?

Theory	Definition
Encrustation	The lipid component of the atheroma is derived from a pre-existing thrombus of the tunica intima.
Imbibition	The lipid component of the atheroma is derived from circulating lipoproteins.
Proliferation	Smooth muscle hyperplasia is stimulated by circulating LDL & PDGF.

Q: What can happen as a consequence of atheroma formation?

- Acute artery occlusion, via rupture, with acute ischaemia e.g. MI
- Aneurysm formation
- Embolism of fat or thrombus, with transient or acute ischaemia
- Gradual progressive occlusion & chronic ischaemia.

Infarction & Ischaemia

Q: What is Infarction & Ischaemia?

Terminology	Definition
Infarction	Tissue or organ necrosis as a sequela of impaired blood supply or venous drainage. Infarction follows ischaemia & results in complete or partial necrosis.
Ischaemia	An abnormal reduction in blood supply to, or venous drainage from, a tissue or organ. Ischaemia may lead to infarction & can be ACUTE or CHRONIC.

Q: How would you classify the causes of infarction & ischaemia?

These may be classified as local or general:

BLOOD VESSEL PROBLEM   * SYSTEMIC *

Local	General
Arterial (Atheroma, Embolus & Thrombus)	Anaemic (All Causes of Severe Anaemia)
Capillary (Sickle Cell, Malaria & Vasculitis)	Hypoxaemic (Post MI)
Venous (Stasis & Thrombus)	V/Q Mismatch (Post PE)

Q: What features influence damage severity due to arterial infarction or ischaemia?

- **Chronicity:** Acute ischaemia is more severe than chronic.
- **Collaterals:** Presence of collaterals reduces severity & is a feature of chronic ischaemia.
- **Co-Morbidity:** This is associated with more severe outcomes e.g. DM & Cardiac Failure.
- **Diameter:** A larger lesion results in a smaller lumen diameter & more severe outcomes.
- **Intervention:** Rapid intervention is associated with less severe outcomes.
- **Oxygenation:** Well oxygenated blood reduces severity.
- **Tissue:** Some tissues are more sensitive e.g. Brain, than others e.g. Skeletal Muscle.

Aneurysm

Q: What is an aneurysm & how can aneurysms be classified?

Abnormal vessel dilation by ≥50% due to vessel wall disease or weakening. They may be classified according to their aetiology, morphology & pathology as follows:

Classification	Example
Aetiology	Congenital or Acquired
Morphology	Saccular or Fusiform
Pathology	True, False or Dissecting

Q: What are the causes of aneurysms?

The causes of aneurysms may be classified as follows:

Classification	Examples
Atheromatous	AAA.
Congenital	Berry aneurysms of the Circle of Willis. 20% of patients with ADPKD develop these saccular aneurysms.
Hypertensive	Charcot-Bouchard aneurysms of the brainstem are associated with chronic hypertension.
Iatrogenic	False aneurysm after femoral artery catheterisation.
Infective	Salmonella, Staphylococcus, Streptococcus & Syphilis.
Ischaemic	Left ventricle aneurysms post-MI.
Traumatic	Penetrating trauma is associated with arterio-venous aneurysm. Rapid deceleration injury is associated with dissecting aortic aneurysm.
Social	Smoking.

Q: What is the difference between a true & false aneurysm?

A true aneurysm involves all 3 layers of the vessel wall e.g. AAA. A false aneurysm therefore does not involve all 3 layers of the vessel wall. Vessel wall trauma or infection may result in localised haematoma that is closely contained to the site of vessel wall injury by surrounding connective tissue. This type of false aneurysm is often termed a 'pulsating haematoma' & may be seen after femoral artery catheterisation.

- Adventitia
- Media
- Intima

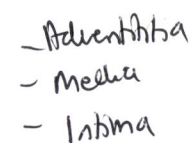

Q: Can you draw a saccular, fusiform & dissecting aneurysm?

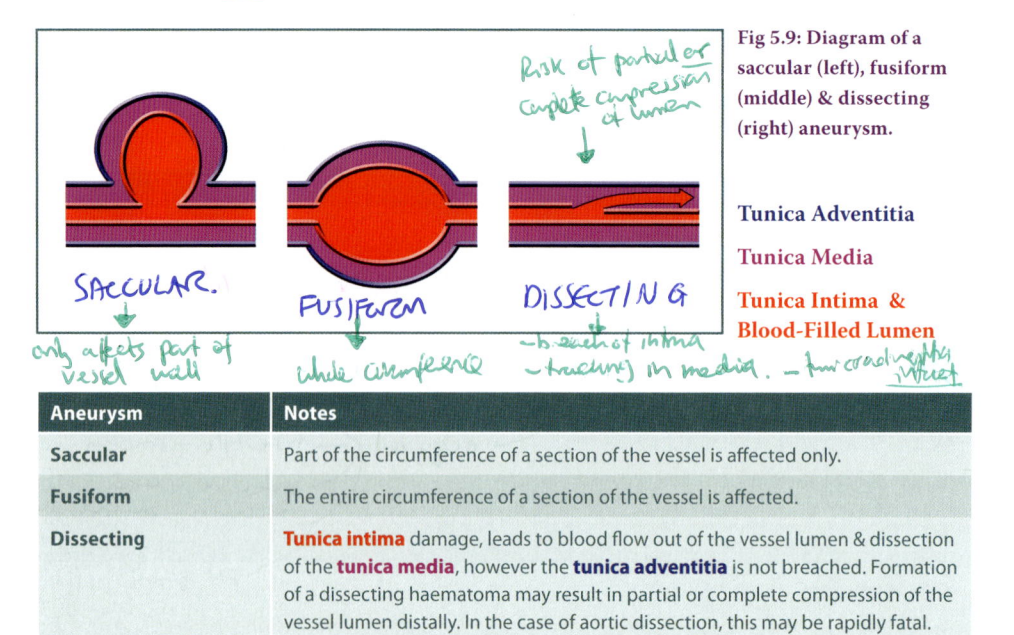

Fig 5.9: Diagram of a saccular (left), fusiform (middle) & dissecting (right) aneurysm.

Tunica Adventitia

Tunica Media

Tunica Intima & Blood-Filled Lumen

SACCULAR — only affects part of vessel wall

FUSIFORM — whole circumference

DISSECTING — breach of intima, tracking in media — fluid travelling in sheet

Risk of partial or complete compression of lumen

Aneurysm	Notes
Saccular	Part of the circumference of a section of the vessel is affected only.
Fusiform	The entire circumference of a section of the vessel is affected.
Dissecting	**Tunica intima** damage, leads to blood flow out of the vessel lumen & dissection of the **tunica media**, however the **tunica adventitia** is not breached. Formation of a dissecting haematoma may result in partial or complete compression of the vessel lumen distally. In the case of aortic dissection, this may be rapidly fatal.

Q: What are the complications of aneurysms?

These may be classified as vascular & due to pressure as follows:

- Compression of local structures
- Thrombosis
- Embolism
- Ischaemia
- Infarction
- Rupture & Haemorrhage
- Death.

SECTION C: SURGICAL SKILLS

CHAPTER 6
OPERATIVE SURGERY & PROCEDURES

W Bhat
S Fraser
Q Bismil
BH Miranda
K Asaad

CHAPTER CONTENTS

Head & Neck

- Thyroidectomy
- Parotidectomy
- Central Venous Access & Central Venous Pressure (CVP) Lines
- Surgical Airways

Trunk & Thorax

- Mastectomy
- Cardiac Pericardiocentesis
- Chest Drains
- Laparotomy
- Principles of Bowel Anastomoses
- Hartmann's Procedure
- Right Hemicolectomy
- Anterior & Abdominoperineal Resection of the Rectum
- Cholecystectomy
- Splenectomy
- Appendicectomy
- Inguinal Hernia Repair
- Femoral Hernia Repair
- Haemorrhoidectomy
- Suprapubic Catheterisation
- Renal Trauma & Nephrectomy
- Testicular Torsion
- Orchidectomy
- Circumcision
- Vasectomy
- Hydrocoele Repair

Limbs, Spine & Vascular

- Carpal Tunnel Decompression
- Approaches to Hip Joint
- Zadek's Procedure & Ingrown Toenail
- Fasciotomy & Compartment Syndrome

- Tendon Repair
- Amputations
- Femoral Embolectomy
- Varicose Vein Surgery
- Abdominal Aortic Aneurysm Repair

Neurosciences
- Burr Hole & Craniotomy
- Intracranial Pressure (ICP) Monitor Insertion
- Lumbar Puncture

HEAD & NECK

Thyroidectomy

Q: What specific measures may be used to prepare the patient pre-thyroidectomy?

- Full history & thorough clinical examination.
- Appropriate investigations e.g. TFT, CXR, USS, Radioisotope Scan.
- Optimise euthyroid state prior to surgery.
- Thyrotoxicosis control with 2-weeks carbimazole & β-blocker e.g. propranolol.
- Lugol's Iodine Solution may additionally help to reduce gland vascularity.
- Laryngoscopy including vocal cord check.

Q: What layers are encountered during the approach to thyroidectomy?

- Skin
- Subcutaneous fat
- Superficial cervical fascia & platysma
- Deep investing layer of cervical fascia
- Strap muscles
- Pretracheal fascia
- Isthmus of thyroid gland.

Q: Outline the steps in performing a total thyroidectomy.

- Full pre-operative assessment including history, examination & appropriate investigations.
- Explain operation to patient & obtain informed consent.
- Patient supine under GA.
- 10–20° of head tilt, with sandbag between shoulder blades.
- Skin preparation & draping.
- Transverse collar incision, 2 fingerbreadths above the suprasternal notch.
- Divide platysma.
- Raise flaps incorporating skin & platysma:
  - Superiorly up to the superior thyroid notch.
  - Inferiorly down to the suprasternal notch.
- Apply Joll's Retractor.
- Incise the deep cervical fascia & retract the strap muscles laterally.
- Mobilise each lobe by ligating & dividing the middle thyroid vein.

- Ligate & divide the superior thyroid artery & vein medially (protecting the external laryngeal nerve).
- Ligate & divide the inferior thyroid artery as inferiorly as possible (protecting the recurrent laryngeal nerve).
- Identify & protect the parathyroid glands.
- Dissect the gland off its posterior attachments (Berry's Ligament) (Fig 6.1).
- Haemostasis.
- Insert 2 suction drains.
- Close strap muscles (prevents trachea tethering to skin).
- Wound closure in layers.

Note: If performing a hemithyroidectomy, confirm the correct side with notes, patient & any radiology.

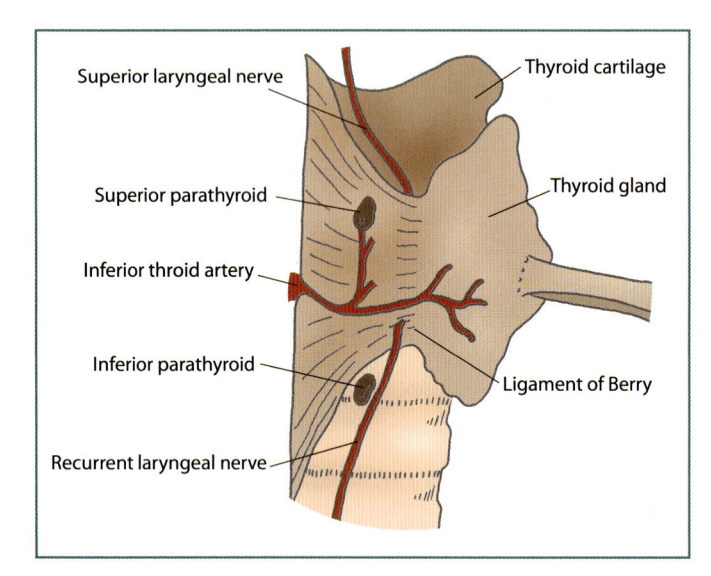

Fig 6.1: Posterior-lateral intra-operative view of the thyroid gland, demonstrating the superior & recurrent laryngeal nerves, inferior thyroid artery & parathyroid glands.

Q: What are the complications of thyroidectomy?

Immediate	Early	Late
Recurrent Laryngeal Nerve Damage (hoarse voice if unilateral / stridor if bilateral)	Thyroid Storm	Scarring (keloid / hypertrophic)
External Laryngeal Nerve Damage (loss of high pitch)	Hypoparathyroidism & Hypocalcaemia (ischaemia / damage to parathyroid glands)	Hypothyroidism
	Constricting Haematoma (may cause tracheal compression)	
	Infection	

Parotidectomy

Q: What are the indications for a superficial parotidectomy?

- Benign Adenomas
- Well Differentiated Tumours
- Chronic Parotitis (any cause)

Q: Describe how you would perform a superficial parotidectomy.

- Full pre-operative assessment including history, examination & appropriate investigations.
- Explain operation to patient, obtain informed consent & confirm correct side.
- Supine under GA with 20° of head-up tilt.
- Skin preparation & draping.
- Make an S-shaped (Fig 6.2) incision with three components:
    - Starting in the pre-auricular region.
    - Extending to the mastoid process.
    - Extending down the anterior border of sternocleidomastoid.
- Deepen incision to bony external auditory meatus, external jugular vein & stylohyoid muscle.
- Raise skin flaps:
    - Superiorly to just above the zygomatic arch.
    - Inferiorly to the anterior border of sternocleidomastoid.
- Identify the facial nerve (VII) using a nerve stimulator & preserve it.
- Ligate & divide the stylomastoid artery.
- Dissect the superficial parotid gland, reflecting it anteriorly.
- Protect the underlying facial nerve (VII) & branches.
- Dissect the parotid duct to the anterior border of masseter, ligate & divide it.
- Remove superficial portion of the gland.
- Haemostasis.
- Place a suction drain in to the parotid bed.
- Wound closure in layers.

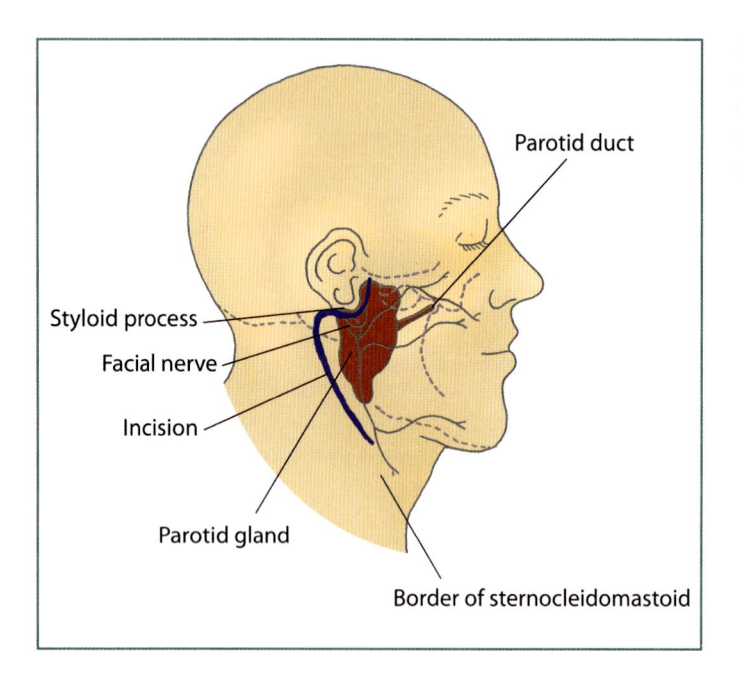

Fig 6.2: Incision for superficial parotidectomy demonstrating relationship to important structures

Q: What are the complications of superficial parotidectomy?

Immediate	Early	Late
Facial Nerve Damage	Haematoma	Parotid Fistula
Great Auricular Nerve Damage	Infection	Frey's Syndrome

Central Venous Access & Central Venous Pressure (CVP) Lines

Q: What are the indications for a CVP line?

- CVP Monitoring
- Infusion of Vaso-Irritant Drugs
- Infusion of Vaso-Active Drugs
- Inadequate Peripheral Access
- Fluid Resuscitation
- TPN Administration.

Q: What are the common sites for CVP line insertion?

- Internal Jugular Vein (IJV)
- Subclavian Vein
- Femoral Vein.

Q: How are CVP lines inserted?

USS guidance is now recommended for CVP line insertion via the IJV, using a Seldinger Technique.

Note: Veins are visibly compressible on USS, compared to arteries where pulsation can be seen.

Q: What are the anatomical landmarks used to locate the common CVP line access veins?

Internal Jugular Vein:
- Identify the 2 heads (sternal & clavicular) of the sternocleidomastoid muscle.
- Lies in front of & lateral to the carotid artery in the lower ⅓ of the neck. It is located on the medial border of sternocleidomastoid's clavicular head, within the triangle formed by its 2 heads & the clavicle.
- When inserting the 'introducer' needle, aim towards the ipsilateral nipple.

Subclavian Vein:
- A continuation of the axillary vein.
- Lies just below the middle ⅓ of the clavicle, running parallel to it in this region, above & deep to the subclavian artery.
- The usual site of insertion is below the junction of the medial & lateral ⅓ of the clavicle.
- When inserting the 'introducer' needle, enter 2cm below the middle of the clavicle, aiming towards the suprasternal notch.

Note: The right subclavian vein is preferred, as the right pleural dome is lower than the left & the thoracic duct is situated on the left side.

Femoral Vein:
- Medial to the femoral artery in the femoral triangle at the top of the thigh.

Q: How is a right IJV CVP line inserted?

- Full pre-procedure assessment including history, examination & appropriate investigations.
- Explain procedure to patient & obtain informed consent.
- Position patient with 30° head down tilt & head rotated to the left.
- Attach cardiac monitor.
- Skin preparation & draping.
- Seldinger Technique.
- Insert introducer needle *(see previous question for anatomical landmarks)* attached to a syringe, advancing & aspirating until flashback occurs.
- Insert the flexible guidewire (USS guided), checking the ECG for cardiac arrhythmias.
- Make a small skin incision using a scalpel.
- Remove introducer needle & use a dilating cannula to enlarge the tract over the guidewire.
- Feed the central line over the guidewire.
- Remove the guidewire, aspirate & flush all lumen.
- Secure with sutures.
- Obtain a CXR to ensure position of CVP line & check for pneumothorax.

Q: What are the complications of CVP line insertion?

Immediate	Early	Late
Pneumothorax	Blockage	Thrombosis
Arrhythmia	Dislodge	Sepsis
Haemorrhage	Infection	
Air Embolism		
Stroke		
Malposition		

Surgical Airways

Q: Do you know of any surgical airways?

- Cricothyroidotomy (needle / surgical)
- Emergency Tracheostomy.

Q: What are the indications for a surgical airway?

These are only required in emergency situations, when all other methods of intubation have failed or cannot be attempted. Common indications include:

- Airway Obstruction
- Maxillofacial Trauma
- Laryngeal Trauma
- Acute Inflammation (allergic reactions, thermal injury)
- Obstructing Masses
- Protection Against Aspiration (decreased conscious level, Guillain-Barré Syndrome, tetanus).

Q: How is a cricothyroidotomy performed?

Needle Cricothyroidotomy:

- Full pre-procedure assessment including history, examination & appropriate investigations.
- Explain procedure to patient & obtain informed consent where possible.
- Identify the cricothyroid membrane (the space between the inferior border of the thyroid cartilage & upper border of the cricoid cartilage).
- If there is time & the patient is awake, infiltrate the area with LA.
- Insert a 12G / 14G cannula through the membrane.
- Attach to high flow oxygen using tubing with a side hole or Y-connector.
- Occlude the side hole or Y-connector for 1 second to allow oxygen to enter the lungs & then release for 4 seconds to facilitate exhalation '*1 on / 4 off*'.

Note: This is a temporary measure that may maintain oxygenation for 30–40 minutes. It should be thought of as a 'time-buyer' only. A more definitive airway must be established as CO_2 retention occurs.

Surgical Cricothyroidotomy:

- Full pre-procedure assessment including history, examination & appropriate investigations.
- Explain procedure to patient & obtain informed consent where possible.
- Identify the cricothyroid membrane *(see above)*.
- Skin preparation & draping.
- If the patient is awake infiltrate the area with LA.
- Make a 3cm transverse incision over the cricothyroid membrane.
- Open the membrane under direct vision.
- Enlarge the hole using artery forceps or designated tracheal dilators if available.
- Insert a cuffed tracheostomy or endotracheal tube into the trachea & inflate the cuff. The cuff should be tested prior to beginning the procedure.

Note: Surgical cricothyroidotomy should not be performed on children aged <12years, due to the risk of subglottic stenosis.

Q: What are the complications of cricothyroidotomy?

Immediate	Early (needle cricothyroidotomy)	Late
Aspiration	Inadequate Ventilation	Subglottic Stenosis
Haemorrhage*	Hypoxia	Permanent Voice Change
Oesophageal Perforation	Hypercarbia	
Recurrent Laryngeal Nerve Damage		
Vocal Cord Damage		
Creation of False Passage		

*Note: There is risk of damage to the anterior jugular vein. If this occurs, apply pressure & secure the airway. If bleeding continues, a formal vein repair is required.

Q: What are the indications for a tracheostomy?

Tracheostomy is usually a planned procedure, typically performed on anaesthetised, ventilated patients. It should only be performed as an emergency if medical personnel have the required specialist skills & training. Indications include:

- Upper Airway Obstruction (trauma, infection, tumour).
- Long-Term Endotracheal Intubation Requirement.
- Improve Respiratory Function.
- Reduce Work of Breathing.
- Lung Toilet.
- Assist Weaning from Ventilation.

Q: How is a tracheostomy performed?

- Full pre-operative assessment including history, examination & appropriate investigations.
- Explain operation to patient & obtain informed consent.
- Patient supine with neck extended under GA.
- Skin preparation & draping.
- Ensure availability of the correct sized tracheostomy tube & ensure cuff is intact.
- Infiltrate LA with adrenaline.
- Make a horizontal incision midway between the cricoid cartilage & supra-sternal notch, between the sternocleidomastoid muscles.
- Divide platysma & separate the strap muscles in the midline (retract / ligate the anterior jugular veins as necessary).
- Divide the thyroid isthmus & ensure meticulous haemostasis.

- Identify the trachea & expose the 2nd–4th tracheal rings (use a tracheal hook under the cricoid cartilage to elevate the trachea if necessary).
- Check tracheostomy tube cuff is undamaged.
- Inform the anaesthetist that you are about to open the trachea.
- Perform tracheal incision between the 2nd & 4th tracheal rings e.g. Bjork flap.
- Suction blood & secretions out of the opened trachea & ask the anaesthetist to withdraw the endotracheal tube just proximal to the tracheal opening.
- Hold the tracheal incision open with dilators & insert the tracheostomy tube.
- Inflate the tracheostomy tube cuff enough to prevent air leakage around it.
- Do not withdraw the endotracheal tube until the tracheostomy tube is confirmed to be in the correct position.
- Approximate the skin loosely around the tracheostomy tube (tight closure will result in surgical emphysema).
- Secure tracheostomy tube with sutures & tracheostomy tape.

Q: What are the complications of tracheostomy?

Immediate	Early	Late
Aspiration	Obstruction	Tracheo-Cutaneous Fistula
Haemorrhage	Dislodge	Tracheomalacia
Malposition	Subcutaneous Emphysema	Trachea / Laryngeal Stenosis
Blockage (more common in single lumen tubes)	Pneumonia	Tracheo-Oesophageal Fistula
Recurrent Laryngeal Nerve Damage	Lung Abscess	Scarring
Oesophageal Perforation	Cellulitis	
Pneumothorax	Tracheal Erosion	

TRUNK & THORAX

Mastectomy
(also see principles of surgery chapter)

Q: What is a total mastectomy & what are the indications?

A total / simple mastectomy involves removal of the whole breast including the nipple & areola complex. This is indicated in the treatment of breast cancer & may also be offered as a prophylactic procedure in high-risk patients.

Q: What other kinds of mastectomy do you know of?

Mastectomy	Description
Skin Sparing	Removal of all breast tissue, but only skin of nipple & areola complex.
Total Skin Sparing	Removal of all breast tissue, leaving all skin behind.
Radical Mastectomy	As for a modified radical mastectomy, but also includes removal of pectoralis major (rarely performed now).
Modified Radical Mastectomy	Simple mastectomy & axillary node clearance.

Q: What is the arterial supply to the breast?

Internal thoracic (mammary), lateral thoracic, thoracoacromial & intercostal (2–4) arteries.

Q: How is a total mastectomy performed?

- Full pre-operative assessment including history, examination & appropriate investigations.
- Explain operation to patient, obtain informed consent & confirm correct side.
- Patient positioned supine, with arm extended, under GA.
- Skin preparation & draping.
- Make an elliptical incision on the breast, including the nipple-areola complex & tumour (skin incision should be ≥3cm from tumour) (Fig 6.3).
- Raise skin flaps between the subcutaneous & mammary fat planes using diathermy.
- Anatomical dissection limits are the sternum (medial), latissimus dorsi (lateral), 2cm below the clavicle (superior), superior border of rectus (inferior).
- Dissect down until pectoralis major muscle is visible.

- Dissect the breast tissue off pectoralis major (removing fascia) from medial to lateral, including the axillary tail of Spence.
- Haemostasis including perforating vessels.
- Suction drain.
- Close skin edges with a subcuticular suture.

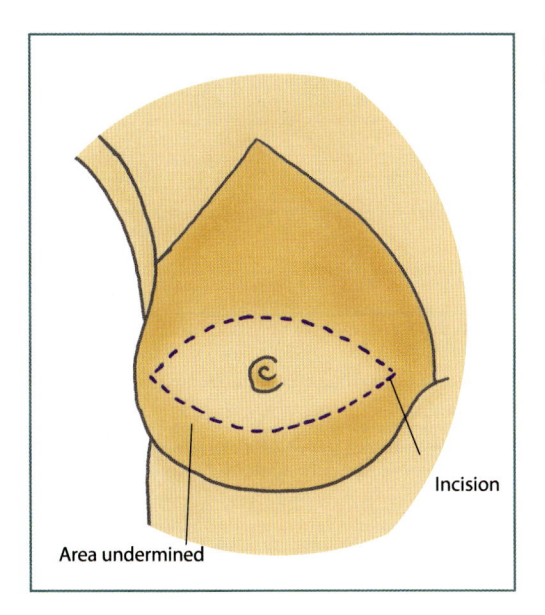

Fig 6.3: Total / simple right mastectomy incision.

Q: What are the complications of mastectomy?

Immediate	Early	Late
Haemorrhage	Infection	Lymphoedema
Intercostobrachial (T2) Nerve Damage	Seroma	Shoulder Movement Limitation
Long Thoracic Nerve of Bell Damage	Skin Flap Necrosis	Psychological
Thoracodorsal Nerve Damage	Cosmetic Deformity	
Medial / Lateral Pectoral Nerve Damage		

Q: What is a wide local excision?

This is a form of breast conserving surgery (previously known as lumpectomy). The aim is to remove the breast cancer with a surrounding margin (≥1cm) of healthy tissue.

Q: What is the lymphatic drainage of the breast?

Axillary (75%), parasternal, posterior intercostal, supraclavicular, contralateral breast.

Q: What is an axillary node clearance?

Axillary node clearance can be defined as removal of the axillary contents (including lymph nodes). The axillary node levels are defined as:

- **Level I:**   Lateral to pectoralis minor.
- **Level II:**   Posterior to pectoralis minor.
- **Level III:** Medial to pectoralis minor.

Note: Axillary node sampling involving level I nodes has largely been superseded by sentinel lymph node biopsy.

Q: What is sentinel lymph node biopsy (SLNB) with respect to breast cancer?

The first lymph node that a breast malignancy drains to in the axilla is termed the sentinel lymph node (SLN). This is followed successively by other lymph nodes further down the chain. If the SLN is positive for metastatic disease there may be other positive nodes further downstream, potentially warranting a full axillary clearance. If negative, the majority of patients do not have axillary lymph node metastases & can forgo a full axillary clearance.

Axillary node status is the most important prognostic indicator for long-term survival. If patients present with palpable axillary nodes, or have abnormal nodes detected on USS, a full axillary clearance should be carried out. If there is no indication of metastatic disease, SLNB can be performed to establish nodal status.

Q: What is the advantage of SLNB over axillary node clearance?

- Axillary node clearance removes all lymph nodes from the axilla, which may be avoided with SLNB.
- SLNB is a much less invasive procedure, usually requiring a shorter hospital stay, smaller incision & less post-operative pain.
- There is substantial reduction in post-operative complications, including lymphoedema, decreased shoulder movement & nerve damage.

Q: What are the operative principles of SLNB?

- The SLN is identified radiologically, by injecting a radioisotope (usually technetium-99m-labelled tin-colloid) several hours before the operation & lymphoscintigram performed.
- Patent blue dye is injected into the breast tissue around the tumour, when the patient is anaesthetised, in order to facilitate the surgeon's location of the SLN.
- Locate the area of maximum radioactivity with a gamma probe.

- Make an incision at this site.
- Open the axilla & dissect down to enter axillary fat.
- Look for blue lymphatics & follow these to locate the SLN, using the gamma probe to confirm the SLN that is 'hot' & 'blue'.
- Excise SLN.
- Haemostasis & wound closure.

Q: What are the reconstructive options in breast cancer surgery?

Reconstructive surgery (Fig 6.4) can be **immediate** or **delayed.** This is influenced by patient choice, co-morbidity & requirement for adjuvant radiotherapy / chemotherapy.

Reconstruction	Description
External	External Prosthesis.
Implant Based	Simple Breast Implant e.g. Silicone.
	Tissue Expander ± Implant.
Regional Flap	Latissimus Dorsi Flap ± Tissue Expander / Implant.
Autologous Tissue	*Fat Transfer:*
	- Fat Harvested from 1 Body Site (similar to liposuction).
	- Fat Centrifuged & Cells Injected (grafted) to Recipient Site.
	Free Flap e.g. DIEP / TRAM:
	- Tissue Flaps Containing Skin, Fat ± Muscle.
	- Harvested from 1 body Site.
	- Anastomosed to Vessels at Recipient Site.
Nipple	Local Skin Flaps & Tattoo.

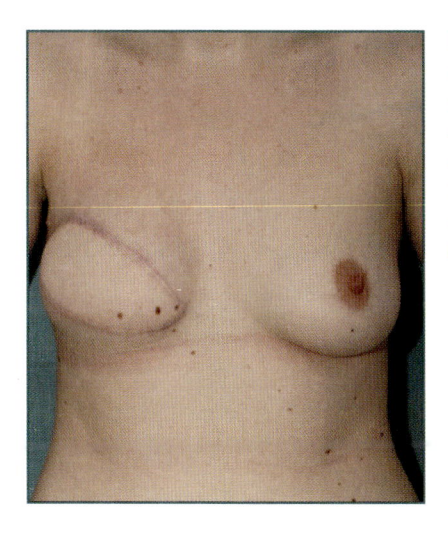

Fig 6.4: Right breast reconstruction. A LD flap is associated with an oblique scar overlying the latissimus dorsi muscle on the back. TRAM & DIEP flaps are associated with a low horizontal abdominal scar.

Cardiac Pericardiocentesis

Q: What are the indications for cardiac pericardiocentesis?

Indications may be thought of as:
- **Diagnostic** or **Therapeutic**
- **Emergency** or **Non-Emergency:**

Emergency (Haemodynamically Unstable Patient)	Non-Emergency (Haemodynamically Stable Patient)
Cardiac Tamponade	Diagnostic
	Palliative
	Prophylactic

Q: What is cardiac tamponade?

Accumulation of fluid occurs in the pericardial space, causing mechanical ventricular obstruction. Diastolic filling is restricted, hence reducing end diastolic volume & subsequent stroke volume. Shock & death may occur rapidly, especially with trauma, if cardiac tamponade is not quickly diagnosed & treated.

Q: How is cardiac tamponade diagnosed?
- There should be a high index of suspicion in chest trauma.
- It should always be considered in trauma patients presenting with PEA & no obvious cause of hypovolaemia or tension pneumothorax.
- The classic signs of cardiac tamponade are Beck's Triad, however other signs may be present:

Beck's Triad	Other Signs
Hypotension	Pulsus Paradoxus
Muffled Heart Sounds	Cyanosis
Raised JVP	Loss of Consciousness

Q: How is pericardiocentesis performed?

- Full pre-procedure assessment including history, examination & appropriate investigations.
- Explain procedure to patient & obtain informed consent.
- Ensure patient has supplemental O_2 & IV access.
- Position patient in semi-recumbent position (30°–45°).
- Attach cardiac monitor.
- Skin preparation & draping.
- Identify xiphoid process & infiltrate LA.
- Insert a wide bore needle just left of the xiphoid process at an angle of 45° to the skin.
- Aim the needle towards the tip of the left scapula.
- Watch for ectopic beats when the myocardium is touched.
- Aspirate whilst advancing the needle.
- If blood is aspirated attach a 3-way tap & syringe to remove larger amounts of blood.

Note: This is not a definitive procedure & blood is often clotted. Virtually all patients who require emergency pericardiocentesis for trauma will also require emergency thoracotomy. Ensure that cardiothoracic surgery & other relevant teams have been contacted well in advance.

Q: What are the complications of pericardiocentesis?

Immediate	Early	Late
Failure of Procedure	Fluid Re-Accumulation	Infectious Pericarditis
Arrhythmias	Coronary Artery Aneurysm	
Coronary Vessel Injury		
Pneumothorax / Haemothorax		
Pneumopericardium		
Myocardial Infarction		
Organ Perforation e.g. Lung, Liver, Stomach		

Chest Drains

Q: What are the indications for chest drain insertion?

Chest drains are inserted when the intrathoracic space has been compromised with reduced volume of the underlying lung. Causes (hence indications for chest drain insertion) include:

- Pneumothorax
- Haemothorax
- Pleural Effusions
- Empyema
- Post-Operative.

Q: What size chest drain should be used?

Small Bore (10–14F)	Large Bore (20–32F)
Limited Pneumothorax	Trauma Patients
Free-Flowing Pleural Effusions	Haemothorax
	Pneumothorax
	Mechanically Ventilated Patients
	Viscous Pleural Fluids

Q: How is a chest drain inserted?

Large Bore Chest Drains:
- Full pre-procedure assessment including history, examination & appropriate investigations.
- Explain procedure to patient, obtain informed consent & confirm correct side.
- Position the patient semi-recumbent at 45° leaning away from the side of the procedure.
- Skin preparation & draping.
- Locate the 5th intercostal space, just anterior to the mid-axillary line.
- Infiltrate local anaesthetic.
- Make an incision on the upper border of the ribs to avoid intercostal nerves & vessels.
- Use blunt dissection to enter the pleural cavity.
- Insert finger & perform a 'sweep' to check that the pleural cavity has been entered.
- Grasp distal end of chest drain with artery forceps & guide into pleural cavity.
- Attach to underwater seal & suture chest drain in place.

Small Bore Chest Drains:
- Full pre-procedure assessment including history, examination & appropriate investigations.
- Explain procedure to patient, obtain informed consent & confirm correct side.
- Position the patient semi-recumbent at 45° leaning away from the side of the procedure.
- Skin preparation & draping.
- Locate the 5th intercostal space, just anterior to the mid-axillary line.
- Infiltrate local anaesthetic.
- Seldinger Technique employed.
- Use a needle & syringe to localise the position for insertion.
- Remove the syringe & insert the guidewire through the needle.
- Remove the needle & enlarge the tract into the pleural cavity using a dilator.
- Pass the small bore drain into the pleural space over the guidewire.
- Attach to underwater seal & suture chest drain in place.

Note: A CXR is required after any chest drain insertion to confirm position. Also ensure that the drain is kept below the level of the patient.

Q: What is the 'safe zone' for chest drain insertion?

A zone bordered by:
- The lateral border of pectoralis major.
- The anterior border of latissimus dorsi.
- A line superior to the horizontal level of the nipple.
- An apex below the axilla.

Q: Why would you site a chest drain just anterior to the mid-axillary line?

To avoid the long thoracic nerve of Bell that runs along the mid-axillary line.

Q: What are the potential complications of chest drain insertion?

Immediate	Early	Late
Haemothorax	Blockage	Infection
Lung Injury	Disconnection	Pneumothorax (after removal)
Diaphragm & Abdominal Cavity Penetration	Dislodge	
	Surgical Emphysema	

Laparotomy

Q: How is a laparotomy performed?

- Full pre-operative assessment including history, examination & appropriate investigations.
- Explain operation to patient & obtain informed consent.
- Patient supine under GA.
- NG tube & urinary catheter.
- Skin preparation & draping.
- Prophylactic antibiotics.
- May place legs in Lloyd Davis support, to provide access to pelvis (if required).
- Long midline incision skirting left of the umbilicus *(see book 2 Fig 4.7)* through skin, fat, fascia, linea alba & extraperitoneal fat.
- Open peritoneum & note any escaping gas, fluid or foul odour.
- A methodical & systematic approach is taken to examine all major structures:
    - Solid viscera & associated organs (liver, gall bladder, spleen, pancreas).
    - Gastrointestinal tract (stomach, duodenum, duodenal flexure, small bowel, ileocecal valve, appendix, caecum, large bowel, rectum & omentum).
    - Retroperitoneum (kidneys, aorta).
    - Pelvis: In females (cervix, uterus, fallopian tubes & ovaries).
      In males (base of prostate felt through the bladder).
      Bladder in both sexes.
- Proceed as appropriate, depending on the indication & findings.

Q: How is the abdomen closed after laparotomy?

Closure is according to Jenkins' Rule:

- Mass closure (including peritoneum & rectus sheath).
- Suture material = looped 1–0 PDS™ on a blunt needle.
- The length of the suture material should be 4 times the length of the wound.
- Sutures are placed 1cm apart with 1cm bites of tissue.
- Skin closure.

Principles of Bowel Anastomoses

Q: What are the methods of bowel anastomosis?
- Sutured / Stapled.
- 1-layer / 2-layers.

Q: What are the principles of successful bowel anastomosis?
- Optimise Patient Co-Morbidities & Nutrition.
- Meticulous Operative Technique.
- No Faecal Contamination of Gut / Peritoneal Cavity.
- Tension Free.
- Well Vascularised Tissue.
- Avoid Twisting the Mesentery.
- Serosa to Serosa.

Q: What types of bowel anastomoses are there?

Anastomosis	Example
End-to-End	Common after small bowel / colon resection to restore continuity.
Side-to-Side	Joining 2 parallel segments of bowel with closed ends / without dividing the bowel.
End-to-Side	Frequently used in Roux-en-Y anastomosis.

Q: How are sutured anastomoses performed?
- The most important aspect is to oppose healthy bowel in a tension-free repair.
- 1-layered / 2-layered technique may be used.
- Continuous / interrupted sutures may be used.
- A continuous suture is appropriate in standard gastric, enteric or colonic anastomoses.
- Interrupted sutures should be considered for technically difficult anastomoses / areas with significant size disparity between bowel ends.
- Sutures placed 5mm apart, ensuring submucosa is taken & inverting the mucosa.

Q: How are stapled anatomoses performed?
- **End-to-End:** Circular stapling devices.
- **Side-to-Side:** Linear stapling devices.

Note: Clean the bowel of all fat & mesentery around site of anastomosis prior to stapling.

Q: What are the potential complications of bowel anastomosis?

Early	Early	Late
Haemorrhage	Anastomotic Leak	Stenosis
	Peritonitis	Adhesions
	Ileus	

Hartmann's Procedure

Q: What are the indications for a Hartmann's Procedure?

- Sigmoid volvulus
- Perforated sigmoid colon
- Obstructing rectosigmoid carcinoma.

Q: How is a Hartmann's Procedure performed?

- Full pre-operative assessment including history, examination & appropriate investigations.
- Explain operation to patient & obtain informed consent.
- Patient supine under GA with slight Trendelenberg tilt.
- NG tube & urinary catheter.
- Skin preparation & draping.
- Prophylactic antibiotics.
- Long midline laparotomy incision & perform a full intra-abdominal assessment *(see above)*.
- Peritoneal lavage.
- Mobilise sigmoid colon (incising sigmoid mesocolon).
- Ligate & divide the sigmoid branches of the inferior mesenteric artery.
- Mobilise the upper ⅓ of the rectum (do not damage the left ureter & gonadal vessels).
- Soft & crushing clamps to distal descending colon & proximal rectum.
- Divide descending colon & rectum.
- Send for histology.
- Close rectal stump in 2 layers.
- Bring descending colon out as end colostomy in RIF.
- Peritoneal lavage.
- Suction drains as required.
- Mass closure of abdomen *(see above)*.
- Skin closure.

Right Hemicolectomy

Q: What are the indications for performing a right hemicolectomy?

These involve disease of the right colon & include:

- Tumour (e.g. caecum / appendix / ascending colon)
- Crohn's Disease
- Bowel Ischaemia / Infarction
- Recurrent Diverticulitis

Q: What incisions could be used for a right hemicolectomy?

- Laparotomy
- Paramedian
- Transverse

(see book 2 Fig 4.7)

Q: How is a right hemicolectomy performed?

- Full pre-operative assessment including history, examination & appropriate investigations.
- Explain operation to patient & obtain informed consent.
- Bowel preparation if elective.
- Patient supine under a GA.
- NG tube & urinary catheter.
- Prophylactic antibiotics.
- Skin preparation & draping.
- Long midline laparotomy incision & perform a full intra-abdominal assessment *(see above)*, noting any co-existing intra-abdominal pathology, hepatic, peritoneal or mesenteric deposits.
- Identify the lesion. **Note: Synchronous tumour occurs in 3% of cases.**
- Mobilise caecum & ascending colon via peritoneal dissection (do not damage the right ureter / gonadal vessels / duodenum).
- Mobilise the hepatic flexure & divide the ileal bands.
- The right colon may be lifted medially off the posterior abdominal wall.
- Identify & ligate the mesenteric vessels: ileocolic, right colic & right branch of middle colic. These should be divided as close to the origin as possible. This facilitates surgical tumour clearance & also adequate mobilisation for reanastomosis.
- Apply soft & crushing clamps:
  - 20–30cm proximal to the ileo-caecal valve (on the terminal ileum).
  - Between the proximal & middle ⅓ of the transverse colon.

- Resect bowel & remove from abdomen.
- Send for histology.
- Clean colon with betadine soaked swabs.
- Ileo-colic anastomosis with 3-0 Vicryl™ sutures.
- Remove soft clamps & achieve haemostasis.
- Close mesenteric window with absorbable Vicryl™ sutures, to prevent internal herniation.
- Suction drains as required.
- Mass closure of abdomen *(see above)*.
- Skin closure.

Q: What should the post-operative care include?

- DVT prophylaxis to continue during hospital stay.
- Monitor fluid input & output.
- On post-operative day 1, can drink free fluids & start light diet as tolerated.

Anterior & Abdominoperineal Resection of the Rectum

Q: What procedures are commonly available for rectal tumours?

Curative	Palliative
Anterior Resection & Primary Anastomosis (>5cm from anal verge)	Stent
Abdominoperineal Resection & Colostomy (≤5cm from anal verge)	Endorectal Diathermy Canalisation
Subtotal Colectomy & Ileostomy (proximal bowel not viable / synchronous tumour)	Radiotherapy
	Diversion Without Resection (loop ileostomy / end colostomy)

Q: How is an anterior resection performed?

- Full pre-operative assessment including history, examination & appropriate investigations.
- Explain operation to patient & obtain informed consent.
- Bowel preparation.
- Patient supine under GA.
- NG tube & urinary catheter.
- Prophylactic antibiotics.
- Place legs in Lloyd Davis support, to provide pelvic access.
- Skin preparation & draping.
- Long midline laparotomy incision & perform a full intra-abdominal assessment *(see above)*, noting any co-existing intra-abdominal pathology, hepatic, peritoneal or mesenteric deposits.
- Place a self-retaining retractor & pack small bowel into the right upper quadrant.
- Mobilise descending colon (incise peritoneum) & sigmoid colon (incise sigmoid mesocolon).
- Mobilise splenic flexure (divide the phrenicocolic ligament).
- Identify & protect the left ureter & gonodal vessels.
- Incise peritoneum over the aorta, identify & divide the inferior mesenteric artery close to its origin.
- The inferior mesenteric vein is ligated & divided close to the inferior border of the pancreas.
- Mobilise rectum (dividing lateral rectal ligaments & mesorectum) & draw out of pelvis, taking care not to damage the autonomic nerves.
- St Marks Pelvic Retractor aids blunt dissection of Devonvillier's Fascia (to protect the bladder & seminal vesicles in males / uterus & vagina in females).
- Divide & remove the rectum & descending colon (soft & crushing clamps are applied to division level) with their mesentary & lymph nodes (clearance is ≥2cm from tumour, however 5cm is preferred).
- Send for histology.
- Washout of stumps.
- Colorectal anastomosis using an end-to-end stapling gun.
- Haemostasis & peritoneal lavage.
- Suction drains as required.
- Mass closure of abdomen *(see above)*.
- Skin closure.

Note: The lower the level of anastomosis, the higher the risk of complications. In such cases a temporary loop ileostomy is formed. This diverts the faecal stream from the large bowel & reduces the incidence of anastomotic leak & sepsis.

Q: How is an abdominoperineal resection performed?

This essentially involves the same abdominal procedure as anterior resection, however additional perineal & colostomy procedures are required. These are outlined below:

Perineal Procedure:

- Perform elliptical perineal incision (from sacrococcygeal articulation posteriorly, around the anus, to the midpoint between the anus & urethral bulb for males / taking the posterior vaginal wall in females).
- Deepen incision & extend until this meets the abdominal operative site. Divide levator ani & mobilise rectum & mesorectum as you continue.
- Deliver rectum, descending colon, mesentary & lymph nodes through the perineal wound.
- Send for histology.

Colostomy Procedure:

- Mark site pre-operatively in LIF.
- Make 3cm circular incision at marked stoma site.
- Deliver cut proximal end of descending colon through wound.
- Suture bowel end flush to skin forming end colostomy.
- Apply clear stoma bag.

Closure:

- Suction drains to abdomen & perineum.
- Abdominal closure as for laparotomy (see above).
- Close perineal wound in layers, oversewing vaginal edges in females.

Note: If a large perineal wound is created, further reconstruction with local / regional flaps may be required e.g. bilateral IGAP (inferior gluteal artery perforator) flaps.

Q: What are the complications of laparotomy with bowel resection for a tumour?

Immediate	Early	Late
Haemorrhage	Anastomotic Leak	Stenosis
Ureter Damage	Ileus	Incisional Hernia
Kidney Damage	Bowel Ischaemia & Perforation	Bowel Obstruction
Pancreas Damage	Peritonitis	Tumour Recurrence
Duodenum Damage	UTI	Wound Dehiscence
	DVT / PE	Fistula
	Pneumonia	Stoma Complications (if present)

Cholecystectomy

Q: What is the anatomy of the gallbladder?

- Lies in the gallbladder fossa (undersurface of liver).
- Has a fundus, body & neck.
- The gallbladder neck becomes continuous with the cystic duct, which is approximately 3–4cm in length.
- The cystic duct joins the right side of the common hepatic duct from the liver to form the CBD. The CBD is roughly 8cm long & joins the main pancreatic duct to enter the 2nd part of the duodenum at the Ampulla of Vater.
- The Sphincter of Oddi prevents reflux of duodenal contents into the biliary system.
- The blood supply to the gallbladder is via the cystic artery, a branch of the right hepatic artery. The cystic vein drains directly into the portal vein.
- The gallbladder also receives small vessels directly from the surface of the liver & so rarely becomes gangrenous.

Q: What is the function of the gallbladder?

- The gallbladder has a 30–50mls capacity.
- It acts as a reservoir to store & concentrate bile.
- The gallbladder absorbs H_2O, selectively absorbs bile salts, excretes cholesterol & secretes mucus.
- Bile is excreted into the duodenum in response to secretin & CCK *(see pathology chapter – gallstone disease for composition & function of bile)*.
- CCK release (synthesised by mucosal intestinal cells & released in response to fatty food entering the duodenum) causes the gallbladder to contract & the Sphincter of Oddi to relax.

Q: What radiological modalities are useful in the diagnosis of gallstone disease?

Radiology	Notes
USS	1st line imaging for gallstones. It may detect stones, estimate gallbladder wall thickness & can identify CBD dilatation. If USS is negative & there is still suspicion of a ductal stone, MRCP may be used as a 2nd line imaging investigation.
MRCP	Non-invasive investigation using MRI. High sensitivity for CBD stones, also allowing biliary, hepatic & pancreatic lesion assessment.
ERCP	Diagnostic & therapeutic for CBD obstruction. If CBD stones are identified, **sphincterotomy** is performed. This allows for relief of obstruction & direct removal of stones in >95% of cases. ERCP also has a role in biliary system biopsy & stent placement for strictures. It is the treatment of choice in acute cholangitis & obstructive jaundice, but has a 10% risk of complications including pancreatitis, haemorrhage, cholangitis & duodenal perforation.

Bleeding   Infection (cholangitis)   Perforation   Pancreatitis

Q: What are the indications for a cholecystectomy?

- Symptomatic gallstone disease.
- To prevent further episodes of gallstone pancreatitis.
- Acute cholecystitis.
- Carcinoma.
- Empyema.
- Perforation.

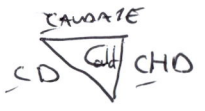

Q: What is Calot's Triangle?

An anatomical space containing the cystic artery.

Border	Description
Superior	Caudate Lobe of Liver
Medial	Common Hepatic Duct
Lateral	Cystic Duct

Q: How is a laparoscopic cholecystectomy performed?

Cholecystectomy may be open / laparoscopic. Laparoscopic cholecystectomy has superseded open cholecystectomy (>90% of patients undergo laparoscopic cholecystectomy) as the 1st line surgical option due to smaller surgical scars, reduced post-operative pain & a shorter recovery time. Laparoscopic cholecystectomy is performed as follows:

- Full pre-operative assessment including history, examination & appropriate investigations.
- Explain operation to patient, obtain informed consent (including conversion to open procedure).
- Patient positioned in Trendelenburg position, with slight left rotation, under GA.
- Skin preparation & draping.
- Obtain pneumoperitoneum under direct vision (Hassan Method) & insert ports (Fig 6.5):
  - Subumbilical (10mm)
  - Epigastric (10mm)
  - Right mid-clavicular line, inferior to the costal margin (5mm)
  - Right anterior axillary line, inferior to the costal margin (5mm).
- Remove adhesions, sweep away omentum, colon or small bowel until the gallbladder is clearly visible.
- Identify Calot's Triangle
- Using the right-sided ports, retract the gallbladder cephalad.

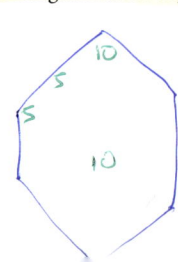

- Keep the gallbladder neck under tension & start dissection of Calot's Triangle.
- Divide the peritoneum, identify & expose the cystic artery & duct.
- Clip the cystic artery & duct, usually double ligating the CBD side. When clipping any structure ensure that both tips of the clip applicator can be seen to avoid inadvertently injuring important adjacent structures.
- Divide the artery & duct using scissors.
- Remove the gallbladder from the liver bed. Blunt & sharp dissection & diathermy may be used.
- Once the gallbladder is removed lift up the gallbladder fossa, check for bleeding & bile leaks.
- Use a bag to remove the gallbladder from the abdomen to prevent bile leakage or stone loss due to gallbladder perforation.
- Remove the gallbladder from either the epigastric or umbilical port.
- Before closing the abdomen do a final check for bleeding, bile leakage or damage to other intra-abdominal structures.
- Remove ports under direct vision.
- Close muscle, fascia & skin of port sites.

Laparoscopic Port Sites Key:

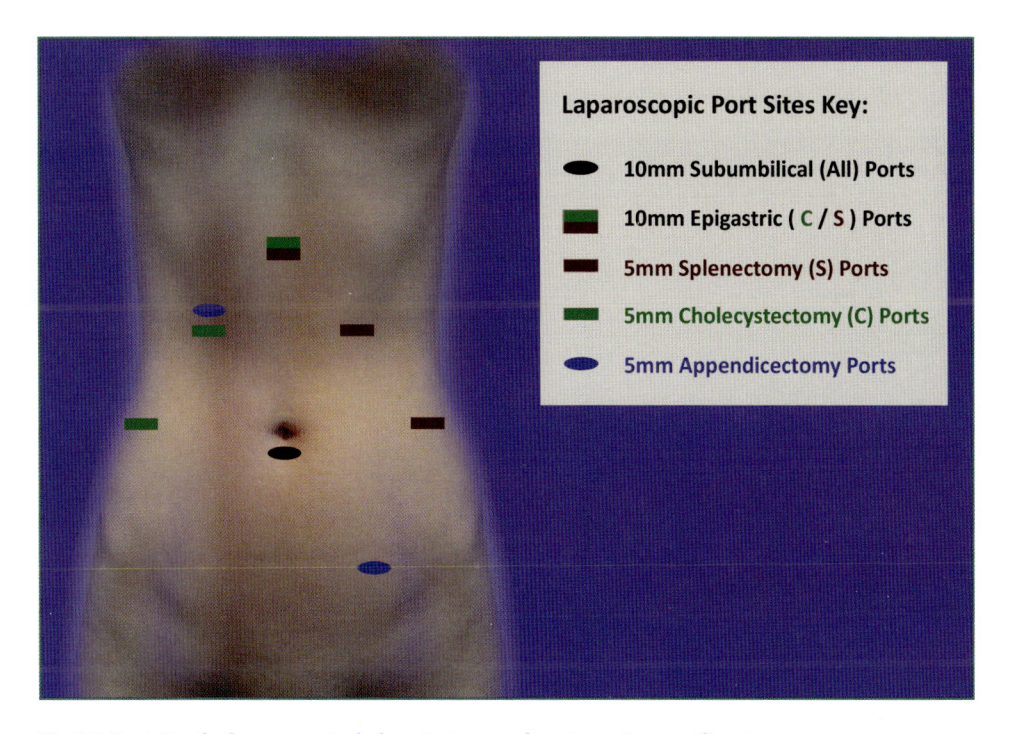

- 10mm Subumbilical (All) Ports
- 10mm Epigastric (C / S) Ports
- 5mm Splenectomy (S) Ports
- 5mm Cholecystectomy (C) Ports
- 5mm Appendicectomy Ports

Fig 6.5: Port sites for laparoscopic cholecystectomy, splenectomy & appendicectomy.

Q: What are the pros & cons of laparoscopy?

Allows detailed examination of the abdominal cavity. This is useful if there is doubt regarding diagnosis, especially in young women with suspected pelvic pathology:

Pros of Laparoscopy	Cons of Laparoscopy
Less Trauma	CO_2 Gas Embolism (minimise with head down tilt)
Less Post-Operative Pain	Pneumothorax
Faster Recovery Time	Pneumomediastinum
Less Adhesions	Perforation
Cosmesis	Longer Procedure
	Conversion to Open (must consent for open procedure)
	Expensive Equipment
	Long Training Times

Q: What are the complications of cholecystectomy?

These include the complications of laparoscopy when relevant *(see above)*.

Immediate	Early	Late
Haemorrhage	Bile Leak (due to clip slipping from cystic duct stump)	Incisional Hernia (after open surgery / laparoscopic port sites)
Bile Duct Injury	Wound Infection	Biliary Stricture
Duodenum Damage		DVT / PE
Bowel Perforation (due to trocar puncture)		

Splenectomy

Q: What is the anatomy of the spleen?

- The spleen lies in the LUQ of the abdomen, below the diaphragm & under the 9th–11th ribs.
- It is intraperitoneal & closely related to the stomach, left kidney & pancreas.
- Arterial supply is from the splenic artery, a branch of the coeliac trunk *(see anatomy chapter)*.
- Venous drainage is via the splenic vein, which joins with the superior mesenteric vein to form the portal vein.

Q: What are the functions of the spleen?

Function	Notes
Cell Filtration & Removal	WBCs, platelets & RBCs. This is part of the reticuloendothelial system.
Storage	30% of Platelets.
Protection	Against Capsulated Organisms.
Synthesis	Antibody & Opsonin.

Q: What are the indications for a splenectomy?

- **Trauma** *(also see radiology chapter – case 14)*
- **Haematological Disorders:** Hereditary spherocytosis, thalassaemia major, ITP, myeloproliferative disorders.
- **Iatrogenic Injury**
- **Parenchyma Pathology:** Abscess, cyst, tumour.
- **Vascular Pathology:** Renal vein thrombosis.

Q: When should splenic trauma be suspected?

The spleen is most commonly injured in blunt abdominal trauma, usually following a RTA. Suspicion should be raised with left hypochondrium pain, shoulder tip pain & the presence of left-sided lower rib fractures.

Q: How is an elective open splenectomy performed?

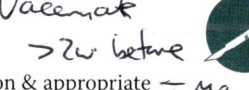

- Full pre-operative assessment including history, examination & appropriate investigations.
- Explain operation to patient & obtain informed consent.
- Patient supine under GA.
- Prophylactic antibiotics.
- Skin preparation & draping.
- Left subcostal incision.
- Systematically assess abdominal contents including the spleen itself, liver, lymph nodes & search for accessory spleneculi.
- Enter the lesser sac through the greater omentum.
- Divide adhesions between the spleen & parietal peritoneum.
- Cut the left leaf of the lienorenal ligament.
- Draw the spleen forward & medially, dissecting it free from the splenic flexure of the colon, diaphragm & tail of the pancreas.
- Incise the gastrosplenic ligament & divide the short gastric vessels.

- Double clamp the splenic vessels at the hilum, ligate & divide the splenic artery, then vein to 'deflate' the spleen.
- Divide any remaining peritoneal attachments & remove the spleen.
- Haemostasis.
- Suction drain.
- Layered closure.

Q: What are the operative principles of laparoscopic splenectomy?

- Full pre-operative assessment including history, examination & appropriate investigations.
- Explain operation to patient & obtain informed consent (including conversion to open procedure).
- Patient position under GA depends on approach e.g. anterolateral / posterior.
- Prophylactic antibiotics.
- Skin preparation & draping.

Anterolateral approach:

- Preferred due to decreased operative time, post-operative stay, transfusions & port sites.
- Obtain pneumoperitoneum under direct vision (Hassan Method) & insert ports (Fig 6.5):
    - Subumbilical (10mm).
    - Epigastric (10mm).
    - Left mid-clavicular line, inferior to the costal margin (5mm).
    - Left anterior axillary line, inferior to the costal margin (5mm).
- Systematically assess abdominal contents including the spleen itself, liver, lymph nodes & search for accessory spleneculi.
- Divide peritoneal reflections & adhesions using a diathermy hook.
- Thin hilar structures to allow placement of an endoscopic stapler to divide the splenic artery & vein.
- Use the endoscopic stapler again to divide the short gastric vessels.
- Free any remaining attachments, place the spleen in a retrieval bag & extract from abdominal cavity.
- Haemostasis.
- Remove ports under direct vision.
- Suction drain as appropriate.
- Close muscle, fascia & skin of port sites.

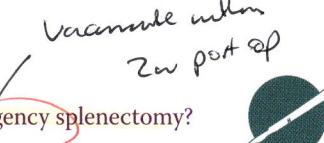

Q: How would you manage a patient who requires emergency splenectomy?

[handwritten note: Vaccinate within 2w post op]

- ATLS resuscitation (trauma situation).
- 4U blood cross match.
- Pre-operative assessment, history, examination & appropriate investigations are performed within the context of ATLS resuscitation.
- Explain operation to patient & obtain informed consent as indicated.
- Patient supine under GA.
- Prophylactic antibiotics.
- Skin preparation & draping.
- Upper midline incision, through skin, fat, fascia, linea alba, extraperitoneal fat & peritoneum.
- Enter the intraperitoneal cavity & confirm the spleen is the source of haemorrhage.
- Evacuate obvious clots.
- Assess whether the spleen may be conserved or requires partial or complete removal:
    - Minor capsular tears may be treated with haemostatic agents alone.
    - Deeper lacerations may be treated with synthetic absorbable sutures, using omentum to prevent sutures cutting through.
    - For partial splenectomy, the spleen is mobilised, the segmental vessels are ligated & divided at the hilum, the capsule is then incised at the point of transection with use of fingers to assist resection of the upper / lower pole. Synthetic absorbable sutures are used to achieve haemostasis.
    - If splenic damage is severe or bleeding continues after repair / partial resection, proceed to total splenectomy. This is performed as for an elective operation, however the splenic vessels are ligated as early as possible.
- Haemostasis.
- Suction drain.
- Layered closure.

Q: List the specific complications of splenectomy?

Operative	Spleen Removal
Haemorrhage	Thrombcytosis & Leukocytosis *↑Plt + WCC*
Injury to Adjacent Organs e.g. Pancreas Tail	Overwhelming Post-Splenectomy Infection
Gastric / Pancreatic Fistula	Portal Vein Thrombosis
Subphrenic Collection / Abscess	

Q: What actions should be taken to avoid overwhelming post-splenectomy infection (OPSI)?

- Vaccination against *Streptococcus pneumoniae*, *Haemophilus influenzae* type B & *Meningococcus* types A & C as follows:
    - **Elective:** ≥14 days pre-operatively.
    - **Emergency:** <14 days post-operatively.
- Immunocompromised patients, with an intact but non-functional spleen, should be vaccinated as soon as the diagnosis is made.
- Life-long prophylactic oral antibiotics are recommended following splenectomy in the UK (phenoxymethylpenicillin / erythromycin if penicillin allergic). There is evidence supporting discontinuation after 2 years, when the risk of OPSI is less.

Appendicectomy

Q: Can you briefly describe the anatomy of the appendix?

- Blind-ended tube.
- Originates from the caecum at the intersection of the 3 taeniae coli.
- Lies 2cm inferior to the ileo-caecal junction.
- Suspended by the meso-appendix, containing the appendicular vessels.

Q: What is appendicitis?

- Obstruction of the appendicular lumen causes include e.g. idiopathic, faeces, faecolith, tumour.
- Inflammation ensues, starting in the mucosa extending out through the submucosal, muscular & peritoneal layers.
- Gangrene & perforation may occur, causing localised (if contained by omentum) / spreading peritonitis.

Q: How is appendicitis diagnosed?

- Full History.
- Thorough Clinical Examination:
    - Central Abdominal Pain → Localising to RIF → Localising to McBurney's Point (⅓ the distance from the ASIS to umbilicus).
    - Associated Nausea, Vomiting, Anorexia, Fever.
    - Bowel Habit Change.
    - Patient Looks Unwell / Septic.
    - Appendix Mass.
- Appropriate Investigations:

Investigation	Notes
Urine	Urinalysis & Preganancy Test (rule out other potential causes)
Blood	FBC & CRP (appendicites rarely present of both are normal)
Imaging	USS (excludes gynaecological pathology)
	CT / MRI (high sensitivity)
Surgical	Exploratory Laparotomy (particularly female patients)

Q: What is the differential diagnosis for appendicitis?

- Crohn's Disease
- Meckel's Diverticulum.
- Urological Pathology.
- Gynaecological Pathology e.g. Ectopic Pregnancy, Ovarian Cyst, PID.
- Caecal Tumour & Diverticulitis (elderly patients).

Note: Young children may present atypically, so a high index of suspicion is required.

Q: How is an open appendicectomy performed?

- Full pre-operative assessment including history, examination & appropriate investigations.
- Explain operation to patient & obtain informed consent.
- Patient positioned supine under GA.
- Skin preparation & draping.
- IV antibiotics.
- Incision over McBurney's Point (transverse / modified Lanz incisions are preferred over gridiron).
- Open the 3 layers of the abdominal wall along the lines of the fibres:
  - External oblique aponeurosis
  - Internal oblique
  - Transversus abdominus.
- Open the peritoneum, swab & send pus for MC+S.
- Locate caecum & follow taeniae coli down to identify the appendix.
- Dunhill's Foreceps to appendix base, ligate & divide the meso-appendix.
- 2 x ties to appendix base, divide appendix between these & remove.
- Insert purse string suture near the appendix base after stump diathermy.
- Peritoneal lavage (for perforation / free pus).
- Close the peritoneum & then close each layer of the abdominal wall, followed by the skin.

Q: How is a laparoscopic appendicectomy performed?

- Full pre-operative assessment including history, examination & appropriate investigations.
- Explain operation to patient & obtain informed consent (including conversion to open procedure).
- Patient positioned supine (slight head down tilt) under GA.
- Skin preparation & draping.
- IV antibiotics.
- Obtain pneumoperitoneum under direct vision (Hassan Method) & insert ports (Fig 6.5):
  - Subumbilical (10mm)
  - Right hypochondrium (5mm)
  - Left iliac fossa (5mm).
- Identify appendix & examine all pelvic / abdominal organs (to exclude differential diagnoses).
- Improve access by placing the patient head down & right side up.
- Grasp the appendix, break down adhesions & divide the mesoappendix using diathermy / clips.
- Secure the base of the appendix with endoloop sutures, place 2 close to the caecum & 1 more distal.
- Divide the appendix & remove through subumbilical port (retrieval bags are necessary if there is evidence of contamination).
- Peritoneal lavage (for perforation / free pus).
- Check pelvis, sub-hepatic & sub-phrenic spaces for fluid collections.
- Remove ports under direct vision.
- Close muscle, fascia & skin of port sites.

Q: What is an appendix mass?

This is usually a late presentation of appendicitis, secondary to appendix perforation & subsequent abscess formation.

Q: What specific treatment options are there for an appendix mass?

After taking a full history & performing a thorough clinical examination, diagnosis may be confirmed with USS / CT. IV antibiotics & percutaneous drainage are usually effective at resolving appendicular abscesses. Open drainage is only required if percutaneous drainage fails & the patient becomes increasingly septic & unwell.

Note: There is currently no consensus on the optimal surgical treatment for an appendicular mass. Conventionally, patients were re-admitted for an interval appendicectomy after 1–2 months (the need for this has recently been questioned). Many patients are now treated entirely with non-operative management & it is uncommon for recurrent appendicitis to develop.

Inguinal Hernia Repair

(also see anatomy chapter)

Q: What are the indications for inguinal hernia repair?

- Incarceration
- Symptomatic e.g. Discomfort, Obstruction, Strangulation
- Patient's Request e.g. Quality of Life Impact.

Q: How is an indirect inguinal hernia repaired using a synthetic mesh (Lichtenstein's Repair)?

- Full pre-operative assessment including history, examination & appropriate investigations.
- Explain operation to patient, obtain informed consent & confirm correct side.
- Patient supine under GA / LA as appropriate.
- Skin preparation & draping.
- Incision 2cm above the medial ⅔ of the inguinal ligament.
- Incise skin, subcutaneous fat, Camper's Fascia & Scarpa's Fascia.
- Carefully open the inguinal canal to the superficial ring, using scissors to cut along the fibres of external oblique.
- Identify & protect the ilioinguinal nerve & spermatic cord.
- Dissect hernial sac free.
- Careful herniotomy, examine bowel contents & transfix the neck of the sac at the deep ring, returning the hernia to the abdominal cavity.
- Lichtenstein's Repair uses a Prolene™ mesh, cut to form a 'fish tail' that is loosely encircled & sutured around the spermatic cord. The mesh is placed on the posterior wall of the inguinal canal & sutured to the pubic tubercle, inguinal ligament & conjoint tendon.
- External oblique is closed, with the remaining wound closed in layers.
- Ensure testis is within scrotum.

Q: What are the complications of inguinal hernia repair?

Immediate	Early	Late
Haemorrhage	Haematoma	Testicular Ischaemia / Atrophy
Ilioinguinal Nerve Injury	Urinary Retention	Recurrence
	Wound Infection	Mesh Infection

Q: What other types of repair do you know?

Repair	Description
Shouldice	Double breasting of transversalis fascia.
Mesh Plug	Simply laying Prolene™ mesh over the deep ring.
Herniotomy	In paediatric patients, sac is transfixed & excised only.
Darn Repair	Uncommon, posterior wall of inguinal canal is reinforced with non-absorbable sutures.
Bassini	Conjoint tendon opposed to inguinal ligament.
Laparoscopic	Particularly for bilateral / recurrent herniae.

Femoral Hernia Repair
(also see anatomy chapter)

Q: What are the indications for femoral hernia repair?

All femoral hernias must be operated due to the risk of incarceration & strangulation.

Q: What common approaches do you know of for repair of a femoral hernia?

Approach	Notes
Lockwood (Low)	Elective cases only.
McEvedy (High)	Emergency cases where there is suspicion of strangulation.

Q: How is a femoral hernia repaired using a low (Lockwood) approach?

- Full pre-operative assessment including history, examination & appropriate investigations.
- Explain operation to patient, obtain informed consent & confirm correct side.
- Patient supine under GA.
- Skin preparation & draping.
- Groin crease incision from mid-inguinal point to symphysis pubis.
- Incise skin, subcutaneous fat, fascia & expose the hernial sac.
- Dissect sac free & examine for bowel contents (anaesthesia may result in spontaneous reduction of incarcerated herniae).
- If the hernia is incarcerated, dilate the ligamentous margins of the sac, enabling reduction.

- Herniotomy.
- Inspect bowel for viability & resect if necessary.
- Transfix sac at neck & excise 1cm distally.
- Protect the femoral vessels laterally.
- Approximate & suture the inguinal & pectineal ligaments, extending 1cm laterally to the defect, using a J-shaped needle.
- Layered closure.

Q: How is a femoral hernia repaired using a high (McEvedy) approach?

The procedure essentially follows the same repair technique, however the incision is different, to allow access to strangulated bowel:

- Full pre-operative assessment including history, examination & appropriate investigations.
- Explain operation to patient, obtain informed consent & confirm correct side.
- Patient supine under GA.
- Skin preparation & draping.
- Oblique incision above the pubic tubercle, crossing the rectus sheath laterally.
- Incise skin, subcutaneous fat, Camper's Fascia, Scarpa's Fascia, anterior rectus sheath, transversalis fascia (note there is no posterior rectus sheath below the arcuate line).
- Retract rectus muscle medially, incise transversalis fascia & peritoneum.
- Herniotomy.
- Inspect bowel for viability & resect if necessary.
- Herniorrhaphy.
- Protect the femoral vessels laterally.
- Suture the inguinal ligament to the pectineal ligament.
- Layered closure.

Q: What is intestinal stenosis of Garre?

Stenosis of the small bowel. Results from healing of a mucosal ulcer by fibrosis during a period of strangulation. It may also result in small bowel obstruction.

Haemorrhoidectomy

Q: What is the pathology & aetiology of haemorrhoids?

Haemorrhoids are excessively dilated anal cushions (3, 7 & 11 o'clock in the lithotomy position) that may compromise the anorectal mucosa, submucosal tissue & blood vessels (small arterioles & veins). There are 3 cushions providing a conforming seal when the internal anal sphincter is contracted. The degeneration of the fibroblastic tissue & smooth muscle results in prolapse.

The most common age of onset is young adulthood & they are more common with:

- Constipation
- Chronic straining
- Obesity
- Previous childbirth.

Diagnosis requires a full history, thorough clinical examination including PR, proctoscopy & rigid sigmoidoscopy. **Note: Rectal bleeding cannot be dismissed as haemorrhoids until thoroughly investigated.**

Q: How can haemorrhoids be classified?

Grade	Symptoms
I	Non-prolapsing. May present with bleeding, pruritis ani & perianal discomfort.
II	Prolapse on defecation, but reduce spontaneously.
III	Prolapse, but require manual reduction.
IV	Prolapse, non-reducible.

Q: What treatments are available for haemorrhoids?

Modality	Treatment
Conservative	• Avoid Constipation. • Avoid Straining. • Dietary Fibre.
Medical	• Topical Preparations. • Bulking Agents. • Laxatives.
Surgical	• **Injection Sclerotherapy:** 5% solution of phenol in almond oil injected into the submucosa of each haemorrhoid. • **Infrared Photocoagulation.** • **Band Ligation:** Best for prolapse symptoms. • **Stapled Anopexy:** Can be used for circumferential prolapsing haemorrhoids. • **Haemorrhoidectomy:** For large haemorrhoids / those not responding to conservative or medical treatment.

Q: How is a haemorrhoidectomy performed?

- Full pre-operative assessment including history, examination & appropriate investigations.
- Explain operation to patient & obtain informed consent.
- Pre-operative bowel preparation with enemas / rectal washout.
- Patient supine in lithotomy position, under GA.
- Skin preparation & draping as appropriate.
- Anal canal inspection & palpation using a Park's Bivalve Anal Speculum.
- Infiltrate LA with adrenaline at the planned incision site.
- Grasp haemorrhoid with forceps & make an external V-incision into perianal mucosa & skin.
- Carefully dissect mucosa & haemorrhoid off of underlying internal sphincter until the pedicle is located.
- Transfix haemorrhoid base to dissected mucosal pedicle to ligate, then divide using diathermy.
- Repeat for additional haemorrhoids.
- Appropriate skin bridges should be left between excision sites in order to prevent stenosis.
- Pack anal canal with suitable dressing.

Note: Post-operatively prescribe bulking agents, laxatives & analgesia to avoid constipation.

Q: What are the complications of haemorrhoidectomy?

Immediate	Early	Late
Haemorrhage	Urinary Retention	Recurrence
Pain	Constipation	Anal Stenosis
		Impaired Continence
		Anal Fissure
		Anal Fistula

Suprapubic Catheterisation

Q: What systems of introducing a suprapubic catheter are available?

- 'Nottingham' Introducer (uses trocar).
- Banano (based on Seldinger technique).

Q: What are the contraindications of suprapubic catheterisation?

Absolute	Relative
Absence of Distended Bladder on Palpation / USS	Clotting Disorders
	Previous Lower Abdominal / Pelvic Surgery
	Pelvic Cancer ± Previous Radiotherapy

Q: How is suprapubic catheterisation performed?

- Full pre-procedure assessment including history, examination & appropriate investigations.
- Explain procedure to patient & obtain informed consent.
- Patient supine (consider sedation).
- Palpate & percuss the abdomen to confirm a full bladder.
- Skin preparation & draping.
- Antibiotic prophylaxis.
- LA infiltration into skin & subcutaneous tissues in the midline, 2cm above the pubic symphysis in the area of dullness to percussion previously identified.
- Introduce a needle 2cm above the pubic symphysis, aiming caudally & aspirate for urine.
- Make a 1cm incision with a scalpel blade over the needle mark.
- Stabilise lower abdominal wall with non-dominant hand.
- Push the trocar & sheath from the suprapubic set through the hole into the bladder (a give is felt as the bladder is entered).
- Remove the trocar, pass the catheter through the sheath & inflate the balloon.
- Remove the sheath & apply a dressing to the entry point of the catheter.
- Connect the catheter to the collection system.

Q: What are the complications of suprapubic catheterisation?

Immediate	Early	Late
Failure	Infection (wound / UTI)	Blockage
Haemorrhage	Haematuria	Calculus
Bowel Perforation		Inflammatory Change
Misplacement		Carcinoma

Renal Trauma & Nephrectomy

Q: What clinical findings suggest renal injury?

- Trauma History
- Penetrating Trauma / Bruising to Loin Region
- Hypotension
- Micro / Macroscopic Haematuria.

Q: How is renal trauma graded?

All trauma must be treated according to ATLS protocol:

Grade	Injury Type	Injury Description	Treatment
I	• Minor Contusion Only.	• Contusion / Contained Subcapsular Haematoma. • Microscopic / Gross Haematuria.	Conservative. Bed Rest until Haematuria Settles.
II	• Minor Parenchyma Laceration. • No Collecting System Involvement.	• Non Expanding Perirenal Haematoma. • Cortical Laceration <1cm Deep. • No Extravasation of Urine.	Bed Rest & Prophylactic Antibiotics.
III	• Major Parenchyma Laceration. • No Collecting System Involvement.	• Parenchyma Laceration Extending <1cm into Renal Cortex. • No Extravasation of Urine.	Do Equally Well with Conservative / Surgical Management.
IV	• Major Parenchyma Laceration. • Collecting System Involvement.	• Parenchyma Laceration Extending >1 cm thorough Renal Cortex, Medulla & Collecting Systems. • ± Contained Renal Pedicle Haematoma.	Surgical Intervention Required. Lacerations to the Parenchyma are Usually Repairable.
V	• Renal Pedicle Injury.	• Multiple Major Lacerations. • Avulsed Renal Pedicle. • Thrombosis of Renal Artery.	Surgical Intervention Required. Renal Pedicle Injuries Usually Require Nephrectomy.

Q: What are the indications for renal trauma surgery?

- Type IV–V injuries.
- Blunt injuries with large renal lacerations & extravasation.
- Haemodynamically unstable patient with major renal injury.

Q: What are the anatomical relations of the kidney?

Relation	Structures
Anterior	**Left Kidney:** Stomach, spleen, pancreas, descending colon. **Right Kidney:** Liver, 2nd part of duodenum, ascending colon.
Posterior	Diaphragm, quadratus lumborum, psoas major, transversus abdominis, 12th rib, subcostal nerve, ilio-hypogastric nerve, ilio-inguinal (L1) nerve.
Medial	Renal hilum (renal vein, artery, ureter & lymphatics).
Lateral	Costodiaphragmatic recess.

Q: What are the indications for different operative approaches for nephrectomy?

Choice is influenced by the indication for nephrectomy & surgeon's preference:

Approach	Indication
Anterior Abdominal	• Renal Trauma. • Large RCC.
Loin	• Non-Functioning Kidney. • Renal Mass.
Laparoscopic	• Benign & Malignant Disease e.g. Cysts, Mass, Non-Functioning Kidney.

Q: What is the difference between a simple & radial nephrectomy?

Nephrectomy	Notes
Simple	Removal of kidney only.
Radical	Removal of kidney, upper ureter, Gerota's Fascia, adrenal glands & lymphatics.

Q: How would you perform a radical nephrectomy using an anterior abdominal approach?

- Full pre-operative assessment including history & examination & appropriate investigations.
- Explain operation to patient, obtain informed consent & confirm correct side.
- Patient supine under GA.
- Patient catheterised.
- Abdomen prepared & draped as for laparotomy.
- Cystoscopy performed & involved ureter circumscribed with diathermy.
- Midline laparotomy incision.
- Divide peritoneal reflection (lies lateral to colon) & retract colon medially to reveal perinephric fat.
- Clamp renal artery.
- Ligate & divide renal vein.
- Transfix & divide renal artery.
- Free ureter along its course by blunt dissection to the distal end.
- Kidney dissected off posterior wall tissue by mobilising it medially.
- Haemostasis.
- Insert suction drains.
- Specimen sent for histology.
- Abdomen closed in layers.

Q: How would you perform a left radical nephrectomy using a loin approach?

- Full pre-operative assessment including history & examination & appropriate investigations.
- Explain operation to patient, obtain informed consent & confirm correct side.
- Patient under GA in right lateral position with table broken (head & feet lowered) to increase access between ribs & pelvic rim.
- Patient catheterised.
- Incision running parallel to the 12th rib on its upper border (from midline to posterior axillary line).
- 12th rib visualised.
- Divide skin, fat, fascia, latissimus dorsi, external oblique, internal oblique & quadratus lumborum to reveal perinephric fat.
- Bluntly dissect perinephric fat to reveal ureter & gonadal vessels.
- Ligate & divide ureter.
- Mobilise kidney, leaving it attached by its pedicle only.
- Clamp, ligate & divide the renal vein, then artery.

- Remove specimen & send for histology.
- Haemostasis.
- Insert suction drains.
- Wound closed in layers.
- Appropriate dressing.

Q: What specific imaging should be ordered prior to performing a nephrectomy?

- CT
- IVU
- Isotope Scan e.g. DMSA / MAG3 (for differential function).

This is to determine if the patient has a contralateral functioning kidney. Many patients may have a single kidney / single functioning kidney either congenitally, due to pyelonephritis or organ donation.

Testicular Torsion
(also see book 2)

Q: Can you describe the operative steps for exploration & repair of testicular torsion?

- Full pre-operative assessment including history, examination & appropriate investigations.
- Explain operation to patient, obtain informed consent & confirm correct side.
- Patient supine under GA.
- Skin preparation & draping.
- Affected testis grasped & pressed against scrotal skin so that tissues are tense.
- Midline scrotal raphe incision (or transverse incision on affected side of hemiscrotum).
- Cut through encountered layers of scrotal approach *(see below)*.
- Open tunica vaginalis & inspect colour, cord, epididymis, testicular & epididymal appendages.
- Affected testis untwisted & wrapped in warm gauze for 10 minutes to assess viability.
- If testis is non-viable, despite detorsion & warming, an orchidectomy is performed.
- If testis is viable, return to scrotum & fix via 1 of the following methods:
    - **3 x Point Fixation:** To scrotal wall / tunica with non-absorbable suture e.g. Prolene™.
    - **Dartos Pouch Formation:** Testis inserted sub-dartos muscle, which obviates need for fixation.
- The contralateral testis should be explored & repaired (the underlying predisposing clapper-bell deformity is likely to be bilateral).
- Haemostasis.

- Skin closure with interrupted absorbable sutures.
- Dress loosely with non-adherent dressing.

Q: What anatomical structures do you pass through during a scrotal approach to the testis (Fig 6.6)?

- Scrotal Skin
- Dartos Fascia
- External Spermatic Fascia (continuation of external oblique)
- Cremasteric Muscle in Cremasteric Fascia (continuation of internal oblique)
- Internal Spermatic Fascia (continuation of transversalis)
- Parietal Tunica Vaginalis (continuation of parietal peritoneum)
- Visceral Tunica Vaginalis (continuation of visceral peritoneum)
- Tunica Albuginea
- Testis.

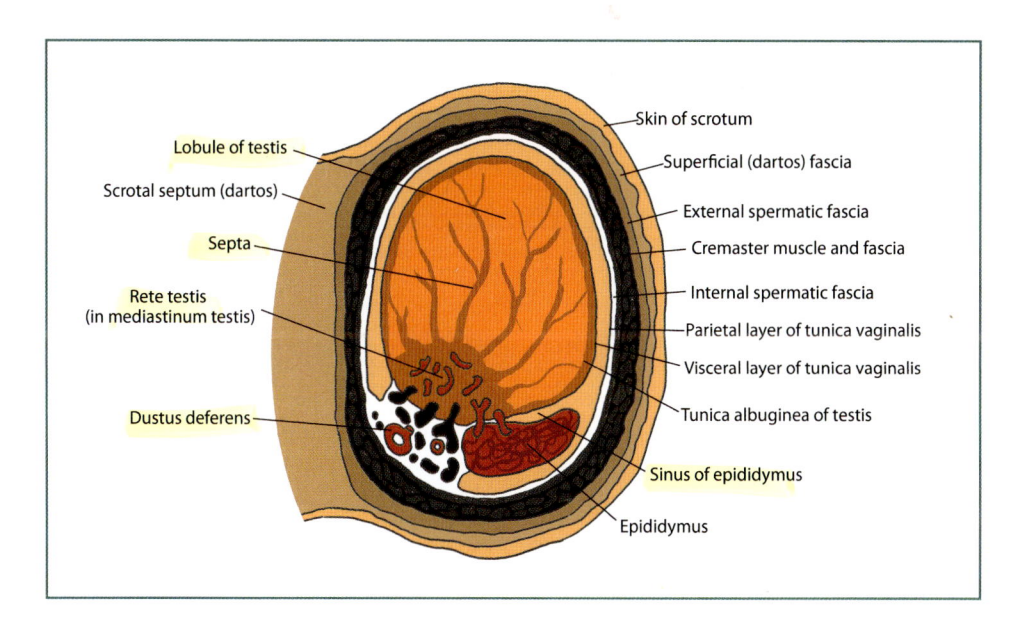

Fig 6.6: Cross section through the scrotum & testis.

Orchidectomy

Q: What is the blood supply to the testis?

- The testicular arteries arise directly from the aorta.
- The artery of the vas deferens is derived from the inferior vesical artery, a branch of the internal iliac artery.

Q: What is the lymphatic drainage of testis & scrotum?

- Testes drain to the para-aortic lymph nodes.
- Scrotal skin drains to the inguinal lymph nodes.

Q: What approach would you use to perform an orchidectomy?

Approach	Example
Scrotal Midline Approach	Exploration for possible testicular torsion.
Inguinal Approach	For testicular tumours: • Testicular tumours spread via lymphatics to the para-aortic lymph nodes, a scrotal approach may result in seeding of tumour cells that may then disseminate to an additional lymphatic field (inguinal lymph nodes). • The inguinal approach allows for cord clamping & prevents the risk of dissemination.

Q: How would you perform an orchidectomy?

- Full pre-operative assessment including history, examination & appropriate investigations.
- Explain operation to patient, obtain informed consent & confirm correct side.
- Patient supine under GA.
- Inguinal region & external genitalia preparation & draping.
- Groin skin crease incision through subcutaneous fat, Camper's & Scarpa's Fasciae.
- Identify external oblique fibres & divide from the superficial to deep inguinal ring.
- Identify spermatic cord, mobilise & cross clamp at the deep inguinal ring.
- The cord & testicle can be dissected free & removed from the scrotum.
- Specimen sent for histology.
- Transfix remaining cord.
- Insert testicular prosthesis into hemiscrotum.
- Haemostasis.
- Wound closure in layers.
- Dress loosely with non-adherent dressing.
- Scrotal support given for comfort.

Q: What are the complications of orchidectomy?

Immediate	Early	Late
Haemorrhage	Scrotal Haematoma	Subfertility
Ilioinguinal Nerve Injury	Infection	Psychological
	Wound Dehiscence	If Bilateral – Testosterone Effects are Lost

Circumcision

Q: What are the indications for circumcision?

Children	Adults
Phimosis	Paraphimosis
Recurrent Balanitis	Recurrent Balanitis
BXO	Prepuce Malignancy
Religious	

Q: Can you describe an operative method of performing circumcision?

- Full pre-operative assessment including history & examination & appropriate investigations.
- Explain operation to patient & obtain informed consent.
- Patient supine under a GA / LA (penile block).
- Skin preparation & draping.
- Retract prepuce, divide adhesions (adhesiolysis) & clean retained secretions.
- Place 2 artery forceps either side of distal prepuce.
- Perform a dorsal slit to a level just below the corona (Fig 6.7).
- Continue incision circumferentially towards frenulum.
- Lift frenulum & excise redundant prepuce.
- Transfixation suture to frenular artery.
- Haemostasis.
- Approximate remaining prepuce & tie with interrupted absorbable sutures.
- Dress loosely with non-adherent dressings e.g. paraffin gauze.

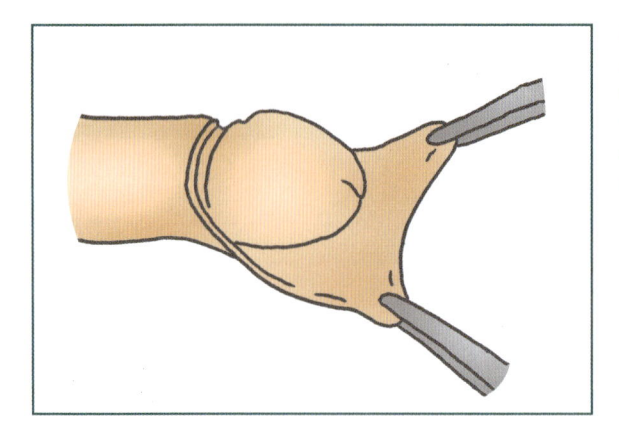

Fig 6.7: During circumcision, a dorsal slit is made in the prepuce, to a level just below the corona, with the incision then continued circumferentially towards the frenulum.

Q: Do you know of an alternative method in children?

The Plastibell Technique can be used safely for outpatient circumcision in children under LA. The Plastibell Circumcision Device is a clear plastic ring with a handle designed for male neonatal circumcision that has a deep groove running circumferentially:

- Full pre-procedure assessment including history & examination & appropriate investigations.
- Explain procedure to patient's parent(s) & obtain informed consent.
- Performed under LA with EMLA cream, penile ring block or dorsal penile nerve block.
- Skin preparation & draping.
- Adhesions between glans & prepuce are divided with a probe.
- The prepuce is cut longitudinally to allow retraction & glans exposure.
- An appropriately sized device is placed over the glans as far as the preputial reflection.
- The ring is then covered over by the prepuce.
- A ligature is tied circumferentially around the prepuce.
- This technique induces tissue necrosis by means of suture compression of the prepuce over a plastic ring that protects the glans.
- Post operatively no dressing is required & the child can be bathed normally.
- The skin sloughs off in 3–7 days & the ring separates.

Q: What are the complications of circumcision?

Immediate	Early	Late
Under Correction	Haemorrhage	External Urethral Meatal Stenosis
Over Correction	Infection	
Damage to Penile Shaft / Glans		

Vasectomy

Q: What are the important points when counselling a patient for vasectomy?

- Considered an irreversible method of sterilisation (reversal has poor results).
- Risk of spontaneous failure (1 in 2000 undergoes recanalisation of the divided vas deferens).
- Post-vasectomy pain syndrome may ensue:
    - Variable intensity genital pain that may be lifelong.
    - Occurs in 5% – 35% of patients.
    - May experience pain on intercourse, ejaculation, physical exertion, or tender epididymides.
- Not immediately effective. Alternative contraception is required until 2 separate samples of semen are negative of spermatozoa. This is usually analysed at 6 & 12 weeks post-vasectomy.

Q: How would you perform a vasectomy?

- Full pre-operative assessment including history & examination & appropriate investigations.
- Explain procedure to patient (Fig 6.8) & obtain informed consent.
- Patient supine under GA / LA.
- Skin preparation & draping.
- Palpate spermatic cord through scrotal skin to identify the vas deferens.
- Infiltrate LA at the incision site.
- Incise scrotal skin in the midline & free the vas deferens from the cord.
- Expose the vas deferens by clearing it of its coverings.
- Excise >2cm of the vas & send for histology.
- The 2 remaining cut ends should be retroflexed & tied separately.
- Repeat the procedure on the contralateral vas deferens.
- Return the ends of the vas deferens to the scrotum.
- Close the incision with a single absorbable suture.
- Apply dressing & scrotal support.

Q: What are the complications of a vasectomy?

Immediate	Early	Late
Haemorrhage	Pain	Post-Vasectomy Pain Syndrome
Damage to Structures e.g. Spermatic Cord	Bruising	Failure
	Oedema	Recanalisation
	Haematoma	Spermatocele
	Epididymitis / Orchitis	Psychological
	Haematospermia	

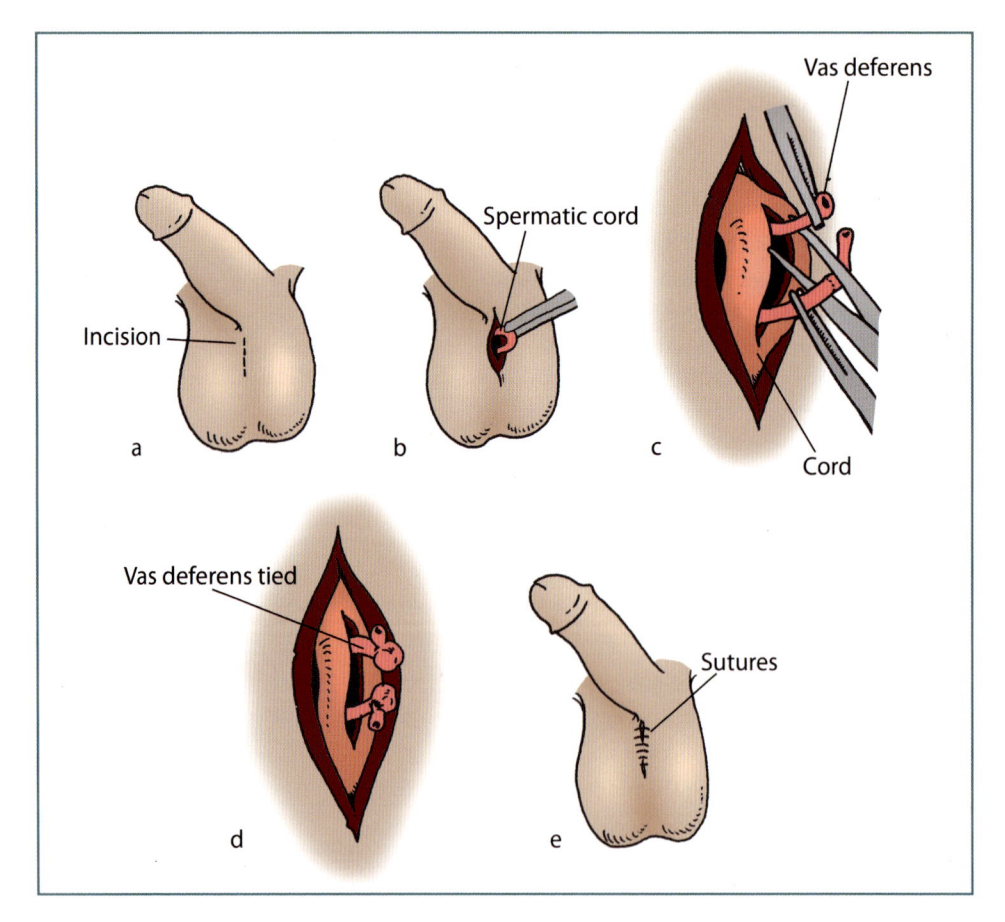

Fig 6.8: Operative steps for vasectomy. A midline incision is made (a), identification of the spermatic cord (b), exposure of the vas & delivery through the incision (c), cutting & retroflexion of the vas (d) & closure (e).

Hydrocoele Repair

(also see book 2).

Q: Can you briefly describe the operative treatment options for a hydrocoele?

- Full pre-operative assessment including history & examination & appropriate investigations.
- Explain operation to patient & obtain informed consent.
- Patient supine under GA.
- External genitalia preparation & draping.
- Incise scrotum over the hydrocoele.
- Incise tunica vaginalis & evacuate fluid.
- Deliver testis through opening in tunica & examine testis.
- Perform repair using absorbable sutures:
    - **Jaboulay's Procedure:** Evert tunica vaginalis edges & suture behind cord.
    - **Lord's Plication:** Plicate tunica vaginalis to epididymo-testicular junction.
- Return testis to scrotum.
- Haemostasis.
- Close scrotum with absorbable sutures.
- Apply non-adherent dressing & scrotal support.

LIMBS, SPINE & VASCULAR

Carpal Tunnel Decompression
(also see anatomy chapter)

Q: What is carpal tunnel syndrome?

Median nerve compression at the wrist as it passes under the flexor retinaculum (Fig 4.18). Symptoms include pain, paraesthesia & numbness in the radial 3½ digits, weakness & atrophy of the thenar muscles. Symptoms may be worse at night & provoked by activities involving prolonged gripping e.g. driving.

Q: What are the causes of carpal tunnel syndrome?

Idopathic	Endocrine / Hormonal	Inflammatory	Mechanical
Unknown	Pregnancy	Rheumatoid Arthritis	Osteophytes (OA)
	Hypothyroidism		Previous Fracture
	Acromegaly		
	DM		

Q: What are the management options for carpal tunnel syndrome?

Modality	Treatment
Conservative	• Address underlying cause
	• Night time splintage (30° wrist extension)
Medical	• Corticosteroid injection
Surgical	• Carpal tunnel decompression (open / endoscopic)

Q: How is open carpal tunnel decompression performed?

- Full pre-operative assessment including history & examination & appropriate investigations.
- Explain operation to patient, obtain informed consent & confirm correct side.
- LA (most commonly).
- Skin preparation & draping (including limb exsanguination & tourniquet inflation).
- Patient supine, arm abducted & placed on arm table.

- Longitudinal incision in line with the radial aspect of ring finger distal to the distal wrist crease, no further than the line of the 1st web space.
- Cut skin, fat, & palmar fascia.
- May insert a McDonald's Dissector under the flexor retinaculum to protect the median nerve.
- Divide the flexor retinaculum under direct vision, ensuring adequate release distally to the fat pad & proximally to antebrachial fascia.
- Observe the median nerve.
- Tourniquet release & haemostasis.
- Suture skin.
- Apply non-adherent dressing, wool & crepe bandage.
- Remove bandage 48 hours post-operatively & mobilise hand & wrist.

Q: What are the complications of carpal tunnel decompression?

Immediate Damage	Early	Late
Median Nerve (recurrent motor branch)	Haematoma	Incomplete Symptom Resolution
Palmar Arch (superficial & deep)	Infection	CRPS
Ulnar Nerve & Artery	Wound Dehiscence	Pillar Pain
		Recurrence of Symptoms

Approaches to Hip Joint

Q: How would you perform a hemiarthroplasty via an anterolateral (Harding) approach?

- Full pre-operative assessment including history & examination & appropriate investigations.
- Explain operation to patient, obtain informed consent & confirm correct side.
- Patient in lateral position under GA.
- Skin preparation & draping.
- Longitudinal skin incision 2.5 cm behind ASIS, to tip of greater trochanter.
- Extend incision vertically down along anterior margin of greater trochanter for 10–15 cm.
- Incise tensor fascia lata & divide gluteus medius.
- Access to femoral neck & capsule is gained. These are divided.
- Cut femoral neck with a power saw.
- Externally rotate leg to allow femoral head to be removed from the acetabulum.
- Measure femoral head size.

- Femoral shaft reamed, trial reduction attempted.
- Hammer in prosthesis to rest on calcar femorale.
- Reduce hip & check stability.
- Repair muscles.
- Close skin.
- Check X-ray in 24h to confirm prosthesis position.

Q: Can you briefly outline the common approaches to the hip joint, indicating those nerves that are at risk of immediate damage?

Anterolateral (Hardinge) Approach *(see previous question)*

Most common approach.

Access between tensor fascia lata & gluteus medius.

Superior gluteal nerve is at risk (supplies gluteus medius & minimus, such that division causes loss of hip abduction & Trendelenberg gait).

Posterior Approach

2nd most common approach.

Skin incision centred on posterior aspect of greater trochanter & curved proximally towards the PSIS.

Dissect through subcutaneous tissue.

Split gluteus maximus along its fibres.

Identify & retract piriformis (the superior gluteal artery is above, the inferior gluteal artery & sciatic nerve are below).

Divide the short external rotator muscles at their insertion at the medial aspect of the greater trochanter (piriformis, gemelli & obturator internus). Repair is then advisable.

Sciatic nerve is at risk.

Anterior (Smith-Peterson) Approach

Used in paediatric orthopaedics to correct congenital dislocation of the hip.

Skin incision from 2cm below midpoint of iliac crest, curved inferiorly to ASIS & extended distally.

Between tensor fascia lata (superior gluteal nerve at risk) & sartorius (femoral nerve at risk).

Divide rectus femoris & anterior ⅓ of the gluteus medius.

Lateral femoral cutaneous nerve of thigh is at risk.

Lateral Approach

Skin incision centred on greater trochanter. Incision extended proximally in line with fibres of gluteus medius & distally in line with the femur.

Involves splitting tensor fascia lata, gluteus medius & minimus (short external hip rotators).

Superior gluteal nerve is at risk.

Medial Approach
Between adductor longus & gracilis.
Then between adductor magnus & brevis.
Posterior branch of obturator nerve is at risk.

Q: What are the complications of hemiarthoplasty?

Immediate	Early	Late
Acetabulum / Femur Fracture	Dislocation	Dislocation
Haemorrhage	Infection	Infection
Neurovascular Damage	DVT/ PE	Loosening
	Fat Embolism	Periprosthetic Fracture
		Leg Length Discrepancy

Zadek's Procedure & Ingrown Toenail

Q: What is an ingrown toenail?

A condition where the nail plate grows into the lateral nail fold. It is often painful & presents with signs of infection or inflammation.

Q: What are the treatments for an ingrown toenail?

Conservative	Surgical
Good Nail Care	Simple Nail Avulsion: • *For acutely infected toenails* • *High incidence of recurrence*
Cut Nail Transversely	Wedge Excision: • *Excision of affected nail segment & nail bed down to periosteum*
Analgesia	Zadek's Procedure: • *Total radical excision of nail & nail bed*
Antiseptic Dressings	

Q: How is Zadek's Procedure performed?

- Full pre-operative assessment including history & examination & appropriate investigations.
- Explain operation to patient, obtain informed consent & confirm correct digit.
- GA / LA ring block with 1% plain lignocaine.
- Skin preparation & draping (including digital tourniquet).
- Remove nail plate from nail bed.
- 2 small incisions are made at the corners of the nail bed, extending to the distal skin crease.
- The skin flaps are raised to expose the germinal matrix.
- Excise germinal matrix & curette the nail bed down to the periosteum.
- 80% phenol may then be used to abate any remaining germinal matrix (wash away with surgical spirit after 2–3 minutes).
- Tourniquet release.
- Haemostasis.
- Suture skin flaps.
- Apply non-adherent dressing.
- Post-operative advice includes leg elevation for 1 day & mobilisation as pain allows.

Q: What are the contraindications to this procedure?

- Acute Infection
- Peripheral Vascular Disease.

Q: What are the complications of surgery?

Early	Late
Pain	Recurrence
Wound Infection	Osteomeylitis (rare)
	Septic Arthritis (rare)

Fasciotomy & Compartment Syndrome

Q: What is compartment syndrome?

Discrete osteofascial compartments exist within the limbs. Pressure may become elevated within these compartments, usually following trauma e.g. tibial fracture. The following events occur:

- Increased compartment pressure.
- Increased venous pressure / reduced venule (not arteriole) diameter.
- Decreased arterio-venous pressure gradient.
- Decreased tissue perfusion.
- Tissue necrosis e.g. nerve & muscle.

It is a surgical emergency, requiring urgent decompression.

Q: What are the clinical features of compartment syndrome?

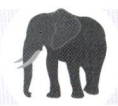

Memory: 6 x P's of compartment syndrome

Clinical Feature	Notes
Pain	Out of proportion to injury & often resistant to potent analgesia e.g. opiates. Pain is worse on passive muscle stretch. These are early signs.
Pressure	A difference of ≤30mmHg between compartment & diastolic pressures.
Paraesthesia / Sensory Loss	May be a useful early sign in nerves crossing involved compartments.
Pallor	Late sign.
Pulselessness	Late sign.
Paralysis	Late sign.

Q: What may present as a diagnostic difficulty?

Unconscious patients / patients with nerve blocks. In these or equivocal cases, consider measuring intra-compartmental pressure.

Q: How would you perform a lower leg fasciotomy?

I would use a 2-incision technique:

- Full pre-operative assessment including history & examination & appropriate investigations.
- Explain operation to patient, obtain informed consent & confirm correct side.
- Patient supine under GA or spinal anaesthesia.
- Skin preparation & draping.
- 2 x Incisions:
    - 2cm posterior to medial border of tibia (decompress superficial & deep posterior compartments).
    - 2cm lateral to anterior border of tibia (decompress anterior & lateral compartments).
- Debride devitalised tissue.
- Haemostasis.
- Do not suture wounds.
- Non-adherent dressing, wool & crepe bandage.
- 2nd look in 48h.

Q: What are the complications of fasciotomy?

Immediate	Early	Late
Haemorrhage	Haematoma	Aesthetic
Nerve Damage e.g. Saphenous Nerve	Inadequate Decompression	Osteomyelitis
Vascular Damage e.g. LSV, Arterial Perforators	Infection	Septic Arthritis
	Open wound	

Note: The complications of untreated compartment syndrome e.g. tissue ischaemia, Volkmann's Ischaemic Contracture, pain syndromes or growth disturbances in children, are extremely serious.

Tendon Repair

Q: What are the salient elements of the history & clinical examination, when assessing soft tissue injuries of the hand?

Assess all trauma cases as per ATLS protocol & consider the following within this framework:

History	Clinical Examination
Age	Posture of Hand / Digits (cascade)
Hand Dominance	Active & Passive Movements of Joints
Occupation	Distal Perfusion
Mechanism of Injury	Sensation
(blunt, sharp, contamination, associated injuries)	
Past Medical History	
Smoking History	
Last Meal	
Allergies	

Q: How would you repair a flexor tendon in a finger?

- Full pre-operative assessment including history & examination & appropriate investigations.
- Explain operation to patient, obtain informed consent & confirm correct digit.
- Patient supine under GA / brachial plexus block.
- Skin preparation & draping (including limb exsanguination & tourniquet inflation).
- Patient supine, arm abducted & placed on arm table, with use of a lead hand.
- Extend wound using Brunner (zig-zag) or mid-axial incision.
- Examine FDS & FDP tendons, radial & ulnar neurovascular bundles for injuries.
- Irrigation.
- Place a core modified Kessler repair suture using e.g. 3-0 or 4-0 Prolene™ / Ethibond™ (Fig 6.9).
- Place a continuos epitendonous repair suture using e.g. 6-0 Prolene™ (Fig 6.9).
- Release tourniquet.
- Haemostasis.
- Skin closure.
- Non-adherent dressing over wound.
- Wool, crepe & extension blocking splint.

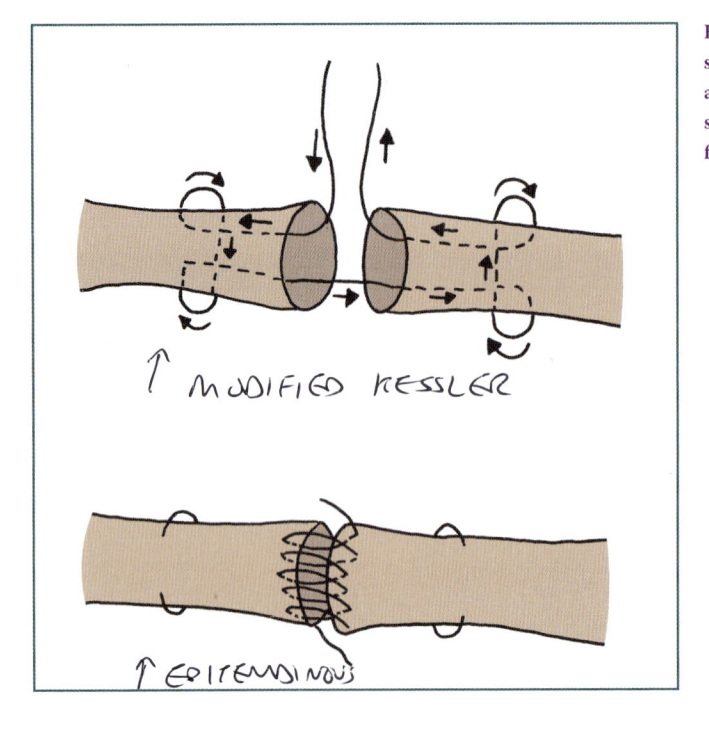

Fig 6.9: Modified Kessler suture (upper image) & an 'over & over' epitendinous suture repair (lower image) for flexor tendon injury.

Q: What post-operative advice would you give the patient?

- Hand therapy referral for early active finger mobilisation
- Protective splint for 6 weeks
- No heavy lifting for 3 months
- Stop smoking

Q: What are the complications of tendon repair?

Immediate	Early	Late
Bleeding	Haematoma	Scar Tenderness / Contracture
Neurovascular Damage	Tendon Rupture	Reduced ROM
	Infection	Adhesions
	Wound Dehiscence	CRPS

Amputations

Q: What are the indications for a lower limb amputation?

Classification	Example
Vascular	• Acute / Critical Ischaemia
	• Intractable Pain
	• Wet Gangrene
	• Non-Healing Ulcers (Particularly in Diabetic Patients)
Trauma	• Crush Injury
	• Unreconstructable Damage
Infection	• Necrotising Fasciitis
Malignancy	• Sarcoma
Function	• Insensate Limb
	• 'Useless' Limb

Q: How would you perform a below knee amputation (BKA)?

- Full pre-operative assessment including history & examination & appropriate investigations.
- Explain operation to patient, obtain informed consent & confirm correct side.
- Patient supine under GA, spinal or epidural anaesthesia.
- Skin preparation & draping.
- Incision for long posterior flap (Fig 6.10):
  - 8cm distal to tibial tuberosity anteriorly
  - 15cm distal to tibial tuberosity posteriorly
  - Extend vertically down the leg on either side & join across the calf, just above the origin of the Achilles tendon.
- Ligate & divide vessels as they are encountered.
- Divide nerves under tension.
- Elevate tibial periosteum & divide tibia with a Gigli saw.
- Bevel the tibial edges anteriorally to prevent 'sharp edge damage' to overlying soft tissue.
- Cut fibula 2cm proximal to the tibia (Fig 6.10).
- File the bone ends to provide smooth surfaces.
- The leg is hinged open to visualise the muscles of the posterior compartment.
- Divide posterior muscles obliquely.
- Ensure adequate haemostasis & insert suction drains as appropriate.

- Suture the posterior flap to the anterior flap & reduce size as necessary if it is too bulky, ensuring a tension free closure.
- Dress with wool & crepe bandages.
- Commence PT as soon as possible to prevent flexion contractures & to optimise mobility with prosthesis.

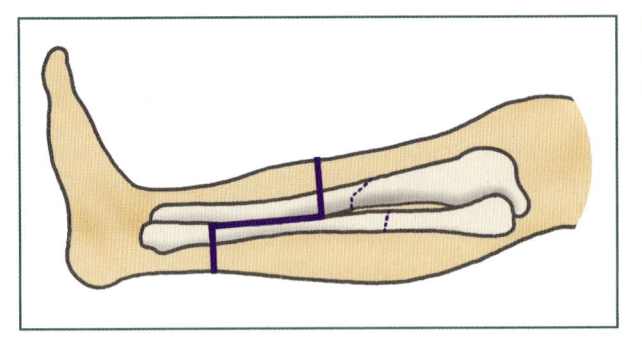

Fig 6.10: Below knee amputation incisions for posterior flap (also see book 2 vascular chapter).

Q: What other BKA flaps may be used?

- Skew Flap
- Equal Length Flap.

Q: What are the specific contraindications to a BKA?

Classification	Notes
Indication for Higher Amputation	Infection, Ischaemia, Malignancy, Insufficient Tissue to Leave Functional Stump >7-8cm.
Knee	OA, Flexion Contracture.
Lower Leg	Infection, Spasticity, Sensory Neuropathy.
Patient	Inability to Mobilise.

Q: How do you perform an above knee amputation (AKA)?

- Full pre-operative assessment including history & examination & appropriate investigations.
- Explain procedure to patient, obtain informed consent & confirm correct side.
- Patient supine under GA, spinal or epidural anaesthesia.
- Skin preparation & draping.
- Mark equal anterior & posterior flaps.
- Bony division must allow for 15 cm clearance from the level of the knee joint.
- Skin incision along the markings (Fig 6.11).
- Divide muscle groups & ligate neurovascular bundles.
- Divide the sciatic nerve as proximally as possible under tension.
- Strip periosteum from the femur at the level of division, >5cm proximal to where the muscle groups were divided.
- Divide the femur transversely & file edges (6.11).
- Ensure adequate haemostasis & insert suction drains as appropriate.
- Approximate anterior & posterior flap muscles over the femoral stump.
- Suture fascia.
- Skin closure.
- Dress with wool & crepe bandages.
- Commence PT as soon as possible to prevent flexion contractures & to optimise mobility with prosthesis.

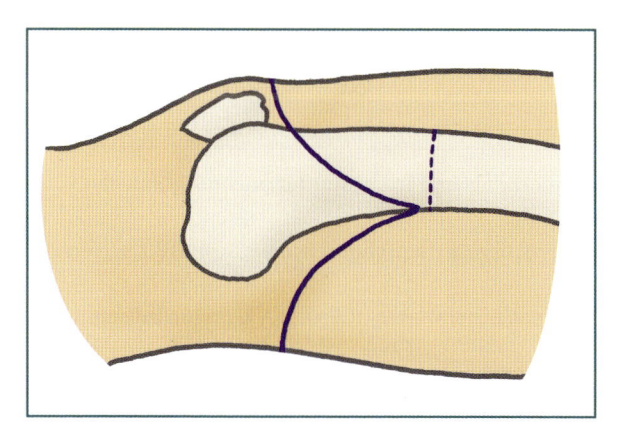

Fig 6.11: Above knee amputation incisions.

Q: What are the complications of amputation?

Immediate	Early	Late
Haemorrhage	Haematoma	Joint Contracture
Neurovascular Damage	Infection	Stump Ulceration
	Wound Dehiscence	Neuroma
	Skin / Flap Necrosis	Stump Oedema
	Difficulty Mobilising	Bony Spur & Osteophyte in Underlying Bone
		Phantom Limb Pain
		Psychological

Femoral Embolectomy

Q: What is the aim of a femoral embolectomy?

To restore circulation through the femoral artery by embolus removal.

Q: Describe the principle steps in performing a femoral embolectomy.

- Full pre-operative assessment including history & examination & appropriate investigations.
- Explain procedure to patient, obtain informed consent & confirm correct side.
- Pateint supine under GA.
- Skin preparation & draping.
- 12–15cm longitudinal incision over the femoral artery, starting proximally near the inguinal ligament.
- Dissect down to the femoral artery & expose the profunda femoris & superficial femoral artery (SFA) (Fig 6.12).
- Put silastic slings around the common femoral artery (CFA), SFA & profunda femoris artery.
- Select correct Fogarty catheter size & test balloon.
- Clamp the 3 main vessels & make an arteriotomy (usually 1cm transverse) in the CFA.
- The embolus is removed by passing the uninflated Fogarty catheter beyond the clot proximally to the aortic bifurcation, inflating the balloon & pulling back.
- Heparinise the vessels & repeat the procedure distally, passing the catheter into the superficial femoral & profunda femoris arteries.
- The arteriotomy is closed with non-absorbable sutures (a patch may be required for closure).
- Ensure adequate haemostasis.

- Wound closure in layers.
- Examine & document reperfusion of the limb.
- Anticoagulate the patient as appropriate.
- Post-procedure arteriography is advisable.

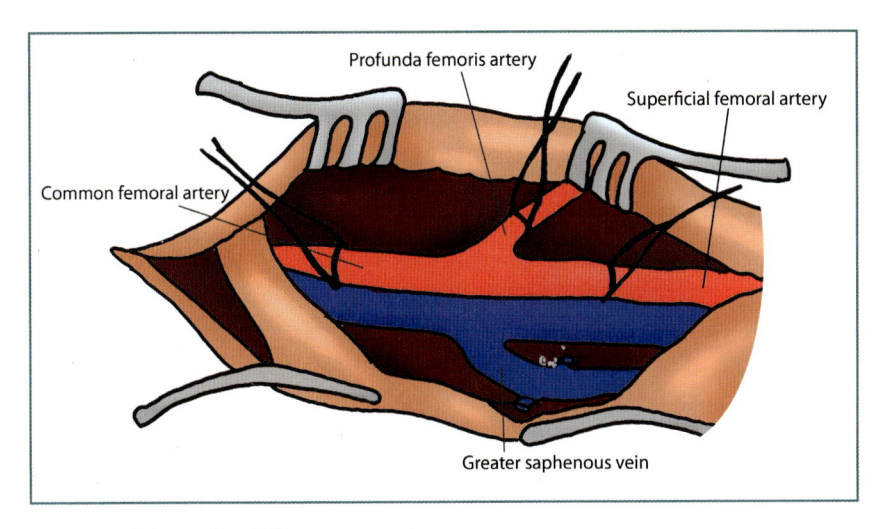

Fig 6.12: Left femoral embolectomy operative exposure.

Varicose Vein Surgery

Q: What are the tributaries of the long saphenous vein in the thigh?

- Superficial Inferior Epigastric Vein
- Medial & Lateral Superficial Circumflex Iliac Veins
- Superficial External Pudendal Vein
- Superficial Circumflex Iliac Vein
- Lateral & Anterior Cutaneous Thigh Veins

Note: There may be anatomical variation between individuals & different names for the same tributaries may appear in different texts.

Q: What are the indications for treating varicose veins?

NICE guidelines advise:

Timeframe	Symptoms
Emergency	Continuous haemorrhage from varicosity eroding skin.
Urgent	Varicosity that has bled & is at risk of re-bleeding.
Soon	Varicose ulcer that is progressive / painful despite treatment.
Routine	Active / healed ulcer or progressive skin changes that may benefit from surgery.
	Recurrent superficial thrombophlebitis.
	Troublesome symptoms attributable to varicose veins.
	Significant impact on quality of life.

Q: What is the treatment of varicose veins?

Conservative	Medical	Surgical
Graduated Support Stockings	Injection Sclerotherapy (1% sodium tetradecyl)	Incompetent SFJ / SPJ Ligation, Vein Stripping & Stab Avulsions of Varicosities 'High Tie & Strip'
Weight Loss		Incompetent Perforating Vessels Ligation (marked with duplex)
Regular Exercise		Subcutaneous Endoscopic Perforator Surgery
		Endovenous Laser Therapy (EVLT) (an alternative to the high tie & strip procedure)

Q: How would you perform surgery for LSV varicosities secondary to SFJ incompetence?

Perform a high tie & strip as follows:
- Full pre-operative assessment including history & examination & appropriate investigations.
- Explain procedure to patient, obtain informed consent & confirm correct side.
- Pre-operatively mark all varicosities with the patient standing.
- Patient in Trendelenberg's Position (20° head down tilt) under GA.
- Skin preparation & draping.

- Groin crease incision, centred 2–5 cm below & lateral to the pubic tubercle.
- Identify, isolate & divide all tributaries to leave SFJ clear.
- Ligate LSV just distal to SFJ.
- Perform a venotomy just distal to the ligature.
- Pass a stripper down the LSV to a level just below the knee.
- Deliver the end of the stripper through a stab incision & attach the stripper head.
- Strip the vein proximally to the groin by applying gentle traction.
- Apply pressure to control bleeding as stripper is withdrawn.
- Multiple avulsions to remaining varicosities can be performed if necessary through stab incisions.
- Ensure adequate haemostasis.
- Close the groin wound.
- Dress with firm elastic bandages.
- Post-operatively : TEDS for 2 weeks.
  Encourage mobilisation, but rest with legs elevated.

Q: What are the complications of varicose vein surgery?

Immediate	Early	Late
Haemorrhage	Haematoma	Recurrence
Femoral Vein Injury	Infection	
Superficial Femoral Artery Injury	Seroma	
Sural ± Saphenous Nerve Injury	DVT	

Abdominal Aortic Aneurysm Repair

Q: What are the indications for AAA repair?

- Symptomatic Patient
- Diameter >5.5cm
- Diameter increasing by 1cm per annum

Note: The UK Small Aneurysm Trial suggests aneurysms 4.0–5.5cm in men are not recommended for surgery as the risks outweigh the benefits. Aneurysms >5.5cm should be operated as the benefits outweigh the risks of surgery. USS Screening for AAA in men aged >60years has survival benefits.

Q: What pre-operative investigations should be ordered for patients prior to elective open AAA repair?

Investigations	Notes
Blood Tests	FBC, U&E, Clotting Profile
Blood Replacement	6U Cross Match
Cardio-Respiratory Assessment	Pulmonary Function tests, Cardiopulmonary Exercise Testing
Cardiac Assessment	ECG, Echocardiogram
Further Imaging	CT (to assess aneurysm morphology)

Q: How is an open AAA repair performed?

- Full pre-operative assessment including history & examination & appropriate investigations.
- Explain operation to patient, obtain informed consent & confirm correct side.
- Pre-operatively mark all varicosities with the patient standing.
- Patient supine under GA.
- Skin preparation & draping.
- Prophylactic broad-spectrum antibiotics given at induction.
- Long mid-line laparotomy incision skirting left of umbilicus.
- Pack small bowel into the right upper quadrant with wet packs.
- Incise peritoneum overlying the aorta.
- Identify the distal extent of aneurysm.
- Give bolus of IV heparin.
- Clamp vessels to achieve distal & proximal control of blood flow.
- Longitudinally incise the aneurysm sac, clearing any debris, clot & atherosclerosis.
- Back bleeding from lumbar or inferior mesenteric vessels should be controlled by over-sewing.
- A straight or bifurcated PTFE graft is measured for size & inserted.
- Suture the proximal & distal ends of the graft with continuous double-ended (2-0 / 3-0 Prolene™) sutures (Fig 6.13).
- Test the proximal, then distal ends of the repair.
- Remove clamps.
- Check bowel for viability (non-viability may necessitate re-implantation of the inferior mesenteric artery).
- Close aneurysm sac over the graft with 2-0 absorbable sutures (Fig 6.13).
- Ensure adequate haemostasis & insert drains as appropriate.

- Layered closure of abdomen.
- Post-operatively:　　Transfer to HDU / ICU.
　　　　　　　　　　　Correct & maintain Hb >10g/dl.
　　　　　　　　　　　Monitor cardiac, respiratory & renal function.
　　　　　　　　　　　Monitor neurological status of patient (CVA / spinal ischaemia).
　　　　　　　　　　　Check for signs of embolism.
　　　　　　　　　　　Check for signs of gut ischaemia.

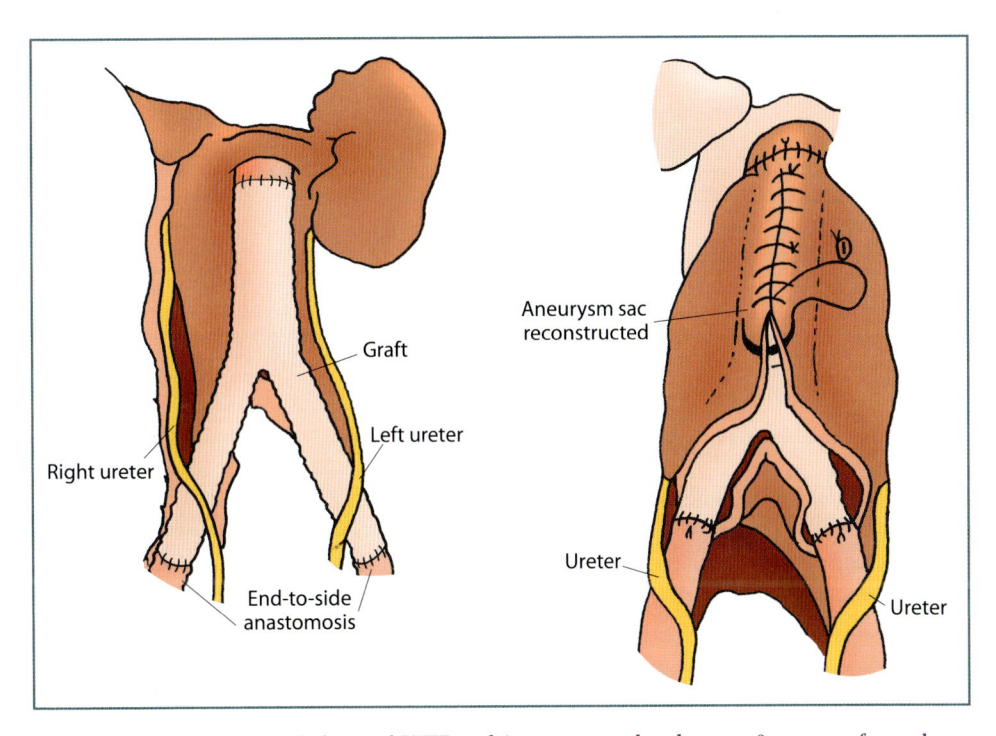

Fig 6.13: Open AAA repair. A bifurcated PTFE graft is anastomosed to the aorta & common femoral arteries (left image). The aneurysm sac is then reconstructed over the graft (right image).

Q: What are the complications of open AAA surgery?

- Mortality of elective AAA repairs <5%.
- Mortality of emergency AAA repairs = 50%.
- Remaining complications may be classified as follows:

Immediate	Early	Late
Haemorrhage	Graft Leak	Aorto-Enteric Fistula
Ureteric Injury	Graft Migration / Kinking	Graft Infection
Bowel Injury	CVA	Impotence
Embolism	ARDS	False Aneurysm
	MI	
	Renal Failure	
	Wound Infection	
	Bowel Obstruction / Ischaemia	
	Incisional Hernia	

Q: Do you know of any alternatives to open repair when treating an AAA?

Endovascular aneurysm repair (EVAR):

- Elective or emergency procedure.
- A PTFE / Dacron™ stent-graft, with a stainless steel supportive mesh, is used.
- Insertion into the aorta, under radiological guidance, is via incisions in femoral arteries.
- The stent acts as a conduit for blood to travel down, preventing it from entering the aneurysm sac, allowing the sac to thrombose over time.
- There is improved mortality compared with open repair.
- EVAR is unsuitable for aneurysms that traverse the major abdominal branches of the aorta (as this would occlude these branches resulting in ischaemia to supplied organs & tissues).

NEUROSCIENCES

Burr Hole & Craniotomy

Q: What is a craniotomy?

An opening of the cranium to facilitate neurosurgical access.

Q: What are the most common indications for performing a craniotomy?

Indication	Example
Trauma	• Evacuation of extradural / subdural / intracerebral haematoma. • Elevation of depressed skull fracture.
Vascular	• Clipping of ruptured or elective aneurysm. • Excision of AVM. • Resection of cavernoma.
Neoplasia	• Decompression of 1° / 2° brain tumour.
Infective	• Excision of intracerebral abscess.
Congenital	• Fenestration / excision of congenital cyst.

Q: How would you perform a craniotomy?

- Full pre-procedure assessment including history, examination & appropriate investigations.
- Explain procedure to patient, obtain informed consent & confirm correct side.
- GA or LA with sedation.
- Hair shave, skin preparation & draping as appropriate.
- Raise a flap of skin & muscle, exposing the pericranium.
- Drill a burr hole(s) *(see below)* through the outer & inner tables of the skull until dura is reached.
- Subsequently use a side cutting electrical saw to create a 'trap door' opening in the skull.
- Replaced bone flap into defect & secure with plates & screws.
- Haemostasis.
- Wound closure in layers.

Q: What are the potential complications related to a craniotomy?

These depend on the underlying reason for the craniotomy & its outcome but include:

Immediate	Early	Late
Haemorrhage	Eyes & Face Swelling & Bruising (due to sub-galeal blood tracking)	Dysphagia (temporalis muscle atrophy)
Brain Tissue Damage	Extradural Haematoma (due to bleeding bone edge)	Weak Forehead Muscles (frontalis branch of facial nerve injury)
	Wound Infection	Neurological Impairment (e.g. deafness, blindness)

Q: When might a non-neurosurgeon consider performing an emergency burr hole?

Clinical	Radiological
'Coning'	Acute Extradural / Subdural Haematoma with Marked Midline Shift
• Rapidly Deteriorating GCS	
• Dilated Pupil(s)	
• Extensor Posturing	
• Cushing Reflex	

Q: How is an emergency burr hole be performed?

- Discuss with a neurosurgeon.
- Full pre-procedure assessment including history, examination & appropriate investigations.
- Explain procedure to patient, obtain informed consent & confirm correct side.
- Shave hair in temporal region.
- Skin preparation & draping.
- LA infiltration & make a 'hockey stick' incision, beginning 1cm anterior to the tragus (Fig 6.14).
- Incise temporalis fascia & muscle, insert self-retaining retractor.
- Place burr hole with high speed electric / mechanical drill in squamous temporal region through outer & inner tables of skull.
- Extend size of skull opening with bone nibblers.
- Control bleeding with electrocautery (from middle meningeal artery) & bone wax for bone edges
- Suction & irrigation of underlying extradural haematoma.
- Close wound, apply sterile dressing & transfer to neurosurgery for formal craniotomy.

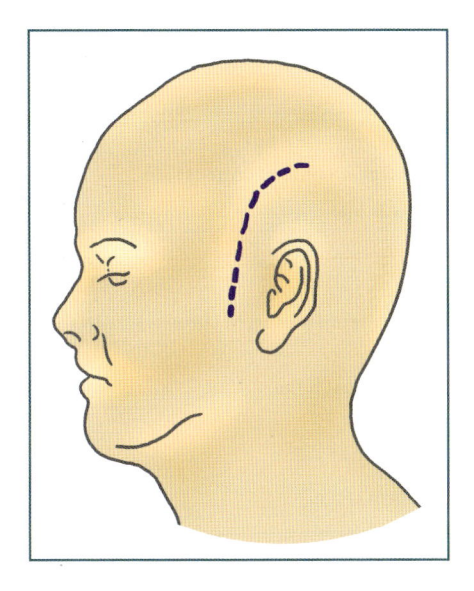

Fig 6.14: Hockey stick incision for burr hole.

Intracranial Pressure (ICP) Monitor Insertion
(also see critical care chapter)

Q: What is ICP monitoring?

Intracranial pressure monitoring directly monitors ICP via placement of a small probe (fibre-optic or strain gauge) into the brain.

Q: What are the indications for ICP monitoring?

- Severe head injury (GCS ≤ 8) with abnormal CT brain.
- Unilateral / bilateral extensor posturing after head injury.
- Consider if significant episode of hypoxia / hypovolaemia after head injury.
- Others e.g. diagnosis of shunt malfunction & benign intracranial hypertension.

Note: Aim is to optimise recovery potential via medical & surgical strategies to maintain:
- CPP > 65 mmHg
- ICP < 25 mmHg

Q: How is an ICP monitor inserted?

- Full pre-procedure assessment including history, examination & appropriate investigations.
- Explain procedure to patient, obtain informed consent & confirm correct side.
- Perform in theatre / ICU with standard cranial access kit.
- Skin preparation & draping as appropriate.
- Infiltrate 2–3mls LA with adrenaline.
- 1–2 cm stab incision (right frontal mid pupillary line, 1cm anterior to coronal suture at Kocher's Point).
- Hand held twist drill burr hole made through right frontal bone.
- Carefully puncture dura with green needle.
- Insert probe 1cm into brain & tunnel 4–5cm under scalp.
- Connect to monitor & ensure adequate ICP waveform trace.
- Suture scalp incision & fix probe.

Q: What are the complications of this ICP monitor insertion?

- Intracerebral haemorrhage   (approximately 2%)
- Infection   (uncommon <1%)
- CSF Leak   (through scalp incision)
- Probe Misplacement / Malfunction

Lumbar Puncture

Q: What is the terminal point of the spinal cord & what are the surface landmarks for performing a lumbar puncture.

The spinal cord ends at the lower edge of the L1 vertebrae. The safest site for performing LP is the L4–5 intervertebral space. This can be easily identified by drawing an imaginary line between the iliac crests, which intersects the spine at the L4 process. The space above & below this can be safely punctured.

Q: What important structures are at the levels L1 to L4?

Level	Structures
L1	*Transpyloric Plane of Addison (midpoint between the jugular notch of the manubrium & the symphysis pubis):* • 9th Costal Cartilage. • Hilum of Spleen & Kidney (with their vascular pedicles). • Neck of Pancreas. • Portal Vein. • Pylorus of Stomach. • Superior Mesenteric Artery. • Fundus of Gallbladder. • 2nd Part of Duodenum.
L2	*Subcostal Plane (lowest points of the thoracic cage):* • Lower margin of 10th rib.
L3	• Umbilicus (slim person).
L4	• Iliac Crests.

Q: What anatomical structures are passed through during lumbar puncture?

- Skin
- Fat
- Superficial Fascia
- Supraspinous Ligament
- Interspinous Ligament
- Ligamentum Flavum
- Areolar Tissue
- Dura Mater
- Arachnoid Mater.

Q: How is a lumbar puncture performed?

- Full pre-procedure assessment including history, examination & appropriate investigations.
- Explain procedure to patient & obtain informed consent.
- Position patient in the left lateral position, with their back at the edge of the bed, neck & back in full flexion & knees tucked into chest.
- Skin preparation & draping.

- Mark L4–5 intervertebral space with a pen *(surface markings described above)*.
- Inject up to 5mls of 1% lignocaine subcutaneously & anaesthetise deeper structures.
- Insert the spinal needle in the midline, aiming towards the umbilicus.
- A 'give' is felt as the needle pierces the spinal ligaments then the dura mater & arachnoid mater to enter the subarachnoid space.
- Withdraw the stylet from the needle & measure the CSF pressure with a manometer (normal = 7–20cm).
- Collect the CSF specimens, taking note of the colour & turbidity.
- Send specimens for MC+S, protein & glucose (where necessary: virology, serology, cytology for malignancy, AFB, oligoclonal bands & fungal cultures).
- Remove needle & apply simple dressing to the site.
- The patient should lie flat for 6 hours.

Q: What are the contraindications of performing a lumbar puncture?

- Focal Neurological Symptoms & Signs of Raised ICP (decreasing level of consciousness, vomiting, papilloedema).
- Cardiorespiratory Compromise.
- Bleeding Diasthesis.
- Local Infection e.g. Sacral Sores.

Q: What are the complications of lumbar puncture?

- Headache.
- Bleeding.
- Infection.
- Coning (herniation of the cerebellar tonsils with medulla compression is rare unless the patient has raised ICP).
- Trauma to Spinal Cord / Nerve Roots.
- Bloody Tap.
- Dry Tap.

Q: What are the normal values for protein, lymphocytes, glucose & opening pressure?

Protein	<0.4g/l.	
Lymphocytes	<4/mm^3	(polymorphs 0mm^3)
Glucose	>2.2mmol/l	(or 70% plasma level)
Opening pressure	<200mm H$_2$O	

SECTION D: PRINCIPLES OF SURGERY & PATIENT SAFETY

CHAPTER 7
BONES & SOFT TISSUES

K Asaad
BH Miranda
SP Kay

CHAPTER CONTENTS

Bones
- Bone Structure
- Fractures
- Osteomyelitis
- Septic Arthritis

Soft Tissues
- The Reconstructive Ladder
- Scars
- Muscle
- Cartilage

BONES

Bone Structure

Q: What types of bone do you know of?

Type	Notes
Woven	Haphazardly organised collagen fibres = mechanically weak. Seen in foetal bones (replaced by lamellar bone from the 3rd trimester) & fracture healing.
Lamellar	Regular parallel alignment of collagen fibres = mechanically strong. Replaces woven bone in the foetus from the 3rd trimester & during fracture healing.
Compact / Cortical	The hard outer layer of bone, composed of tightly packed osteons. Osteons consist of lamellae, surrounding a central Haversian canal. Turnover is slow.
Cancellous / Trabecular	The porous central layer of bone, composed of a network of irregular bony rods & plates. Cancellous bone is less dense than compact bone, although turnover is much faster.

Q: What is the composition of bone?

Composition	Notes
Cellular	Osteoprogenitor Cells, Ostoblasts, Osteoclasts, Osteocytes, Lining Cells
Matrix	• **Inorganic (60%):** Calcium Hydroxyapatite, Osteocalcium Phosphate • **Organic (40%):** Collagen (type I), Proteoglycans, Proteins, Cytokines, Growth Factors

Fractures

Q: How are fractures classified?

These may be classified according to cause, extent, pattern, displacement & structural involvement as follows (Fig 7.1):

Classification	Example	Interpretation
CAUSE	Traumatic	Due to strong deforming force.
	Stress	Occur in normal bone subjected to repeated trauma.
	Pathological	Occur when bone is weakened by pre-existing disease, such that minimal insult results in fracture e.g. metastasis, osteoporosis.
EXTENT	Partial	Only part of the cortex is involved.
	Complete	Both cortices are involved.
	Transverse	Fracture lies 90° to long axis of bone.
	Oblique	Fracture lies off the long axis of bone (>30°).
	Spiral	Due to twisting around the long axis of bone.
	Comminuted	>2 bone fragments produced.
	Avulsion	Fractured segment is pulled off e.g. by inserting tendon.
	Butterfly	Force to 1 side of bone blows out a triangular wedge on the other side.
PATTERN	Segmented	Force to 1 side of bone blows out a complete bone segment.
	Crush	Compressive forces result in bone collapse e.g. vertebral column in patients with osteoporosis.
	Wedge	Flexion-extension injuries may produce a V-shaped bone defect, such that 1 cortex side appears wider than the other at radiography.
	Burst	Compressive forces may result in many fragments of bone bursting away from the area of greatest force.
	Greenstick	1 cortex side is broken & the other undergoes plastic deformation. Affects children.
	Subluxation	Partial loss of contact between 2 joint surfaces that usually articulate.
	Dislocation	Complete loss of contact between 2 joint surfaces that usually articulate.
DISPLACEMENT	Translation	Fracture displacement is in the same plane e.g. medial, lateral, superior, inferior.
	Angulation	May be anterior, posterior, varus, valgus etc.
	Rotation	May be external, internal etc.
STRUCTURAL INVOLVEMENT	Simple	Fracture does not communicate with the outside & no additional structural damage.
	Open / Compound	Fracture communicates with the outside e.g. open wounds, skull fractures communicating with air sinuses.
	Complicated	Additional structural damage present e.g. nerve, vascular, visceral.
	Intra-Articular	Fracture involves an articulating joint.

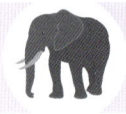

> **Memory:** When describing fractures, consider the above classification system in order to structure your answer.

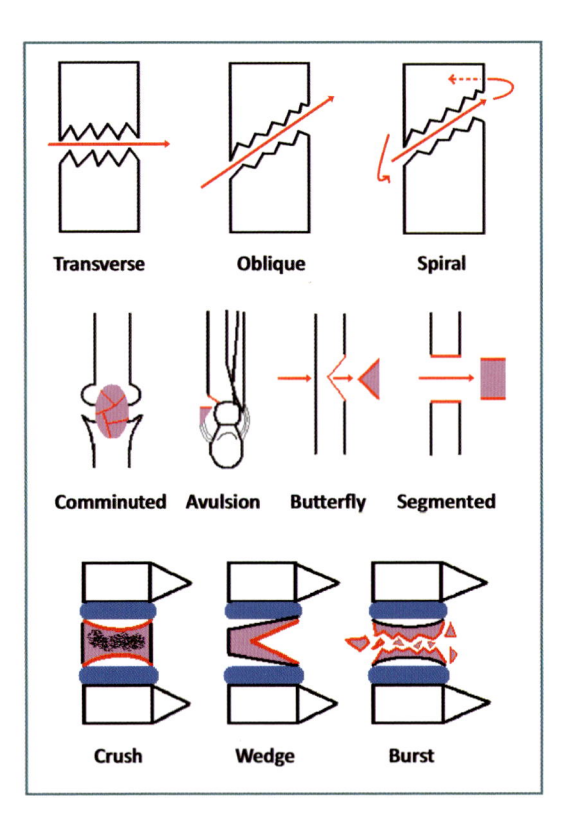

Fig 7.1: Diagrammatic representation of various fracture patterns.

Q: What is the Salter-Harris fracture classification?

A classification system for fractures involving the epiphyseal growth plate in children (Fig 7.2). A higher class implies a more severe fracture.

> **Memory:** **SALT CRUSH**
>
> | | | |
> |---|---|---|
> | S | = Separated from growth plate | (Class I) |
> | A | = Above growth plate | (Class II) |
> | L | = Lower than growth plate | (Class III) |
> | T | = Together both above & below growth plate | (Class IV) |
> | CRUSH | = Impacted growth plate | (Class V) |

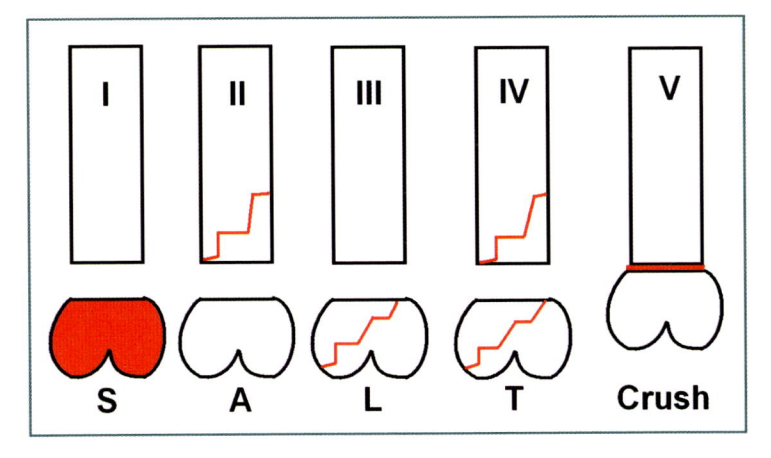

Fig 7.2: Salter-Harris classification. Note: This diagrammatic representation only works with the growth plate orientated inferiorly.

Q: What are the phases of fracture healing?

There are 3 major phases that may be further sub-classified as follows (Fig 7.3):

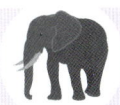

Memory: 3 x **R**s of fracture healing.

Phase	Sub-Classification	Description
REACTIVE	Inflammation	Haemorrhage & tissue destruction with haematoma formation. Necrosis of osteocytes at the fracture ends.
	Granulation	Fibroblast proliferation & capillary growth at the site of haematoma. Granulation tissue is formed.
REPARATIVE	Callus	Periosteal cells transform into chondroblasts (forming hyaline cartilage) & osteoblasts (forming bone). These tissues grow & bridge the fracture.
	Lamellar Bone Formation	Lamellar bone replaces woven bone & cartilage. This bone is trabecular & has most of the original bone strength.
REMODELLING	Remodelling	Compact bone substitutes trabecular bone. Bone shape returns to normal as influenced by stress forces encountered during rehabilitation.

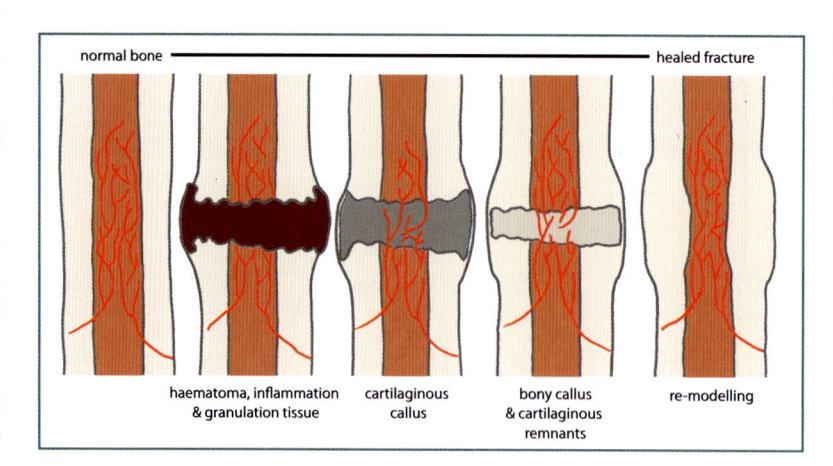

Fig 7.3: Diagram of fracture healing.

normal bone — haematoma, inflammation & granulation tissue — cartilaginous callus — bony callus & cartilaginous remnants — re-modelling — healed fracture

Q: What are the principles of fracture treatment?

This requires ATLS resuscitation (with appropriate history & clinical examination) & includes:

Principle	Interpretation
Reduce	The fractured ends of bone need to be realigned. This may be done either in the acute setting or under general anaesthetic. Open reduction involves surgical exposure prior to fracture reduction.
Hold	Immobilisation times are governed by the fracture type, location & extent. This may be achieved by a number of fixation methods: • **Internal Fixation** — Screw, Plate, Intramedullary Nail • **External Fixation** — External Fixation Device, Pin-Traction • **Non-Invasive Stabilisation:** — Cast, Splint, Strap **Note: K-wires may be used as internal / percutaneous fixation.**
Rehabilitate	Involves physiotherapy & occupational therapy. Rehabilitation protocols are governed by evidence-based research & must be adhered to in order to maximise recovery. Protocols are highly variable depending on fracture type, location & extent.

Q: What factors affect bone healing?

General Factors	Local Factors
Age	Blood Supply
Co-Morbidities	Infection
Nutrition	Injury Severity
Smoking	Stabilisation
Drugs (NSAIDs, Steroids)	Site
	Soft Tissue Interposition

Q: What are the complications of fractures?

Complication	Local	General
EARLY	Haemorrhage	Hypovolaemic Shock
	Structural Damage e.g. Nerve, Vessel, Viscera	Urinary Retention
	Loss of Function	DVT
	Tetanus	Pneumonia
	Wound Infection & Gangrene	Fat Embolism
	Compartment Syndrome	Crush Syndrome
LATE	Delayed Union	Pulmonary Embolism
	Non-Union	Pneumonia
	Mal-Union	Immobility
	Sudek's Atrophy	PTSD
	Myositis Ossificans	
	Avascular Necrosis	
	Joint Stiffness / Contracture	
	Osteomyelitis	

Osteomyelitis

Q: What is osteomyelitis?

An inflammatory lesion due to infection of bone or bone marrow. It may be classified as acute or chronic, by route of infection or causative organism.

Q: What are the most common causative organisms of osteomyelitis, relating to age group?

Age	Organism
<4 Months	*Staphylococcus aureus, Streptococcus* Groups A & B, *Enterobacter, Escherichia coli.*
4 Months–Late Teenager	*Staphylococcus aureus, Streptococcus* Group A, *Haemophilus influenzae, Enterobacter.*
Adult	*Staphylococcus aurues, Enterobacter,* Streptococcus Group B, *Pseudomonas, Escherichia coli.*

Q: Are any causative organisms of osteomyelitis related to specific diseases?

There are many important causes e.g. MRSA. The remainder may be classified according to disease:

Disease	Organism
Diabetes Mellitus	Anaerobes
Immunocompromise	*Aspergillus fumigatus, Candida albicans, Mycobacterium Avium-Intracellulare Complex*
HIV	*Mycobacterium tuberculosis*
Sickle Cell Anaemia	*Salmonella*

Q: What is the pathogenesis of osteomyelitis?

- A focus of acute inflammation develops around capillaries in the bone metaphysis.
- As this progresses, capillaries & other vessels become compressed, blood supply to bone trabeculae is compromised & osteonecrosis ensues.
- Dead bone fragments separate from healthy bone, forming a **sequestrum**.
- If the lesion persists, a new surrounding bone layer may form beneath the periosteum. This is the **involucrum**.
- Pus & debris may drain to the skin's surface via sinus formation.

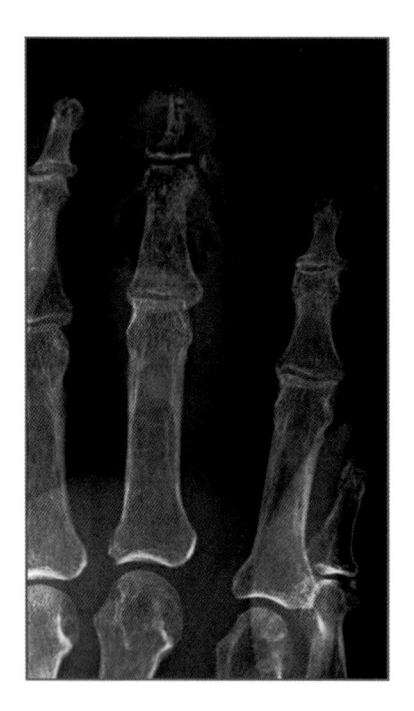

Fig 7.4: Radiograph illustrating an acute abscess of the left hand middle finger tip, with associated osteomyelitis & distal phalanx destruction.

Q: What are the complications of osteomyelitis?

- Sinus Formation
- Overlying Soft Tissue Infection
- Metastatic Infection e.g. Brain (abscess), Joints (septic arthritis), Lungs (abscess)
- Septicaemia
- Limb Length Discrepancy
- Pathological Fractures
- Chronic Osteomyelitis.

Q: What would your management of a patient with osteomyelitis be?

- **Full History**
- **Thorough Clinical Examination**
- **Appropriate Investigations:**

Investigation	Examples
Blood Tests	FBC, U&E, LFT, CRP.
Microbiology	Blood cultures & wound swabs.
Radiographs	AP & true lateral long bone radiograph.
Other	More complex scans as appropriate.

- **Treatment:**

Treatment	Examples	Interpretation
MEDICAL	**Dressings**	These may be biological or synthetic, adherent or non-adherent.
	Analgesia	According to analgesic ladder.
	High Dose (IV) Antibiotics	This may be for weeks, with continued oral treatment in the community after hospital discharge.
SURGICAL	**Debridement**	Of necrotic & infected tissue.
	Reconstruction	After infection cleared.
	Amputation	May be required.

Septic Arthritis

Q: What is septic arthritis?

Suppurative inflammation of a joint due to an infectious organism. It is usually caused by bacteria, but may also be due to a virus or fungus.

Q: What are the routes of infection?

- **Iatrogenic**
- **Penetrating Trauma**
- **Haematogenous Spread** e.g. Abscess, Wound Infection
- **Dissemination** e.g. Osteomyelitis.

Q: What are the bacterial causes of septic arthritis?

- *Staphylococcus aureus* & *epidermidis*
- *Streptococcus*
- *Pseudomonas*
- *Gonococcus*
- *Escherichia coli.*

Q: What are the clinical features of septic arthritis?

Only 1 joint is usually affected. Severe joint pain with even the smallest movement is characteristic. Clinical features may be classified as local or general as follows:

Local	General
Severe Joint Pain	Fever
Erythema	Anorexia
Joint Swelling	Toxaemia
Joint Immobility	Underlying Cause

Q: How would you manage a patient with suspected septic arthritis?

- **Full History**
- **Thorough Clinical Examination**
- **Appropriate Investigations:**

Investigation	Examples
Blood Tests	FBC, U&E, LFT, CRP.
Microbiology	Joint aspiration for MC+S is diagnostic. Blood cultures.
Radiographs	Remember that by the time radiological changes for septic arthritis are present, irreparable joint damage has already occurred.
Other	More complex scans as appropriate.

- **Treatment:**

Treatment	Examples	Interpretation
CONSERVATIVE	Physiotherapy	Rehabilitation as necessary.
	Occupational Therapy	Rehabilitation as necessary.
MEDICAL	Analgesia	According to analgesic ladder.
	High Dose (IV) Antibiotics	Empirical treatment until bacterial sensitivities known.
SURGICAL	Drainage	Drainage & joint irrigation should be repeated as necessary.
	Reconstruction	After infection cleared.
	Amputation	May be required.

Q: What are the complications of septic arthritis?

- Joint Stiffness
- Fibrosis
- Ankylosis
- Recurrent Infection
- Osteomyelitis
- Early Onset Osteoarthritis.

SOFT TISSUES

The Reconstructive Ladder

Q: What is the reconstructive ladder?

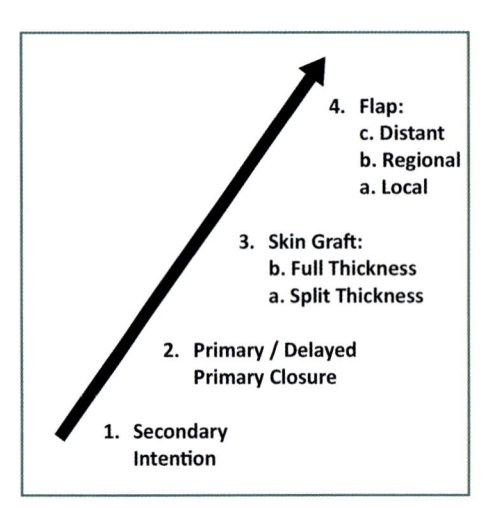

Fig 7.5: Reconstructive ladder.

A term to describe different techniques of wound management, escalating them in increasing complexity.

4. Flap:
   c. Distant
   b. Regional
   a. Local
3. Skin Graft:
   b. Full Thickness
   a. Split Thickness
2. Primary / Delayed Primary Closure
1. Secondary Intention

Q: Are there any adjuncts to these procedures?

- **Tissue Expansion:** An increase in a tissue's surface area is mechanically induced. This is usually with a tissue expander, an inflatable device implanted e.g. subcutaneously, that is periodically injected with saline until the tissue e.g. skin is at the required size.
- **Negative Pressure Therapy** (e.g. VAC™): Gauze or foam is placed on the wound bed & connected to a vacuum pump, under an occlusive dressing. The vacuum draws out excess fluid & cellular waste.

Q: What is the difference between a graft & flap?

- **Graft:** Tissue is transferred from a donor site & establishes a new blood supply at the recipient site. e.g. skin, cartilage.
- **Flap:** An area of tissue is transferred from a donor site to a recipient site with its own blood supply & intrinsic circulation. It may contain ≥1 tissue type e.g. skin, fat, fascia & muscle.

Q: What is the difference between a full thickness & split thickness skin graft?

- **Split Thickness:** Takes the epidermis & only a portion of the dermis.
- **Full Thickness:** Takes the epidermis & all of the dermis.

Q: What are the advantages & disadvantages of split vs. full thickness skin grafts?

These may be considered according to clinical factors relating to the graft type as follows:

Clinical Factor	Split Thickness	Full Thickness
Colour / Texture Match	Poor	More Similar to Normal Skin
Contraction	Significant	Reduced
Donor Site	Any Body Area e.g. Thigh / Buttocks	Aim for Primary Closure so Size Limited
Graft Take	More Likely Under Less Favourable Conditions	Requires Well Vascularised Bed

Scars

Q: What is a scar?

The end-product of wound healing by repair (as opposed to regeneration).

Q: How do you classify the complications of scarring?

Cosmetic	Functional	Sensory
Distortion of Tissue	Flexion Contracture	Pain
Erythema	Growth Disturbance	Pruritis
Hypertrophic Scar	Reduced Movement	Psychological
Keloid Scar		
Depressed scar		
Trap Door Appearance		

Q: What factors affect scarring?

- Body Site
- Genetic e.g. Skin Colour
- Nature of Injury
- Orientation Relative to Relaxed Skin Tension Lines
- Surgical Technique
- Wound Management
- Local & Systemic Factors e.g. Infection, Nutrition, Smoking & Steroids.

Q: What is the spot diagnosis?

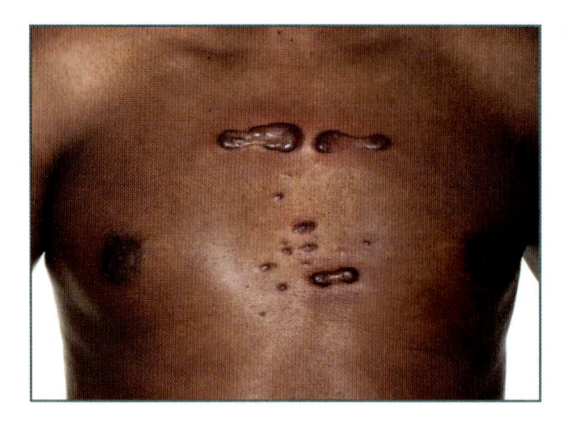

Fig 7.6: Sternal keloid scarring.

Q: What are the differences between keloid & hypertrophic scarring?

Hypertrophic	Keloid
Thick & Raised	Thick & Raised
Remains Within Wound Borders	Extends Beyond Wound Borders
Appear in Weeks	Appear over Months – Years
All Races Affected	More Prevalent in Asian / Afro-Caribbean Races
No Proven Immunological Component	IgG, IgM, C3 & ANA Involvement
Normal Rate of Collagen Synthesis	Increased Rate of Collagen Synthesis
Naturally Regresses	No Natural Regression

Q: How are keloid scars managed?

Conservative	Medical	Surgical
Scar Massage	Steroid Injections	Intralesional Excision ± Steroid / Radiotherapy
Silicone Therapy		
Pressure Device / Garment		
Scar Camouflage		

Muscle

Q: What types of muscle do you know of & what are their differences?

Classification	Notes
Skeletal	• Striated & Voluntary • Located at Joints • Summation Possible • Triads of 1 x T-Tubule & 2 x Lateral Cisternae • Troponin is the Calcium Binding Protein
Cardiac	• Striated & Voluntary • Located in Myocardium • No Summation Possible • Intercelated Discs with Desmosomes & Gap Junctions • Troponin is the Calcium Binding Protein
Smooth	• Haphazard Fibre Arrangement & Involuntary • Located in Vessels & Viscera • Prolonged Contraction & Greater Stretch vs. Skeletal Muscle • Gap Junctions Present, T-Tubules Absent • Calmodulin is the Calcium Binding Protein

Q: What types of skeletal muscle fibres do you know of?

Classification	Notes
Type I	• Slow Twitch • Red (Myoglobin Rich) • Mitochondria Rich • Aerobic e.g. Long Distance Running (Slow Fatigue)
Type II	• Fast Twitch • White • Glycogen Rich • Anaerobic e.g. Sprinters (Rapid Fatigue)

Q: What is the structure of skeletal muscle?

Skeletal muscle is comprised of:

1. **Bundles** of fascicles (surrounded by) Epimysium
2. **Fascicles** of muscle fibres (surrounded by) Perimysium
3. **Fibres** of myofibrils (surrounded by) Endomysium

Note: Muscle fibres represent the cellular unit. They contain the sarcolemma (the calcium storage structure for muscular contraction). Myofibrils are comprised of myosin (thick / heavy) & actin (thin / light) myofilaments, arranged into structures known as sarcomeres (Fig 7.7).

Q: Can you draw a sarcomere?

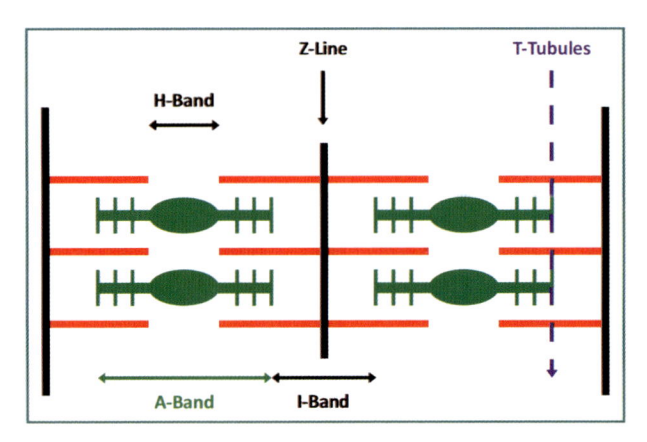

Fig 7.7: Sarcomere.

Sarcomeres are characterised by **myosin (thick)** & **actin (thin)** myofilaments. The sarcomere arrangement produces characteristic **lines** & **bands**.

T-Tubules are invaginations of sarcolemma (muscle cell membrane), located at the junction of A & I bands, near the sarcoplasmic reticulum. They allow rapid transmission of the action potential & rapid Ca^{2+} release from the sarcoplasmic reticulum.

Q: Can you describe the phenomenon of excitation–contraction coupling, using skeletal muscle as an example?

This is the process of conversion, within muscle, of an action potential to a mechanical response as follows:

- Delivery of the action potential to the motor end plate.
- Spread of the action potential through T tubules.
- Mobilisation of Ca^{2+} from sarcoplasmic reticulum stores.
- Binding of Ca^{2+} to troponin C on actin chains = tropomysin displacement & myosin-binding site exposure.
- Myosin chains form cross-links with actin (on myosin-binding sites).
- ATPase dephosphorylation of ATP, to ADP + Phosphate = active sliding of myosin chains & contraction.

Cartilage

Q: What is cartilage?

Strong & flexible connective tissue that is distributed throughout the body. It is avascular & composed of:

Composition	Notes
Water	For diffusion of nutrients & lubrication.
Chondrocytes	Cells that synthesise proteins, proteoglycans & ground substance.
Collagen	Protein fibres providing tensile strength providing protein fibres.
Elastin	Elastic protein fibres.
Proteoglycans	Protein polysaccharides providing compressive strength.
Ground Substance	Gel-like amorphous component of the extracellular matrix.

Q: What types of cartilage do you know of?

Type	Notes
Fibrocartilage	Composed of type I collagen & provides high tensile strength. Present in areas subject to frequent stress e.g. symphysis pubis, tendon & ligament insertions.
Hyaline	Composed of type II collagen & is hard, forming a smooth articular surface for joint movement (overlying bone). Also found in the ear, larynx, sternum & between ribs.
Elastic	Composed of large amounts of elastin fibres. It is stiff but elastic, preventing collapse of tubular structures & providing shock absorption e.g. Eustachian tube, pinna, epiglottis & trachea.
Fibroelastic	Has the properties of fibrocartilage & elastic cartilage, providing minimal movement between joints, but with shock absorption properties e.g. intervertebral discs & knee menisci.
Physeal	Found at growth plates. Growth plates are composed of 1 calcification zone & 3 cartilagenous zones; resting, proliferating & maturation.

Q: How does cartilage repair after damage?

Cartilage is avascular, with chondrocytes bound in lacunae. This means that regenerative capabilities are limited, a feature that contributes to the common degenerative clinical condition OA. Where repair is possible, this is achieved by replacement with fibrocartilagenous scar tissue.

CHAPTER 8
ENDOCRINOLOGY

K Asaad
BH Miranda
SP Kay

CHAPTER CONTENTS

Multiple Endocrine Neoplasia (MEN)

Gynaecomastia

Hyperparathyroidism

Cushing's Disease / Syndrome

Carcinoid Syndrome

Hypo / Hyperthyroidism

MULTIPLE ENDOCRINE NEOPLASIA (MEN)

Q: Do you know of any inherited syndromes causing tumours of the endocrine system?

Multiple endocrine neoplasia. A rare group of syndromes, inherited in an autosomal dominant manner, comprising tumours of endocrine glands.

Q: What are the different syndromes?

Type	Notes
MEN I	Memory: 3 x **P**'s • **Pancreatic Islet Cell Tumour** • **Pituitary Adenoma** • **Primary Hyperparathyroidism**
MEN IIa	Memory: 3 x **C**'s • **Catecholamines** (Phaeochromocytoma) • **Calcitonin** (Thyroid Medullary Carcinoma) • **Calcium** (Primary Hyperparathyroidism)
MEN IIb	Same features as MEN IIa without parathyroid involvement. Also: • Marfanoid Habitus • Multiple Neuromas

GYNAECOMASTIA

Q: What is gynaecomastia?

Benign enlargement of the male breast.

Q: What are the causes of gynaecomastia?

Physiological	Pathological	Pharmacological
Idiopathic	Cirrhosis	Cimetidine
Neonatal	Hyperthyroidism	Digoxin
Puberty	Hypogonadism	Spironolactone
Old Age	Kleinfelter's Sydrome	Steroids
	Renal Disease	Tetrahydrocannibinol (marijuana)
	Testicular Tumours	

Q: How do you classify gynaecomastia?

Simon's Classification:

Grade	Description
I	Small enlargement & no skin excess.
IIa	Moderate enlargement & no skin excess.
IIb	Moderate enlargement & minor skin excess.
III	Marked enlargement & skin excess, resembling female pendulous breasts.

Q: What are the surgical options to treat gynaecomastia?

Treatment of the underlying cause is vital, remembering that most pubertal gynaecomastia resolves within 2 years. If gynaecomastia persists or causes psychological distress, surgical options include:

- Liposuction
- Excision of Breast Tissue   (peri-areolar / transverse incision)
- Reduction Mammoplasty   (longstanding macromastia)

HYPERPARATHYROIDISM

Q: What are the parathyroid glands?

- There are usually 4 glands (2 sets of pairs – superior & inferior), on the posterior aspect of the thyroid gland, that secrete PTH.
- Superior glands arise from the 4th pharyngeal pouch, adjacent to the upper central portion of the thyroid gland where the inferior thyroid artery crosses the recurrent laryngeal nerve.
- Inferior glands arise from the 3rd pharyngeal pouch & vary in position.

Q: How is hyperparathyroidism classified?

Classification	Cause
Primary	• Single Parathyroid Adenoma (85%) • Parathyroid Hyperplasia (12%) • Multiple Parathyroid Adenomata (2%) • Parathyroid Carcinoma (<1%)
Secondary	This is a physiological response to chronic hypocalcaemia e.g. CRF.
Tertiary	Autonomous hyperactive parathyroid glands. This follows prolonged untreated secondary hyperparathyroidism, even once the cause has been removed e.g. post renal transplant.

Q: What are the clinical features of hyperparathyroidism?

Features	Description
Asymptomatic	Chance finding of hypercalcaemia on blood testing.
Cardiovascular	Arrhythmias, hypertension, vascular calcification.
Hypercalcaemia	"Bones, stones, groans & moans".
Osteoporosis	Bone pain, pathological fractures, vertebral column collapse.

Note: Secondary hyperparathyroidism does not result in clinical features that are related to hypercalcaemia.

Q: How does serum PTH & calcium relate to hyperparathyroidism?

Classification	Calcium	PTH
Primary	High	High
Secondary	Low / Normal	High
Tertiary	High	High

Q: What are the specific treatment principles of hyperparathyroidism?

- Fluid resuscitation is vital in the acute setting to address dehydration & hypercalcaemia.
- Parathyroidectomy is the treatment for primary hyperparathyroidism. Patients may become hypocalcaemic post-operatively & require calcium / vitamin D supplementation.
- Investigate & treat the cause e.g. calcimemetics for patients with secondary hyperparathyroidism on dialysis.

CUSHING'S DISEASE / SYNDROME

Q: What is Cushing's Syndrome?

A collection of stereotypical clinical features, caused by high levels of circulating glucocorticoids.

Q: What is Cushing's Disease?

A benign, ACTH secreting pituitary adenoma, causing over-stimulation of the adrenal cortex.

Q: How are the causes of Cushing's Syndrome classified?

Most cases are iatrogenic, due to steroid therapy. Of the remaining causes, Cushing's Disease = 70% & ectopic ACTH producing tumours = 10% of causes. Classification is as follows:

ACTH Dependent	ACTH Independent	Pseudo-Cushing's
Cushing's Disease	Iatrogenic Steroids	Alcohol Abuse
Ectopic ACTH Producing Tumour • Small Cell Lung Carcinoma • Carcinoid Tumour	Adrenal Cortex Neoplasm	
Iatrogenic ACTH Administration		

Q: How are the clinical features of Cushing's Syndrome classified?

Classification	Features
Bone	Osteoporosis
Brain	Depression, Anxiety
Cardiovascular	Hypertension
Fat	Buffalo Hump, Moon Face, Weight Gain, Truncal Obesity & Limb Thinning (lemon on stick appearance)
Hair	Hirsutism
Hyperglycaemic	Diabetes
Muscle	Atrophy
Skin	Acne, Eccymosis, Striae

Q: How is Cushing's Syndrome diagnosed?

After taking a **full history** & performing a **thorough clinical examination**, I would first order investigations to confirm Cushing's Syndrome, then order investigations to elucidate the cause.

Investigations for Cushing's Syndrome	Notes
Low Dose Dexamethasone Suppression Test	Administer dexamethasone & monitor ACTH & cortisol levels. Non-suppression of plasma cortisol at 48h = Cushing's Syndrome present.
24h Urinary Cortisol	Raised.
Circadian Cortisol	09:00h plasma cortisol is normal, but is elevated at 24:00h.

Investigations to Elucidate Cause	Notes
Plasma ACTH	If low (<10ng/l) on ≥2 occasions = ACTH independent cause likely.
	If very high (>300ng/l) = ectopic cause likely.
High Dose Dexamethasone Suppression Test	Failure to suppress plasma cortisol = ectopic cause, adrenal cortex neoplasm. 80% of patients with Cushing's Disease display partial suppression (>50%).
CXR	Ectopic cause e.g. small cell lung carcinoma.
Adrenal CT	Adrenal neoplasm.
Pituitary MRI	Pituitary neoplasm.

Q: How is Cushing's Syndrome treated?

Treatment is dependent on the underlying cause:

Cause	Treatment
Pituitary Neoplasm	• Transsphenoidal / transfrontal pituitary surgery. • Irradiation is useful when surgery is unsuccessful, contraindicated or unacceptable.
Ectopic ACTH Secretion	• Surgery. • Chemotherapy. • Radiotherapy.
Iatrogenic Steroids	• Adjust steroids accordingly. • Manage symptoms.
Adrenal Neoplasms	• Adrenalectomy is the treatment of choice. • Post-operative chemotherapy & radiotherapy is required for carcinoma. • Post-operative glucocorticoid & mineralocorticoid replacement therapy may be required.

CARCINOID SYNDROME

Q: What is a carcinoid tumour?

- Tumour arising from APUD cells.
- May be intestinal or extra-intestinal.
- Common intestinal sites include appendix & small intestine.
- Extra-intestinal sites include lung, ovary & testis.

Q: How do carcinoid tumours present?

- Classical Carcinoid Syndrome   (affects 10% of patients)
- Abdominal Mass / Bowel Obstruction (gastrointestinal)
- Appendicitis   (appendix)
- Pelvic Mass   (ovary)
- Respiratory Symptoms   (lung)
- Testicular Mass   (testis)

Q: What is carcinoid syndrome?

A collection of clinical features seen in approximately 10% of patients with carcinoid tumours that include:

- Abdominal Cramps & Diarrhoea
- Bronchoconstrictive Episodes
- Skin Flushing   (after e.g. alcohol, coffee, drugs, food)
- Cardiac Failure   (due to plaque-like thickenings of endocardium & valves)
- Nausea & Vomiting

These features are primarily due to serotonin secretion, but other products are secreted e.g. kallikrein, histamine & secretin.

Q: How would you make a diagnosis of carcinoid syndrome?

After taking a **full history** & performing a **thorough clinical examination**, I would consider the following investigations:

Investigation	Notes
24h Urinary 5-HIAA Excretion	5-HIAA is a metabolite of serotonin, with increased excretion in patients with carcinoid syndrome (>25mg / day).
OctreoScan™	Radiolabelled octreotide, a somatostatin anaologue, is administered intravenously. Single photon emission computed tomography is performed at 4 hours & 24 hours. Octreotide has an affinity for somatostatin receptor-bearing neuroendocrine tumours & detects approximately 89% of tumours.
CT & MRI	Detection rates are approximately 80%.

Q: How is carcinoid syndrome treated?

Symptomatic	Potentially Curative
Octreotide	Surgical Excision of Tumour
Antihistamine	Chemotherapy e.g. 5-Fluorouracil & Doxorubicin

HYPO / HYPERTHYROIDISM

(also see book 2 head & neck chapter)

Q: Which hormones are produced by the thyroid gland?

Hormone	Source
T3 (Tri-Iodothyronine)	Colloid
T4 (Thyroxine)	Colloid
Calcitonin	Parafollicular Cells

Note: Significantly more T4 (than T3) is released by the thyroid gland. This is later converted to the more active form T3 by de-iodination.

Q: How are thyroid hormones controlled?

Negative feedback affecting the following pathway:
- TRH is released by the hypothalamus.
- TSH is released by the anterior pituitary.
- TSH acts on the thyroid gland after delivery via the bloodstream.
- Increased T3 & T4, results in decreased TRH & TSH release (negative feedback).

Q: How are the effects of thyroid hormones classified?

Classification	Effects
Foetus	Brain Development, Muscle Development.
Adrenergic	Increased Stimulation of β-Adrenergic Receptors.
Bone	Increased Catabolism.
Cardiovascular	Positive Ionotropic Effect & Tachycardia.
Gastrointestinal	Increased Motility.
Metabolic	Increased Glycogenolysis, Glucose Absorption & Lipolysis.
	Increased Basal Metabolic Rate.

Q: What factors affect thyroid function?

Hyperthyroid	Hypothyroid	Euthyroid
Iodine Excess	Iodine Deficiency	Multinodular Goitre (mostly)*
Graves' Disease	Hashimoto's Disease	Malignant Thyroid (mostly)*
Toxic Nodule	Thyroidectomy	*Note: may become toxic
Subacute Thyroiditis	Radioiodine	
High Dose Thyroxine		
Amioderone		

Q: What would you expect to see on the thyroid function tests of a patient with hyperthyroidism?

- Low TSH
- Increased T3 ± T4

CHAPTER 9
ONCOLOGY

K Asaad
BH Miranda
SP Kay

CHAPTER CONTENTS

Oncological Principles
- Screening
- Staging & Grading

Skin Cancer
- Basal Cell Carcinoma (BCC)
- Squamous Cell Carcinoma (SCC)
- Malignant Melanoma

Thyroid

Salivary Glands

Breast

Liver

Pancreas

Renal Tract
- Renal Cell Carcinoma (RCC)
- Transitional Cell Carcinoma (TCC)
- Wilms' Tumour

Intestinal Polyps & Colorectal Carcinoma

ONCOLOGICAL PRINCIPLES

Screening

Q: What is screening?

A strategy to detect a disease, present in a population without clinical features, thereby improving morbidity & mortality from that disease.

Q: What are the principles of a screening programme?

These are based on World Health Organisation guidelines as follows:

- The disease should be an important health problem.
- The natural history of the disease should be adequately understood.
- There should be a latent stage of the disease.
- Facilities for diagnosis & treatment should be available.
- There should be a test for the disease.
- The test should be acceptable to the population being screened.
- There should be a treatment for the disease.
- Early treatment should improve prognosis.
- There should be an agreed policy on whom to treat.
- The total cost of finding a case should be economically balanced in relation to medical expenditure as a whole.
- Case finding should be a continuous process & not an isolated event.

Q: What types of bias are associated with screening?

Bias	Interpretation
Lead	Earlier detection & treatment does not increase survival.
Lag	Treatment of slowly evolving disease, with a longer latent phase, gives the impression of creating a better prognosis e.g. slow growing cancer.
Selection	Populations may tend towards or away from participation in screening programmes for various reasons, creating an incorrect impression of the success of the screening test: • If the screening test is offered at a far location, it may be harder for elderly / severely ill populations to participate. This would produce more positive outcomes (due to a younger / healthier population) & incorrectly create a better view of the screening test. • In cases of patients with a family history of cancer, participation in screening may be more likely. This would produce more negative outcomes (due to family history as a risk factor for cancer) & incorrectly (perhaps) create a poorer view of the screening test.
Over Diagnosis	Identification of abnormalities that may not cause the patient a problem in their lifetime e.g. slow growing cancer.
Avoidance	The most accurate way of assessing a screening test is via a randomised controlled trial. These may be costly to run, such that they may be avoided in favour of other methodology.

Q: What is sensitivity & specificity?

- **Sensitivity:** True Positives ÷ (True Positives + False Negatives) x 100%
  % of patients with disease who test positive.
- **Specificity:** True Negatives ÷ (True Negatives + False Positives) x 100%
  % of patients without disease who test negative.

Q: What screening programmes do you know of in the UK?

Screening Program	Notes
Bowel	• FOB test every 2 years. • Men & women aged 60–69 years. • Abnormal tests – repeat +/- colonoscopy.
Breast	• 3 yearly mammography. • Women aged 50–70 years.
Cervix	• Liquid based cytology of cervical cells. • Women aged 25–49 years, 3 yearly. • Women aged 50–64 years, 5 yearly.

Staging & Grading

Q: What is staging & grading of cancer?

These help to guide both prognosis & treatment & may be described as follows:

- **Staging:** *Relates to degree of spread*:
    - Accurate staging requires clinical, pathological & radiological data.
    - TNM is a commonly used staging system.
    - Some cancers may use specific staging systems e.g. Dukes for colorectal cancer.
- **Grading:** *Refers to degree of differentiation of a cancer from its parent tissue*:
    - Poorly differentiated cancers are high grade.
    - Well differentiated cancers are low grade.
    - Higher grades are associated with a poorer prognosis.

Q: What is the TNM staging system?

Primary Tumour Extent (T)		Regional Lymph Nodes (N)		Metastasis & Distant Lymph Nodes (M)	
Tx	Primary tumour cannot be evaluated.	Nx	Regional nodal status cannot be evaluated.	Mx	Distant metastasis & lymph nodes cannot be evaluated.
T0	No evidence of primary tumour.	N0	No regional lymph node involvement.	M0	No distant metastasis or lymph node involvement.
Tis	Carcinoma *in situ*.	N1-3	Levels of regional lymph node involvement.	M1	Distant metastasis present.
T1-4	Size & extent of primary tumour.				

- Values for these 3 criteria vary according to cancer type.
- When combined, a stage (e.g. I–IV) may be assigned to the cancer.
- Each stage may be subdivided e.g. IIA, IIB & the prognosis varied accordingly.

SKIN CANCER

Basal Cell Carcinoma (BCC)

Q: What is a BCC?

A basal cell carcinoma (or rodent ulcer) is a malignant, locally infiltrative, neoplasm of the basal cells of the epidermis. It is the most prevalent form of skin cancer. Metastasis is very rare, but aggressive when present.

Q: How are BCCs classified?

Histologically there are many different sub-types. BCCs may be classified as:

Classification	Examples
Localised	- Nodular (most common) - Nodulocystic - Pigmented
Superficial	- Superficial Spreading - Multifocal
Infiltrative	- Morphoeic - Morpheaform

Q: How are BCC risk factors classified?

Congenital	Acquired
Fitzpatrick Skin Type I	UV Exposure
Gorlin's Syndrome	Increased Age

Q: What are the clinical features of BCCs?

- More common on sun-exposed sites e.g. head & neck.
- Appearance may be variable.
- Nodular is the most common sub-type.

Sub-type	Description
Nodular (Fig 9.1)	• Raised Lesion • 'Rolled Edges' with 'Pearly Sheen' • Central Depression / Ulceration • Superficial Telangiectasia
Superficial	• Erythematous Patches
Infiltrative	• Flat Pale Areas

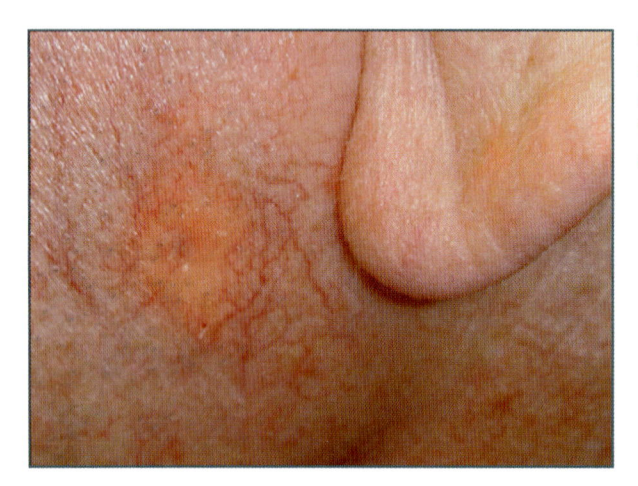

Fig 9.1: Nodular basal cell carcinoma. The lesion is raised with central depression & telangiectasia. The edges are 'rolled' with a 'pearly sheen'.

Q: What are the treatment options for BCCs?

This depends on the BCC sub-type, location, patient co-morbidities, patient wishes & should be discussed within an MDT environment. In addition to excision, reconstruction may be required.

Medical	Surgical
Chemotherapy e.g. 5-FU Cream	Curettage & Cautery
Cryotherapy	Excision
Phototherapy	Moh's Micrographic Surgery
Radiotherapy	

Q: What excision margins are suitable for excision of a BCC?

BCC	Excision Margins		
Primary	Small (<2cm):	3mm	= 85% Clearance (e.g. Face)
		4–5mm	= 95% Clearance
	Large (>2cm) / Morphoeic:	5mm	= 85% Clearance
		13–15mm	= 95% Clearance
Recurrent	5-10mm		
	Consider Moh's Micrographic Surgery		
Incomplete Excision	Re-excison		
	Consider surveillance		

Q: What is Moh's Micrographic Surgery?

- Sequential horizontal tumour excision with immediate frozen section examination.
- If the margins are not adequately clear, more is removed from the patient & re-examined.
- This is repeated until clear margins are achieved.

Squamous Cell Carcinoma (SCC)

Q: What is a cutaneous SCC?

A cutaneous squamous cell carcinoma is a malignant skin cancer arising from keratinising cells of the epidermis. It is the 2nd most prevalent form of skin cancer & has metastatic potential.

Q: How are SCC risk factors classified?

Congenital	Exposure Related	Acquired
Fitzpatrick Skin Type I	UV Exposure	Immunosuppression e.g. HIV, Iatrogenic
Xeroderma Pigmentosum	Chemicals e.g. Arsenic, Organic Hydrocarbons	Chronic Wounds e.g. Marjolin's Ulcer
	HPV Infection	Increased Age

Q: Do you know of any pre-malignant lesions of SCC?

Lesion	Description
Actinic Keratosis	• Rough White Patches 'Stuck Onto' Erythematous Base • 10–15% Progress to SCC
Bowen's Disease	• Red, Scaly Patch • Considered as SCC *in situ* • 5% progress to SCC
Leukoplakia	• White Patch on Oral / Other Mucosal Surface • 15% Progress to SCC

Q: What is the clinical appearance of SCC?

This is variable, but the classic appearance is an ulcerated lesion, with hard raised edges (Fig 9.2).

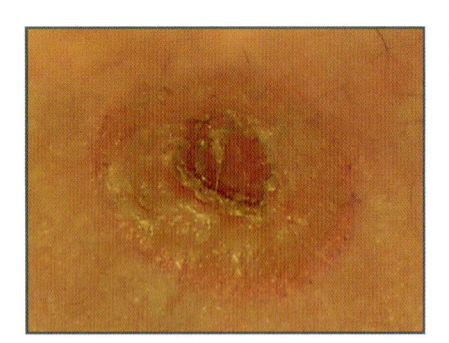

Fig 9.2: Squamous cell carcinoma. The lesion has central ulceration & raised edges.

Q: How is cutaneous SCC staged?

Primary Tumour Extent (T)		Regional Lymph Nodes (N)	
Tx	Primary tumour cannot be evaluated.	Nx	Regional nodal status cannot be evaluated.
T0	No evidence of primary tumour.	N0	No regional lymph node involvement.
Tis	Carcinoma *in situ*.	N1	Regional lymphadenopathy present.
T1	Primary tumour longest axis ≤2cm.	**Metastasis & Distant Lymph Nodes (M)**	
T2	Primary tumour longest axis >2cm & ≤5cm.	Mx	Distant metastasis & lymph nodes cannot be evaluated.
T3	Primary tumour longest axis >5cm.	M0	No distant metastasis / lymphadenopathy.
T4	Primary tumour extension into deep extradermal structures e.g. bone, muscle cartilage.	M1	Distant metastasis present.

Q: What are the treatment options for cutaneous SCC?

These should be considered within an MDT environment & include:

Medical	Surgical
Cryotherapy	Excision ± Reconstruction
Radiotherapy	Moh's Micrographic Surgery

Q: What excision margins are suitable for excision of a SCC?

SCC	Excision Margins	
<2cm Diameter	4mm	= 95% Cure
>2cm Diameter	≥6mm	= 95% Cure
	Consider Moh's Micrographic Surgery	

Malignant Melanoma

Q: What is a malignant melanoma?

A malignant neoplasm of melanocytes, predominantly in the skin, but also occurring in the leptomeninges, eyes, gastrointestinal tract, oral & genital mucous membranes. It has the greatest mortality of all skin cancers.

Q: What are the risk factors for malignant melanoma?

Congenital	Exposure Related	Acquired
Family History	UV Exposure	Immunosuppression
Fitzpatrick Skin Type I		
Xeroderma Pigmentosum		
Dysplastic Naevus Syndrome		

Q: What clinical features make you suspicious of malignant melanoma?

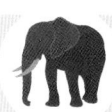

Memory: **ABCDE** for suspicious features of malignant melanoma

Asymmetry
Border Irregularity
Colour Variegation
Diameter >6mm
Evolving e.g. Size, Shape, Symptoms

Q: What sub-types of malignant melanoma do you know?

Sub-Type	Notes
Superficial Spreading (Fig 9.3)	• 50% of all sub-types. • Presents as a flat / slightly raised brown lesion with heterogeneous (irregular) pigmentation & irregular borders. • Usually affects the trunk (males) or legs (females).
Nodular	• 15–30% of all sub-types. • Presents as a blue-black nodule, with smooth borders, that may ulcerate / bleed. • 5% are amelanotic.
Lentigo Maligna Melanoma	• 10–15% of sub-types. • Presents on sun-damaged skin of elderly patients. • The precursor lesion is known as Hutchinson's Freckle / lentigo maligna.
Acral Lentiginous	• 30–70% of sub-types in dark skinned & 5% in fair skinned races. • Lesions present on the palms & soles or subungual (below the nail plate). • Hutchinson's Sign describes extension of an acral lentiginous melanoma to the nail folds.
Amelanocytic	• <5% of sub-types. This refers to an unpigmented melanoma. • Commonly affects nodular melanomas / metastases (due to incapability of poorly differentiated cells to synthesise melanin).

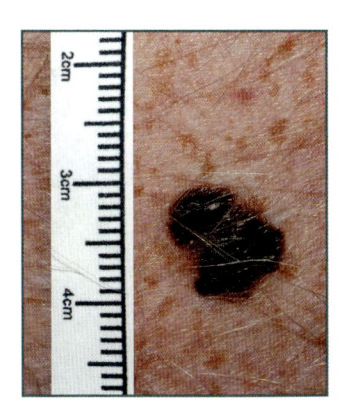

Fig 9.3: Superficial spreading malignant melanoma.

Q: What is the surgical management of suspected malignant melanoma?

- Excision biopsy (2mm margin) to confirm diagnosis & Breslow thickness.
- Consider incisional biopsy for large lesions.
- Wider local excision is performed for positive biopsies, with margins based on Breslow thickness.
- SLNB may also be considered at the time of wider local excision.

Q: What is Breslow thickness & why is it important?

The depth of penetration (mm) of the melanoma, from the statum granulosum. It is important as it guides excision margins & prognosis as follows:

Breslow Thickness (mm) (malignant melanoma)	Excision Margins (cm) (malignant melanoma)	5 Year Survival (%)
In situ	0.5	95
<1	1	95
1–2	1–2	80
2.1–4	2–3	65
>4	2–3	50

Q: What do you understand by Clark's Levels?

This is an anatomical measure of tumour depth.

Level	Notes
I	Confined to epidermis.
II	Extends to papillary dermis.
III	Extends to junction between papillary & reticular dermis.
IV	Extends into reticular dermis.
V	Extends into subcutaneous fat.

Q: How would you stage malignant melanoma?

Primary Tumour Extent (T)		Regional Lymph Nodes (N)	
Tx	Primary tumour cannot be evaluated.	Nx	Regional nodal status cannot be evaluated.
T0	No evidence of primary tumour.	N0	No regional lymph node involvement.
Tis	Carcinoma *in situ*.	N1	**N1a:** 1 enlarged regional lymph node & micro-metastases present.
T1	**T1a:** ≤1mm depth, without ulceration. **T1b:** ≤1mm depth, with ulceration.		**N1b:** 1 enlarged regional lymph node & macro-metastases present.
T2	**T2a:** 1.01–2mm depth, without ulceration. **T2a:** 1.01–2mm depth, with ulceration.	N2	**N2a:** 2–3 enlarged regional lymph nodes with micro-metastases present.
T3	**T3a:** 2.01–4mm depth, without ulceration. **T3b:** 2.01–4mm depth, with ulceration.		**N2b:** 2–3 enlarged regional lymph nodes with macro-metastases present.
T4	**T4a:** >4mm depth, without ulceration. **T4b:** >4mm depth, with ulceration.	N3	≥4 enlarged regional lymph nodes / matted nodes / in-transit metastases / satellite lesions.

Metastasis & Distant Lymph Nodes (M)			
Mx	Distant metastasis & lymph nodes cannot be evaluated.	M1a	Distant skin metastases present.
		M1b	Distant lung metastases present.
M0	No distant metastasis / lymphadenopathy.	M1c	Other visceral / distant metastases present. Any melanoma with elevated LDH.

Q: When would you perform a sentinel lymph node biopsy for malignant melanoma?

- At the time of wider local excision.
- Patients with thick melanomas.
- Presence of >1 malignant melanoma.
- Consider in melanomas with adverse features e.g. ulceration, lymphovascular invasion, mitotic rate ≥1mm^2.
- Role in melanomas <1mm thick remains controversial.

Q: Who makes up the malignant melanoma multidisciplinary treatment team?

This will vary according to each unit, but should comprise of:

- Dermatologist
- Plastic Surgeon
- Clinical Oncologist
- Pathologist
- Clinical Nurse Specialist
- Psychologist

THYROID

(also see book 2 head & neck chapter)

Q: What is the epidemiology of thyroid cancer?

- Rare.
- Accounts for approximately 0.5% of cancer related deaths.
- 2–3 times more common in females.

Q: What are the common thyroid cancers?

Thyroid Cancer	%	Notes
Papillary Adenocarcinoma	70	Common in children. 90% have lymphatic metastases at presentation.
Follicular Carcinoma	20	Common around 50 years. Blood-borne spread.
Medullary Carcinoma	5	Parafollicular C cell origin. Produce calcitonin. 90% are sporadic, 10% are MEN related.
Anaplastic Carcinoma	<5%	Common in older patients.
Lymphoma	<5%	Core biopsy best for diagnosis. Treat with radiotherapy & chemotherapy.

Q: How is thyroid malignancy investigated?

After taking a **full history** & performing a **thorough clinical examination**, I would consider the following investigations:

Investigations	Notes
Blood Tests	FBC, U&E, LFT, CRP, TFT, Ca^{2+} & Clotting.
USS & FNA	USS defines dimensions of tumour, if it is diffuse / solitary nodule / multinodular / cyst. Cytology from FNA can reveal diagnosis.
Core Biopsy	Useful particularly if FNA is inconclusive.
CT / MRI	Defines complex anatomy, retrosternal extension, airway deviation or compression & oesophageal compression.
Radioisotope Scan	Identifies whether a nodule is **'hot & functioning'** (takes up isotope) or **'cold & non-functioning'** (no isotope uptake). Hot nodules are rarely malignant.

Q: Can you differentiate between follicular adenoma & carcinoma using FNAC?

No, their cytology is identical. Histological evidence of capsular invasion is required.

SALIVARY GLANDS

(also see book 2 head & neck chapter)

Q: What is the epidemiology of salivary gland neoplasms?

- 5% of all head & neck tumours.
- 80% arise in the parotid gland.
- 15% arise in the submandibular gland.
- 5% arise in the sublingual & minor salivary glands.

Q: What are the common parotid & submandibular salivary gland neoplasms?

Gland	%	Salivary Neoplasm
Parotid	80	Pleomorphic Adenoma
	10	Mucoepidermoid Carcinoma
	5	Warthin's Tumour
Submandibular	35	Pleomorphic Adenoma
	25	Adenoid Cystic Carcinoma
	10	Mucoepidermoid Carcinoma
	5	Adenocarcinoma

Q: What is a pleomorphic adenoma?

- Commonest of all salivary gland neoplasms.
- 80% of parotid tumours (35% of submandibular).
- Peak incidence in 5th decade of life.
- Histologically contains stromal & epithelial elements.
- Presents as a slow-growing & benign painless mass.
- Commonly in the superficial lobe of the parotid gland & treated by superficial parotidectomy.
- Small proportion may undergo malignant transformation.

Q: What are the features of Warthin's Tumour?

- Also known as a papillary cystadenoma.
- 5% of parotid tumours.
- 10% are bilateral.
- Peaks during 7th decade of life & 7 times more prevalent in males.
- Histologically is an adenolymphoma with cystic spaces surrounded by eosinophilic columnar cells.
- Presents as a slow-growing & benign painless mass of the parotid gland & treated by surgery.
- Malignant change is extremely rare.

BREAST

Q: What is the epidemiology of breast cancer?

- Commonest cancer in females (after skin).
- 500,000 deaths / year worldwide.
- 1% occurs in males.

Q: What are the risk factors for breast cancer?

General	Oestrogen Exposure Related
Age	Early Menarche & Late Menopause
Family History	1st Pregnancy >30 years
BRCA1 & BRCA2 Genes	Non-Breast-Feeding Mothers
Previous Breast Malignancy	OCP / HRT

Q: What investigations should be ordered to guide management of breast disease?

Triple assessment is vital:

Triple Assessment	Notes
1. Clinical Examination	Full history & thorough clinical examination.
2. Imaging	Mammogram / USS.
3. Tissue Sampling	FNAC / Core Biopsy / Open Biopsy.

To assess metastasis, the following investigations are useful:

- **LFTs & Liver USS** (liver)
- **CXR** (chest)
- **Radioisotope Bone Scan** (bone)
- **CT Brain** (brain)

Q: What types of breast cancer do you know of?

Non-Invasive Lesions	Invasive Carcinoma
Ductal Carcinoma *in situ*.	Invasive Ductal Carcinoma (70%).
Lobular Carcinoma *in situ*.	Invasive Lobular Carcinoma (20%).
	Other (10%): Microinvasive, Tubular, Medullary, Mucinous, Papillary.

Q: How is breast cancer staged?

According to the TNM classification as follows:

Primary Tumour Extent (T)		Regional Lymph Nodes (N)	
Tx	Primary tumour cannot be evaluated.	Nx	Regional nodal status cannot be evaluated.
T0	No evidence of primary tumour.	N0	No regional lymph node involvement.
Tis	Carcinoma *in situ*.	N1	Mobile ipsilateral axillary nodes.
T1	**Primary tumour longest axis ≤2cm:** T1a: ≤0.5cm. T1b: >0.5cm & ≤1cm. T1c: >1cm & ≤2cm.	N2	Fixed ipsilateral axillary nodes or ipsilateral internal mammary nodes.
		N3	Ipsilateral supra/infraclavicular nodes or presence of both ipsilateral axillary & internal mammary nodes together.
T2	Primary tumour longest axis >2cm & ≤5cm.		
T3	Primary tumour longest axis >5cm.	**Metastasis & Distant Lymph Nodes (M)**	
T4	**Primary tumour extension:** T4a: Extension to chest wall.	Mx	Distant metastasis & lymph nodes cannot be evaluated.
	T4b: Oedema, skin ulceration or satellite nodes present.	M0	No distant metastasis or lymph node involvement.
	T4c: T4a & T4b together. T4d: Inflammatory carcinoma.	M1	Distant metastasis present.

Q: What are the medical / surgical treatment options for breast cancer?

This depends on the site & size of tumour, patient co-morbidities, patient wishes & must be discussed with an MDT environment.

Treatment	Notes
Hormonal Therapy	• Tamoxifen (selective oestrogen receptor modulator for receptor positive cases). • Aromatase Inhibitors e.g. Anastrozole.
Chemotherapy	• Neo-Adjuvant (shrinks tumour before surgery). • Adjuvant (reduces recurrence risk post-operatively). • To Treat Recurrence. • Drugs Include: Fluorouracil, Cyclophosphamide, Doxorubicin
Surgical *(also see operative surgery chapter)*	• Breast Conserving Surgery. • Mastectomy (including prophylactic contralateral mastectomy). • Sentinel Lymph Node Biopsy (staging). • Axillary Lymph Node Sampling / Dissection. • Breast Reconstruction. **Note: Breast cancer surgery is mostly undertaken for curative purposes.**
Radiotherapy	• Primarily used after surgery to decrease recurrence risk.

LIVER

Q: What is the epidemiology of liver cancer?

- 1% of all cancers in the UK.
- Highest incidence in Africa & Asia.
- Lowest incidence in America & Europe.
- Hepatic metastases are the most common type in the UK.

Q: What benign hepatic tumours do you know?

Tumour	Description
Haemangioma	• Most common benign liver tumour. • Vascular neoplasm of endothelial cells. • Mainly affects middle-aged females. • Often small & solitary. • Usually incidental finding. • Treatment is conservative & monitoring. • Surgical excision indicated if rupture / rapid change in size occurs.
Focal Nodular Hyperplasia	• 2nd most common benign liver tumour. • Solitary stellate lesion. • Numerous small bile ducts within fibrous tissue. • May become vascular & enlarge. • No malignant potential. • Often resected as difficult to distinguish from hepatic adenoma.
Adenoma	• Well differentiated & circumscribed nodule. • Mainly affects females aged 20–40 years. • Increased risk with oestrogenic medications & anabolic steroids. • May spontaneously bleed. • Large lesions may present with hepatomegaly. • Small risk of malignant transformation. • Treatment is surgical excision.

Q: What malignant hepatic tumours do you know?

Tumour	Example	Description
PRIMARY	**Hepatocellular Carcinoma (HCC)**	• More common in Africa & Asia, with a younger presentation. • Large, heterogeneous, vascular & haemorrhagic malignancy. • Risks include HBV, HCV, cirrhosis & aflatoxin. • Produces α-fetoprotein tumour marker. • Never biopsy HCC as there is a risk of seeding. • Treatment is preventative e.g. HBV vaccination or curative e.g. partial hepatectomy / liver transplant.
	Cholangiocarcinoma	• Rare. • Aggressive adenocarcinoma of bile duct epithelium. • May present with obstructive jaundice. • Risks include liver fluke infestation & PSC. • Treatment is surgical excision ± chemotherapy & radiotherapy.
	Angiosarcoma	• Rare endothelial vascular malignancy. • Highly malignant.
	Hepatoblastoma	• Uncommon malignancy. • Occurs in infants & children. • Presents with abdominal mass. • Prognosis poor unless associated with α-fetoprotein production. • Treatment is neoadjuvant chemotherapy & surgical excision.
SECONDARY	**Metastasis**	• The most common hepatic malignancy. • Underlying primary tumour is frequently breast, gastrointestinal, lung, ovarian, prostatic or renal. • Features are of hepatic involvement & of the underlying primary. • Prognosis is generally poor & related to the underlying primary. • Treatment is surgical resection & of the underlying primary.

PANCREAS

Q: What is the epidemiology of pancreatic carcinoma?

- 3rd most common gastrointestinal cancer.
- Increasing incidence in developed countries.
- Accounts for approximately 5% of all cancer deaths.
- Uncommon in patients aged <50 years.
- 3 times more prevalent in males.
- 1 year survival = 10%.

Q: What are the pathological features of pancreatic carcinoma?

- 80% are adenocarcinomas of the exocrine pancreas.
- 60% occur at the head of the pancreas.
- Rarely due to endocrine tumours e.g. insulinoma & glucagonoma.

Q: What are the risks for pancreatic adenocarcinoma?

Congenital	Acquired
Male	Smoking
Family History	High Fat Diet
	Chronic Pancreatitis
	DM

Q: How does pancreatic carcinoma present?

- Often presents late.
- Painless jaundice (if carcinoma obstructs CBD).
- Anorexia & weight loss.
- Epigastric mass.
- Epigastric pain radiating to back.
- Ascites.

Q: What is Trousseau's Sign?

Thrombophlebitis migrans associated with malignancy e.g. lung & pancreas. This occurs due to a malignant hypercoagulable state. Clusters of tender blood clots appear in succession, along & within the lumen of the affected vessel(s) e.g. superficial veins throughout the body, deep limb veins & portal vein.

Note: Trousseau also described carpal spasm, caused by arm compression above systolic pressure, as a sign of hypocalcaemia.

Q: What specific treatments are available for pancreatic adenocarcinoma?

- 15% are resectable & therefore potentially curable.
- The most common procedure is Whipple's Procedure (pancreaticoduodenectomy) for carcinoma of the head of the pancreas.
- Other procedures include distal pancreatectomy (tail carcinoma) & total pancreatectomy (diffuse carcinoma).
- Patients may develop diabetes or require pancreatic supplements post-operatively.
- Chemotherapy has some role as adjuvant, neo-adjuvant or palliative therapy.
- Radiotherapy is only useful for palliative therapy.

Q: What endocrine tumours of the pancreas do you know?

Endocrine pancreatic tumours are associated with MEN I & may be classified as follows:

Tumour	Description
Insulinoma	• Tumour of β-islets of Langerhans. • 75% of all endocrine pancreatic tumours & 10% are malignant. • Presents with episodic hypoglycaemia, increased appetite & weight gain. • Curative treatment is with surgery & chemotherapy.
Glucagonoma	• Tumour of α-islets of Langerhans. • Hypersecretion of glucagon ensues. • 75% are malignant & 90% have hepatic / lymphatic metastases at presentation. • Presents with hyperglycaemic attacks, anaemia, rash & diarrhoea. • Also causes secondary diabetes mellitus. • Curative treatment is with surgery & chemotherapy. • Insulin & octreotide may be useful.
VIPoma	• Tumour of PP (pancreatic polypeptide producing) cells. • Hypersecretion of vasoactive intestinal polypeptide ensues. • Causes profuse watery diarrhoea, hypokalaemia, achlorhydria. • Curative treatment is surgical. • Corticosteroids & octreotide may be useful.
Gastrinoma	• Often found in pancreas but also gastric antrum & small intestine. • 60% are malignant & 10% are multiple. • Clinical features are due to overproduction of gastrin e.g. peptic ulcer disease. • Can result in Zollinger-Ellison syndrome. • Curative treatment is surgical. • Proton pump inhibitors & octreotide may be useful.

RENAL TRACT

Q: How are renal tumours classified?

Benign	Malignant	
Fibroma	*Primary:*	*Secondary:*
Cortical Adenoma	Renal Cell Carcinoma (RCC)	Metastases
Oncocytoma	Nephroblastoma / Wilms' Tumour	
Angiomyolipoma	Transitional Cell Carcinoma (TCC)	

Q: How would you investigate a patient with a suspected renal tract tumour?

After taking a **full history** & performing a **thorough clinical examination**, I would consider the following investigations:

Investigation	Notes	
Blood Tests	FBC, U&E, LFT & CRP.	
Urine Dipstick	Haematuria.	
Histology	May be USS guided e.g. RCC (although in RCC, biopsy is rarely required for diagnosis). May be taken at cystoscopy e.g. TCC bladder.	
Imaging	**Radiography:**	AXR / KUB may show malignant opacity.
		CXR may show cannonball metastases.
	USS Renal Tract:	Defines solid / cystic lesions.
		Defines local invasion e.g. RCC into IVC.
	IVU:	Space occupying lesions & filling defects visible.
		Distortion of renal tract outline.
	Flexible Cystoscopy:	Direct vision of bladder & urethra.
		Histological biopsy obtainable e.g. TCC bladder.
		Treatment possible e.g. TCC bladder.
	CT:	Assess local spread & metastasis e.g. RCC into IVC.
	Bone Scan:	Assess bone metastasis.

Renal Cell Carcinoma (RCC)

Q: What is RCC?

- Most common primary malignancy of the kidney parenchyma.
- Histologically an adenocarcinoma.
- Uncommon in patients aged <50 years.

Q: What are the risk factors for developing RCC?

- Male : Female (2:1)
- Family History
- Smoking
- Von Hippel-Lindau Syndrome.

Q: What are the clinical features of RCC?

- Classically presents with a triad of haematuria, abdominal mass & loin pain.
- May be an incidental finding on CT.
- May present with paraneoplastic syndromes e.g. hypertension (renin), polycythaemia (EPO) & hypercalcaemia (PTHRP).
- May present with features of metastasis e.g. bone pain, hepatomegaly, respiratory symptoms & confusion.

Q: How is RCC staged?

Either by TNM or Robson's Staging. Robson's Staging is as follows:

Stage	Explanation
I	Tumour Confined to Kidney.
II	Extension to Perinephric Fat.
III	Metastasis to Renal Vein.
IV	Metastasis to Adjacent / Distance Organs.

Q: Why may RCC present as a left varicocoele?

The tumour may invade the left renal vein & obstruct the left testicular vein (which drains into the left renal vein). This is uncommon with a right-sided RCC as the right testicular vein drains directly into the IVC.

Q: What are the treatment options for RCC?

Chemotherapy	Surgery	Radiotherapy
Progesterone	Nephrectomy	Palliative e.g. Bone Metastasis Pain
IFNα		
IL-2		
VEGF / PDGF Inhibitors		

Transitional Cell Carcinoma (TCC)

Q: What types of bladder carcinoma do you know?

- **TCC:** Most common type in the UK.
- **SCC:** Develops due to chronic inflammation from e.g. calculi / schistosomiasis.
- **Adenocarcinoma:** Also develops in remnants of the urachus.

Note: Schistosomiasis is the most common cause of bladder cancer worldwide.

Q: What is TCC of the renal tract?

- Malignant tumour of the transitional epithelium of the renal tract.
- 4 times more prevalent than RCC.
- Uncommon in patients aged <50 years.

Q: How does TCC of the renal tract present?

- Classically with painless haematuria.
- May present with features of metastasis.

Q: What are the risk factors for renal tract TCC?

- Male : Female (3:1).
- Smoking.
- β-Naphthylamine e.g. Dye & Rubber Industries.
- Nitrosamines e.g. Smoked Fish.

Q: What is field change?

Transitional cell epithelium lines the renal tract from the renal pelvices to the proximal urethra. Exposure to a carcinogen will increase the risk of TCC throughout this entire 'field' of transitional cell epithelium. This is the concept of field change.

Q: By what common routes may renal tract TCC spread?

Spread	Examples
Local	Prostate & Rectum (males), Uterus & Vagina (females).
Lymphatic	Iliac & Para-Aortic Lymph Nodes.
Haematogenous	Bone, Brain, Liver & Lungs.

Q: What are the treatment options for renal tract TCC?

Treatment options depend on site, grade & stage of disease. This should be discussed within an MDT environment. Treatment options include:

Chemotherapy	Radiotherapy	Surgery
Intravesical Cytotoxic Chemotherapy (bladder)*	Curative (early presentation)	Nephroureterectomy & Bladder Cuff Removal (ureter)
Intravesical BCG Immunotherapy (bladder)*	Palliative (late presentation)	Cystectomy (bladder)
		Cystoscopic Excision (urethra)

*Note: These require regular cystoscopy follow up.

Wilms' Tumour

Q: What is the epidemiology of Wilms' Tumour?

- Most common renal malignancy in children.
- Most common intra-abdominal malignancy in patients aged <10 years.
- Peak incidence ages 1–4 years.

Q: What is the pathology of Wilms' Tumour?

- Also known as a mixed nephroblastoma.
- Composed of metanephric blastema, stroma & epithelium elements with varying differentiation.
- Histology reveals abortive glomeruli & tubules surrounded by stroma.
- Stroma may contain bone, cartilage, fat & muscle.
- Aggressive & rapidly growing.

Q: How does Wilms' Tumour present & what is a common surgical treatment option?

- Abdominal mass, haematuria, hypertension, abdominal pain & intestinal obstruction.
- <5% are bilateral.
- Treatment depends on stage & involves nephrectomy ± chemotherapy & radiotherapy.

INTESTINAL POLYPS & COLORECTAL CARCINOMA

Q: What are intestinal polyps?

Benign protuberant neoplasms in the intestinal lumen, most commonly affecting the colon / rectum.

Q: How are intestinal neoplasms classified?

Type	Example	
Epithelial	*Benign:* • Tubular Adenoma • Tubulovillous Adenoma • Villous Adenoma	*Malignant:* • Polypoid Adenocarcinoma • Carcinoid Polyp
Mesenchymal	*Benign:* • Fibroma • Leiomyoma • Lipoma	*Malignant:* • Sarcoma • Lymphomatous Polyp
Hamartomatous	• Juvenile Polyp • Peutz-Jegher's Syndrome • Haemangioma • Neurofibroma	
Inflammatory	• Ulcerative Colitis Pseudopolyp	

Q: What is the malignant potential of a colorectal adenoma?

Most colorectal adenocarcinomas arise within benign adenomas. Malignant potential relates to degree of dysplasia, adenoma type & size as follows:

Type	Malignant Change
Tubular Adenoma	5%
Tubulovillous Adenoma	20%
Villous Adenoma	40%

Size	Malignant Change
<1cm	1%
1–2cm	10%
>2cm	40%

Q: What is the epidemiology of colorectal cancer?

- Represents 10% of all cancers.
- 3rd most common cause of cancer related death.
- Uncommon in patients aged <50 years.
- More common in the western world.

Q: What are the risk factors for colorectal cancer?

Congenital	Acquired
Family History	Age
Familial Adenomatous Polyposis (FAP)	Western Diet (high fat & low fibre)
Hereditary Non-Polyposis Colorectal Carcinoma (HNPCC)	Colorectal Polyps
	Ulcerative Colitis

Q: What is familial adenomatous polyposis (FAP)?

- Rare autosomal dominant condition.
- Mutations of APC gene on chromosome 5q21.
- Patients develop hundreds of colorectal polyps that carpet the colon & rectum (seen at endoscopy), around the age of 20–30 years.
- Colorectal carcinoma develops in patients aged <40 years if untreated.
- Screening high risk patients from their early teens involves 6–12 monthly colonoscopy.
- Treatment is by colectomy.

Q: What is hereditary non-polyposis colorectal carcinoma (HNPCC)?

- Rare autosomal dominant condition.
- 80% lifetime risk of developing colon cancer.
- Mutations of genes involved in the DNA mismatch repair pathway.
- 90% of mutations occur in MLH1 (3p21) & MSH2 (2p21) genes.
- Amsterdam criteria identifies patients suitable for genetic testing.
- Screening high risk patients aged >25 years involves 6-12 monthly colonoscopy.
- Treatment is by colectomy.

Q: What is the adenoma-carcinoma sequence?

The stepwise pattern of mutational activation of oncogenes & inactivation / loss of tumour suppressor genes, resulting in the transition from normal epithelium to adenoma, then carcinoma (Fig 9.4).

Normal Epithelium ⇨ Hyperproliferation ⇨ Adenoma ⇨ Carcinoma

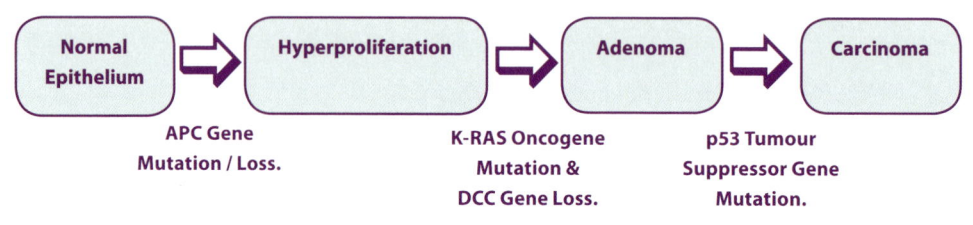

- APC Gene Mutation / Loss.
- K-RAS Oncogene Mutation & DCC Gene Loss.
- p53 Tumour Suppressor Gene Mutation.

Fig 9.4: Diagram illustrating the steps of the adenoma-carcinoma sequence.

This also explains the **multi-hit hypothesis** as progression to carcinoma is due to the accumulation of multiple genomic alterations. The order of events that occur in the adenoma-carcinoma sequence may not be as important as the accumulation of genomic alterations.

Q: What are the clinical features of colorectal carcinoma?

Most are clinically silent for years. Features depend on the site of the cancer & may be classified as local, systemic or metastatic as follows:

Local	Systemic	Metastatic
Abdominal / Rectal Mass	Anorexia	Hepatomegaly
Abdominal Pain (unlikely if left sided)	Weight Loss	Jaundice
Altered Bowel Habit	Anaemia	Respiratory Symptoms
PR Bleeding	Paraneoplastic Syndromes	
Bowel Obstruction		
Bowel Perforation		
Tenesmus (rectal involvement)		

Q: What investigations would you order for a patient with suspected colorectal cancer?

Modality	Tests
Blood Tests	• FBC, U&E, CEA
Imaging	• CXR
	• USS Liver
	• CT Abdomen / Pelvis
	• Double Contrast Barium Enema
Procedures	• Rigid Sigmoidoscopy
	• Flexible Sigmoidoscopy / Colonoscopy
	Note: Biopsies should also be taken.

Q: How is colorectal carcinoma staged?

Dukes' Staging:

Stage	Description	5 Year Survival
A	Tumour confined to intestinal wall & no invasion into muscle layer.	90%
B	Invasion into muscle layer.	60%
C	Lymph node involvement.	40%
D	Distant metastasis.	<5%

TNM Staging:

Primary Tumour Extent (T)		Regional Lymph Nodes (N)	
Tx	Primary tumour cannot be evaluated.	Nx	Regional nodal status cannot be evaluated.
T0	No evidence of primary tumour.	N0	No regional lymph node involvement.
Tis	Carcinoma *in situ*.	N1	1–3 regional lymph nodes involved.
T1	Primary tumour confined to submucosa.	N2	≥4 regional lymph nodes involved.
T2	Primary tumour invades muscularis propria.	**Metastasis & Distant Lymph Nodes (M)**	
T3	Primary tumour invades subserosa.	Mx	Distant metastasis & lymph nodes cannot be evaluated.
T4	Primary tumour invades through bowel wall into adjacent tissues / organs.	M0	No distant metastasis or lymph node involvement.
		M1	Distant metastasis present.

Q: What are the surgical options for a patient with colorectal cancer?

Surgery for colorectal cancer may be palliative, e.g. faecal diversion procedures, or curative. Curative surgery depends on the site of the cancer (Fig 9.5). The aim is to get clear resection margins 5cm proximal & 2cm distal to the cancer. Surgical procedures therefore include:

Site	Operation
Caecum to Hepatic Flexure	Right Hemicolectomy *(see operative surgery chapter)*
Transverse Colon	Extended Right Hemicolectomy
Splenic Flexure to Sigmoid Colon	Left Hemicolectomy
Sigmoid Colon	Sigmoid Colectomy
Upper Rectum (>5cm from anal verge)	Anterior Resection *(see operative surgery chapter)*
Lower Rectum (≤5cm from anal verge)	Abdominoperineal (AP) Resection *(see operative surgery chapter)*

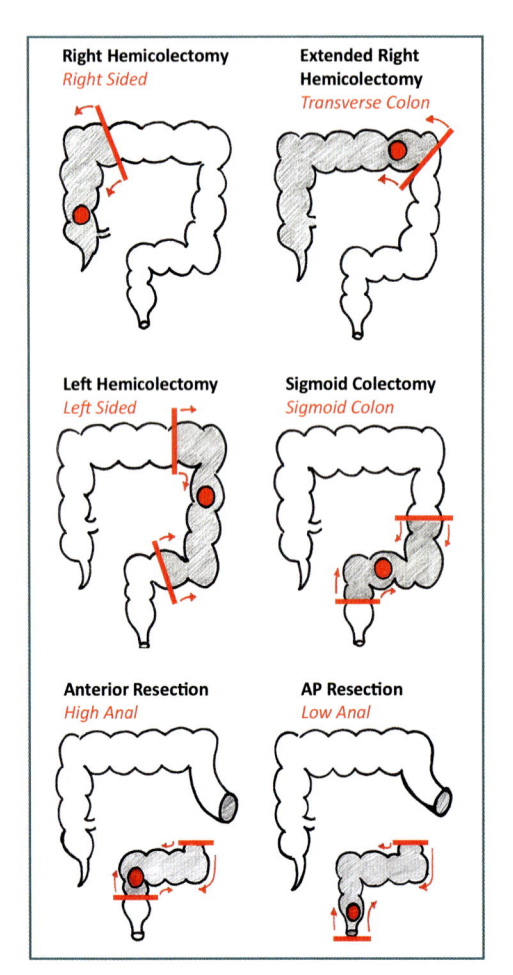

Fig 9.5: Surgical treatment options for colorectal carcinoma, according to tumour location.

CHAPTER 10
PERIOPERATIVE CARE & SURGICAL TECHNOLOGY

K Asaad
BH Miranda
SP Kay

CHAPTER CONTENTS

Perioperative Care
- Clinical Trials
- Thromboprophylaxis
- Patient Positioning
- Patient Safety for Theatre

Surgical Technology
- Theatre Design
- Disinfection & Sterilisation
- LASER
- Tourniquets
- Diathermy
- Suture Materials
- Drains
- Dressings

PERIOPERATIVE CARE

Clinical Trials

Q: What is the purpose of clinical trials?

Clinical trials are required to show safety & efficacy of new drugs, therapies or devices. They invariably address a clinical question e.g. is drug a better than drug b?

Q: What must take place before a clinical trial can begin?

- Research & Development Funding
- Study Design Protocol
- Ethics Committee Approval
- Pre-Clinical Studies.

Q: What are the phases of clinical trials?

Phase	Description
I	Initial study on a small (20–50) group of healthy volunteers ± patients to identify safety, metabolism, dose range & side effects.
II	Controlled clinical study on a larger (50–300) group. Assesses drug effectiveness, side effects & risks.
III	Randomised, controlled multicentre trial (300–3000). Assesses risk-benefit relationship of drug.
IV	Post marketing studies. Fully ascertains drug risks, benefits & optimal use.

Q: What is randomisation?

Participants are randomly allocated into treatment groups within the trial.

Q: What is blinding?

Blinding (also called masking) aims to eliminate bias by concealing if a participant is in the experimental or control arm of the trial.

- **Single Blinding:** Only 1 party, either the investigator or participant, does not know which arm of the trial the participant is in.
- **Double Blinding**: Neither the investigator nor the participant knows which arm of the trial the participant is in.

Q: What levels of clinical evidence do you know of?

Level	Explanation	
1	1a:	Systematic review or meta-analysis of RCT
	1b:	Individual RCT
	1c:	All or none
2	2a:	Systematic review of well designed non-randomised control trials
	2b:	Individual cohort study
	2c:	Outcome study
3	3a:	Systematic review case control studies
	3b:	Case control study
4	Case series	
5	Expert opinion	

Q: What strengths of evidence-based recommendations do you know of?

These are graded A–D according to level of evidence as follows:

Grade	Description
A	Based on level 1 evidence
B	Based on level 2 evidence or extrapolated from level 1 evidence
C	Based on level 3 evidence or extrapolated from level 2 evidence
D	Based on level 4 evidence or extrapolated from level 3 evidence

Thromboprophylaxis

Q: What methods of reducing DVT & VTE risk in surgical patients do you know of?

Risk factors for deep vein thrombosis (DVT) are discussed in the pathology chapter of this book. Reducing DVT & venous thromboembolism (VTE) risk in surgical patients may be classified by intervention method as follows:

Conservative	Mechanical	Medical	Surgical
Maintain Good Hydration	Intermittent Pneumatic Compression Devices	COCP – Stop 4 Weeks Prior to Elective Surgery	Avoid GA Where Possible
Leg Exercises		LMWH Prophylaxis	Vena Cava Filters
Thromboembolic Deterrent Stockings		(IV) Fluids	
Early Mobilisation After Surgery			

Q: What pressure should be produced by thromboembolic deterrent stockings?

This follows the Sigel profile:

- 8 mmHg: Thigh
- 14 mmHg: Mid-Calf
- 18 mmHg: Ankle.

Q: How would you decide on the DVT / VTE prophylactic strategy for a patient?

I would follow NICE guidelines (outlined below).

- **Assess Patient Risk Factors**
- **Assess Patient Bleeding Risk Factors**   e.g. Anticoagulants, Haemophilia, Thrombocytopaenia.
- **Implement Conservative Measures**
- **Consider Prophylaxis According to Surgery:**

Surgery	Prophylaxis
• Hip Fracture	• Mechanical Prophylaxis & 4 Weeks LMWH post-op.
• Hip Replacement	• Mechanical Prophylaxis & LMWH.
	• Continue 4 Weeks LMWH post-op if ≥1 Risk Factor.
• Other Orthopaedic	• Mechanical Prophylaxis & LMWH.
• Cardiac	• Mechanical Prophylaxis.
• General	• Add LMWH if ≥1 Risk Factor.
• Gynaecological (Excluding Caesarean)	
• Thoracic	
• Neurosurgery (Including Spinal)	
• Urological	
• Vascular	

Patient Positioning

Q: What is the importance of correct patient positioning?

- Prevent Iatrogenic Harm
- Surgical Access
- Allow Stable Position to Prevent Patient Moving or Lines Being Dislodged
- Allow Intra-Operative Monitoring.

Q: How are the complications of poor positioning classified?

Category	Example
Cutaneous	Skin necrosis e.g. over bony prominences (pressure sore).
Embolic	Air embolus in sitting position e.g. neurosurgery.
Musculoskeletal	Joint dislocation.
Neurological	Ulnar / peroneal nerve injury from pressure or traction.
Ocular	Eye compression in prone position.
Respiratory	FRC & TLC reduced in supine position especially in obese patients.
Vascular	Compartment Syndrome in Lloyd Davies position.

Q: How are pressure sores classified?

Grade	Description
I	Superficial, non-blanching erythema of intact skin.
II	Breach in skin no deeper than dermis.
III	Breach in skin beyond dermis, into subcutaneous fat.
IV	Full thickness breach in skin with exposed muscle, tendon or bone.

Q: Which nerves are most at risk in the anaesthetised patient?

Nerve Injury	Explanation
Ulnar	Commonest nerve injury. Compression often between medial epicondyle & arm board / bed. More likely if elbow flexed or forearm pronated.
Brachial Plexus	Plexus stretched or compressed between clavicle & 1st rib. More likely if head rotated & arm extended posteriorly.
Radial	Compressed against spiral groove of humerus & other object.
Common Peroneal	Lateral aspect of leg compressed against stirrup.
Sciatic	Stretched by excessive hip flexion or damage due to direct compression.
Saphenous	Medial condyle compressed against stirrups.
Obturator	Excessive thigh flexion, compresses nerve as it exits obturator foramen.

Patient Safety for Theatre

Q: How is patient safety for surgery maintained?

Admission	Pre-Operative	Intra-Operative	Post-Operative
Full History & Examination	Patient Identifiers e.g. Identity Bracelet	Equipment Well Maintained, Functioning & Used Appropriately	Analgesia & Medications
Check for Metal Valves, Pacemakers, Prosthetics & Dentures	Patient Notes Available	Staff Trained on Equipment Use	Post-Operative Review
Pre-Operative Work Up Satisfactory e.g. Blood Tests & Imaging	Correct Operation & Side with Patient, Notes, Images & List	Adequate Staff for Patient Handling	Patient Observations Adequate
Mark Patient & Check Operative Side	Informed Consent	Appropriate Positioning	Accurate Fluid Balance
Book ICU / HDU (If required)	Allergies e.g. Latex, Iodine & Elastoplast™	Padding to Bony Prominences or High Risk Areas	Drains Open & Working
	Place Appropriately on List e.g. Latex Allergic, Diabetic, MRSA	Diathermy Pad (if monopolar) & Fluid Pooling Avoided	Instructions for Ward
	DVT Prophylaxis	Meticulous Operative Technique	Ward Transfer
	Blood Units Available in Fridge (if ordered)	Drains, Lines & Dressings Secure	Post-Operative Review
	Surgical Timeout	Note with Post-Operative Instructions	Handover to 'On-Call' Team

SURGICAL TECHNOLOGY

Theatre Design:

Q: What are the components of an operating theatre suite?

- Patient Reception
- Changing Room
- Anaesthetic Room
- Operating Theatre
- Scrub Room
- Clean Utility Room
- Dirty Utility Room
- Staff Rest Area.

Q: What are the different zones in an operating theatre suite?

Zone	Description
Outer	General access areas e.g. patient reception.
Limited Access	Clean area between reception & within theatre suite.
Restricted Access	Properly clothed personnel only e.g. anaesthetic room & scrub room.
Aseptic	The operating theatre.

Q: Can you describe the air flow system in theatres?

- Air is maintained under pressure to allow outflow from theatre & inflow of filtered air.
- Normal air flow is turbulent (random movement of gas particles).
- Laminar (directional) air flow can be horizontal or vertical, allowing for an increased rate of air exchange.
- Most theatres have 20–40 air changes per hour.
- This can increase to 400–600 air changes per hour in a Charnley Tent.

Q: What level of bacteria counts are acceptable in theatre air?

- <35 per m^3 of bacteria carrying particles.
- <1 colony per m^3 of *Clostridium* or *Staphylococcus aureus*.

Disinfection & Sterilisation:

Q: Can you define asepsis, antisepsis, disinfection & sterilisation?

Term	Definition
Asepsis	Prevention of contamination to a body area from another site.
Antisepsis	Use of solutions e.g. iodine / alcohol, to disinfect an object or surface.
Disinfection	Removal of some or all microorganisms, but not necessarily viruses or spores.
Sterilisation	Total destruction of all viable microorganisms, including spores, viruses & mycobacteria, on an object.

Q: What methods of disinfection do you know of?

Method	Explanation
Low Temperature Steam	Used at 73°C for 20 mins, to clean instruments prior to sterilisation.
Boiling Water	Used at 100°C for 5 mins e.g. speculae & proctoscopes.
Formaldehyde	Used as a gas at 50°C, for heat-sensitive equipment e.g. ventilators & incubators.
Glutaraldehyde	2% solution decontaminates endoscopes.
Other Methods	Iodine, chlorhexidine & cetrimide.

Q: What sterilisation methods do you know of?

Method	Explanation
Steam	Used at 120°C for 20 mins / 134°C for 3 mins, for surgical instruments that have been cleaned first.
Dry Heat	Used at 160°C for ≥2 hours.
Ethylene Oxide	Use for heat-sensitive equipment e.g. endoscopes. Also used for industrial processing of single use equipment.
Low-Temp Steam & Formaldehyde	Useful for heat sensitive equipment. Not suitable if contaminated with body fluids (protein deposits harden) or in narrow bore tubing (condensation).
Irradiation	Industrial process e.g. large batches of syringes.

LASER

Q: What does LASER stand for?

Light Amplification by Stimulated Emission of Radiation

Q: How is LASER light created?

- This requires an active medium (gas, liquid or solid) inside a reflective cavity (≥2 mirrors).
- The medium is excited by energy.
- Electrons are dropped to a less excited state by interaction with a photon, causing the release of another photon.
- This 2nd photon is created with the same phase, frequency & direction as the 1st photon.
- 1 of the mirrors is partially reflective (the output coupler) & the LASER beam is emitted through it.

Q: How are LASERs classified?

According to the level of potential damage caused by exposure. There are 7 classes, ranked in ascending order according to risk of damage:

Class	Damage Information	Example Use
1	Safe for normal use.	CD players & laser printers.
1M	These are divergent / large diameter beams. Safety is as for class 1, unless passed through magnifying optical devices.	Fibre-optic communication systems.
2	Safe as the eye blink reflex prevents damage.	Barcode scanners & some laser pointers.
2M	These are divergent / large diameter beams. Safety is as for class 2, unless passed through magnifying optical devices.	Civil engineering applications.
3B	Small risk of eye damage within the blink reflex time.	CD & DVD burners.
3R	Can cause immediate severe eye damage with exposure.	Building industry alignment devices.
4	Can cause immediate severe eye & skin damage. Also a fire hazard.	Industrial, medical & scientific LASERs.

Q: What types of LASERs are used in medicine?

These may be classified according to their active medium as follows:

Active Medium	Colour	Use
CO_2	Invisible	Haemostasis, Lesion Removal
NdYAG	Invisible	Tumour Ablation
Argon	Blue-Green	Photocoagulation
Ruby	Red	Tattoo Removal

Tourniquets

Q: What is a tourniquet?

A temporary compressing device used to control arterial or venous circulation, on an extremity, for a period of time.

Q: What uses do tourniquets have in medicine?

These may be classified according to specialty:

Specialty	Use
Anaesthesia	Facilitate regional anaesthesia e.g. Bier's Block.
Oncology	Isolated limb perfusion.
Surgery	Prevent blood flow to a limb in order to achieve 'bloodless surgery'.
General	Facilitates venepuncture & IV access.

Q: How would you ensure the safe use of tourniquets?

Timing	Action
Pre-operative	• Equipment Maintenance • Cleaning • Appropriate Cuff Size • Padding Under Cuff
Intra-Operative	• Limb Exanguination • Appropriate Limb Occlusion Pressure • Monitor Tourniquet Time • Check Haemostasis
Post-operative	• Check Limb Vascularity

Q: What are the contra-indications for tourniquet use?

Category	Example
Vascular	• Peripheral Vascular Disease • Raynaud's • DVT in Involved Limb • Sickle Cell Disease
Infective	• Severe Limb Infection
Musculoskeletal	• Severely Injured / Traumatised Limb • Poor Skin Condition of the Involved Limb
Neurological	• Peripheral Neuropathy
Mechanical	• Lack of Appropriate Equipment

Q: What are the complications of tourniquet use?

Complication	Explanation
Skin Trauma	• Inadequate padding causing bruising, abrasions, blistering • Burns may occur when preparatory solutions seep under the cuff
Volume Overload	• Limb exsanguination autotransfuses blood into the central circulation • May not be tolerated if poor cardiac reserve
Metabolic / Blood Gas Changes	• Decreased pH • Decreased P_aO_2 • Increased P_aCO_2 • Increased K^+ • Increased lactate
Tourniquet Pain	• May occur despite adequate anaesthesia
Tourniquet Failure	• Inadequate pressure • Inadequate exsanguination • Faulty equipment
Post-Tourniquet Syndrome	• Swollen, stiff, pale limb with weakness but no paralysis • Several weeks duration • Post-operative oedema is the main aetiology
Haematoma / Bleeding	• Bleeding vessels not identified intra-operatively • Delayed blood flow after tourniquet release
Muscle Injury	• Ischaemia related
Nerve Injury	• Nerve compression (radial nerve most commonly)
Compartment Syndrome	• Rare

Diathermy

Q: What is diathermy?

The passage of high frequency alternating current (400kHz-10 MHz) through body tissue. This produces high temperatures (1000°C) to allow coagulation or cutting.

Q: Why are such high frequencies used?

- Low frequency AC e.g. mains electricity at 50Hz, may cause stimulation of neuromuscular tissue.
- 5–10mA may cause muscle contraction, 80–100mA may cause ventricular fibrillation.
- At frequencies >50kHz, this response disappears & 500mA can safely be passed through the patient.

Q: What are the differences between monopolar & bipolar diathermy (Fig 10.1)?

Monopolar	Bipolar
High power required (400W).	Low power required (50W).
Current is delivered from a generator to an active electrode...	Current passes from a diathermy generator to a pair of forceps...
... & spreads throughout the body, returning to the generator via a patient plate electrode.	... & passes from 1 limb of the forceps, through tissue, to the other limb of the forceps.
Patient plate electrode required with good skin contact area >70cm^2.	No patient plate electrode required.
Can touch other instruments to pass current through to operating field.	Safer for use on end arteries, structures with narrow pedicles & patients with pacemakers.

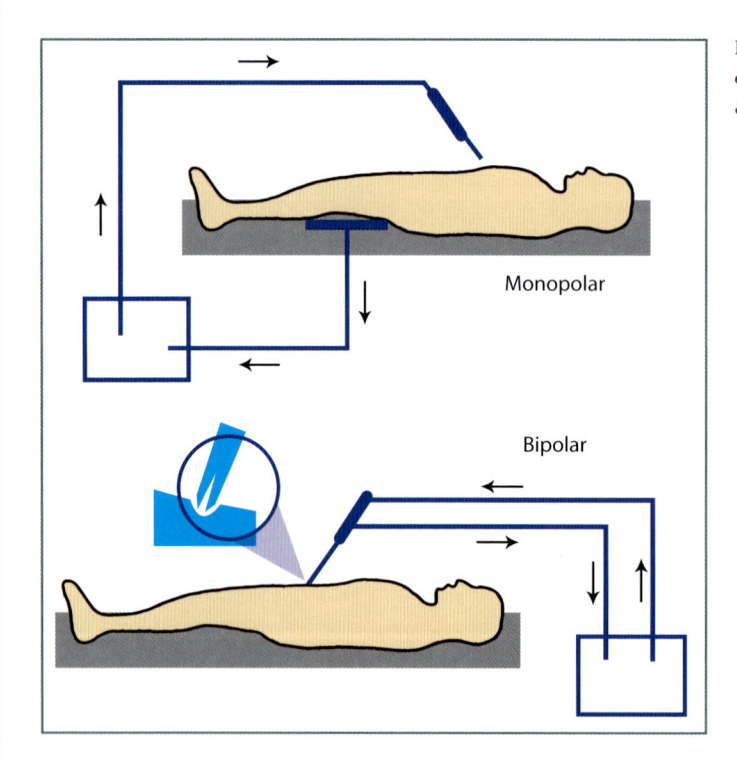

Fig 10.1: Diagram of current flow in monopolar & bipolar diathermy.

Q: What are the complications of diathermy?

Complication	Explanation
Burns	• Inadvertent contact with tissue or instruments.
	• Inadvertent foot pedal operation.
	• Retained heat in electrode.
	• Incorrect application of patient plate electrode.
	• Nearby flammable liquid / gas.
	• Pooling of flammable liquid e.g. skin preparation fluids.
Electrocution	• Faulty insulation.
Explosion	• Due to ignition of gas in a hollow viscera e.g. bowel.
Channelling	• Thrombosis of vessel with narrow pedicle.
Capacitor Coupling	• If an electrode is inside an insulator, which is within a conductor, an electrostatic field may form inducing current in the conductor e.g. metal laparoscopic ports.
Direct Coupling	• May occur when inadvertently touching an instrument with monopolar diathermy.
	• This is often used intentionally, as it also allows coagulation of tissues that are grasped with forceps.
Pacemakers	• High frequency currents may reprogram pacemakers, resulting in pacing irregularities.
	• Pacemaker wires may conduct nearby current towards the heart, resulting in a myocardial burn.

Q: How would you ensure safe use of diathermy?

- Equipment maintenance & staff training.
- Patient plate electrode correctly applied.
- Check dial settings.
- Alarm sound when switched on.
- Meticulous operative technique.
- Avoid accidentally touching uninsulated objects.
- Electrode placed in quiver when not in use.
- Bipolar diathermy best when operating on appendages & patients with pacemakers.
- If using monopolar diathermy, use short, low power bursts.
- Contact cardiologist about possible pre & post-operative pacemaker reprogramming.

Suture Materials

Q: How are suture materials classified?

Classification	Explanation
Composition	**Natural** e.g. silk v. **Synthetic** e.g. Prolene™.
Structure	**Braided** e.g. Vicryl™ v. **Monofilament** e.g. Monocryl™.
Absorption	**Absorbable** e.g. PDS™ v. **Non-Absorbable** e.g. Nylon.

Q: Can you list some common suture materials & describe their properties?

Suture Material	Composition	Structure	Absorption	Example
Collagen	Natural	Monofilament	Absorbable	Catgut
Silk	Natural	Braided	Non-Absorbable	Silk
Poliglecaprone	Synthetic	Monofilament	Absorbable	Monocryl™
Polydioxanone	Synthetic	Monofilament	Absorbable	PDS™
Polyproprlene	Synthetic	Monofilament	Non-Absorbable	Prolene™
Nylon	Synthetic	Monofilament	Non-Absorbable	Ethilon™
Polyglactin	Synthetic	Braided	Absorbable	Vicryl™

Q: Can you list some essential suture characteristics?

- Sterile
- Hypoallergenic
- Irritant, Impurity & Carcinogen Free
- Uniform Diameter
- Pliability for Ease of Handling & Knot Security
- Uniform High Tensile Strength
- Predictable Absorption Profile
- Cost Effective.

Q: How are sutures absorbed?

There are 2 principle methods, proteolytic enzyme degradation & hydrolysis.

Q: What range of suture sizes are used?

Conventional suture sizes are designated by the United States Pharmacopeia. These range from 11-0 to 5, with increasing diameter as follows:

USP Designation	Diameter (mm)
11-0	0.01
10-0	0.02
9-0	0.03
8-0	0.04
7-0	0.05
6-0	0.07
5-0	0.1
4-0	0.15
3-0	0.2
2-0	0.3
0	0.35
1	0.4
2	0.5
3	0.6
4	0.6
5	0.7

Q: How would you classify suture needles?

By shape or point geometry as follows:

Shape	Point Geometry
Straight	**Taper:** Round body that smoothly tapers to a point.
Half Curved	**Cutting:** Triangular body, sharp cutting edge on inside.
1/4 Circle	**Reverse Cutting:** Cutting edge on outside.
3/8 Circle	**Trocar Point:** Small triangular cutting point & round, tapered body.
1/2 Circle	**Blunt:** Blunt tip.
5/8 Circle	
Compound Curve	

Q: What alternatives to sutures exist?

- Healing by Secondary Intention
- Steristrips
- Tissue Adhesive
- Clips / Staples.

Drains

Q: What is a Drain?

A drain is a device that facilitates removal of gas or liquid from a wound or body cavity.

Q: How are drains classified?

Classification	Example
Mechanism of Action	**Active:** Actively maintain drainage using suction drains.
	Passive: Relies on a pressure differential between the body cavity & exterior.
Construction	**Open** e.g. Penrose drain.
	Closed e.g. Redivac™ drain.
Material	**Silastic:** Relatively inert with minimal tissue reaction.
	Rubber: Can induce tissue reactions & allow tracts to form e.g. biliary T-tube.

Q: What are the complications of drain use?

Immediate	Early	Late
Tissue / Organ Damage (during insertion)	Blockage	Infection
Vessel Damage	Inadequate Drainage	Erosion into Adjacent Structures
Nerve Damage	Disconnection	
Incorrect Placement	Dislodge	

Dressings

Q: What are the functions of dressings?

Function	Example
Mechanical	• Absorb • Pressure • Protection • Seal
Cleaning	• Antisepsis • Debridement
Healing	• Granulation Promotion • Haemostasis
Analgesia	• Padding • Pain Relief

Q: How are dressings classified?

No classification system is ideal, however the following are commonly used:

Occlusive		Non-Occlusive	
Granuflex™	(hydrocolloid)	Jelonet™	(paraffin gauze)
Tegaderm™	(polyurethane membrane)	Mepitel™	(silicone gauze)
Permeable		**Impermeable**	
Allevyn™	(foam)	Granuflex™	(hydrocolloid)
Kaltostat™	(alginate)	Tegaderm™	(polyurethane membrane)
Intrasite™	(hydrogel)		
Biological		**Non-Biological**	
Allograft		Jelonet™	(paraffin gauze)
Xenograft		Mepitel™	(silicone gauze)
Cultured Cells		Granuflex™	(hydrocolloid)
Dermal Substitutes		Tegaderm™	(polyurethane membrane)

Q: Can you list some suitable dressings for common wound types?

Wound	Dressing	Example
Granulating / Epithelialising (Low Exudate)	Non-Adherent Hydrocolloid	Jelonet™ Duoderm™
Granulating / Epithelialising (High Exudate)	Hydrofibre	Aquacel™
Sloughy (Low Exudate)	Hydrogel	Intrasite™
Sloughy (High Exudate)	Hydrofibre	Aquacel™
Necrotic (Low Exudate)	Hydrogel Hydrocolloid	Intrasite™ Granuflex™
Necrotic (High Exudate)	Hydrofibre Capillary Action	Aquacel™ Vacutex™
Malodorous Wounds	Charcoal	Actisorb Silver™
Cavity	Simple Packing	Ribbon Gauze

Note: This list is by no means exclusive or exhaustive as new dressings appear on the market continually & guidelines vary between hospitals.

Q: What organisms may be used in wound care?

Organism	Notes
Leeches	Secrete substances, resulting in anaesthesia, anticoagulation & vasodilation.
Maggots	Secrete proteolytic enzymes that digest necrotic & sloughy tissue.

Q: What is a negative pressure dressing?

Application of controlled levels of negative pressure to a wound may accelerate debridement & promote granulation. Such dressings often comprise of a foam / gauze dressing over the wound, covered by an occlusive dressing. This is then connected to a suction device via tubing e.g. VAC™.

Q: What level of pressure is used?

- -125mmHg commonly
- This may be continuous or intermittent.

Q: What are the contraindications to negative pressure therapy?

- Fistula
- Malignancy in Wound
- Necrotic Tissue / Eschar in Wound (when debridement has not been attempted)
- Osteomyelitis (untreated).

SECTION E: ADDITIONAL OSCE PRACTICE

CHAPTER 11
ADDITIONAL OSCE QUESTIONS

E Ewart
BH Miranda

CHAPTER CONTENTS

Burns Assessment:
- Case 1:   Lund & Browder Chart

General Surgery:
- Case 2:   Epigastric Pain & Vomiting
- Case 3:   Painful Groin Lump
- Case 4:   Duodenal Ulcer Perforation
- Case 5:   Necrotising Fasciitis
- Case 6:   Dysphagia
- Case 7:   Referral to Coroner

Trauma & Orthopaedics:
- Case 8:   Acute Gout
- Case 9:   Scaphoid Fracture
- Case 10:   Fractured Neck of Femur
- Case 11:   Osteoarthritis
- Case 12:   Fractured Tibia

Urology:
- Case 13:   Acute Testicular Pain
- Case 14:   Haematuria
- Case 15:   Renal Trauma
- Case 16:   Intravenous Urography (IVU)

Cardiorespiratory:
- Case 17:   Preoperative Assessment
- Case 18:   Post-Operative Chest Pain
- Case 19:   Pneumothorax
- Case 20:   Mediastinal Mass

BURNS ASSESSMENT:

Case 1: You are the CT2 on call for burns & plastic surgery. You are called to see a 75kg adult male who sustained severe flame burns as shown below. Please study the Lund & Browder chart (Fig 11.1) below & answer the following questions:

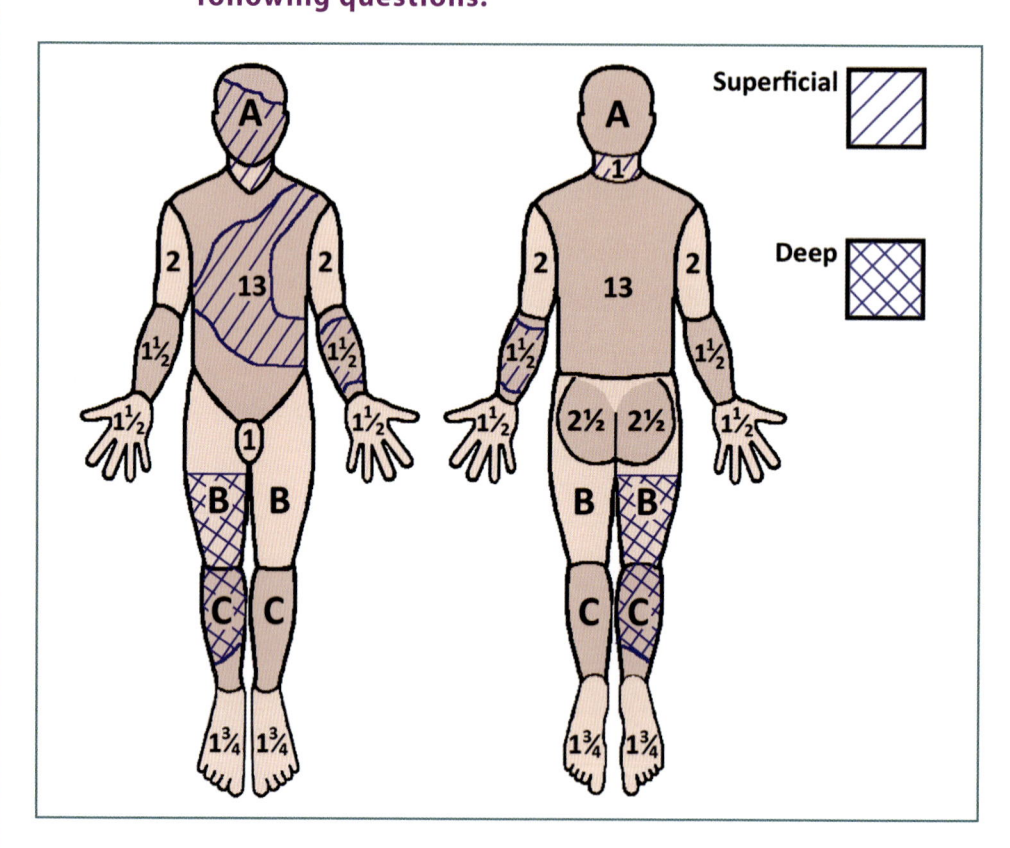

Area	Age 0	1	5	10	15	Adult
A = ½ Head	9½	8½	6½	5½	4½	3½
B = ½ Thigh	2¾	3¼	4	4½	4½	4¾
C = ½ One Lower Leg	2½	2½	2¾	3	3¼	3½

Note: This is the relative % body surface area by age.

Q: What is the total percentage burn?

- Head = 2.5%
- Neck = 1 + 1 = 2%
- Anterior Trunk = 6.5%
- Left Arm = 1.5 + 1.5 = 3%
- Thigh = 4.75%
- Leg = 6%
- Total = 24.75%

Note: There will always be some variability between clinicians when calculating the total percentage burn due to the subjective nature of recording & interpreting the burn pattern on the Lund & Browder chart.

Q: How much fluid would you administer to the patient & over what time period?

- This is governed by Parkland's Formula as follows:
  Total Fluid Requirement / 24h = % Burn Surface Area x Weight (kg) x 4ml
- Therefore: 24.75% x 75kg x 4ml = 7425ml
- The 1st half (3712.5ml) should be given over 8 hours (from the time of the initial burn).
- The 2nd half (3712.5ml) should be given over the following 16 hours.

GENERAL SURGERY

Case 2: A 68 year old man is referred by A&E with epigastric pain & vomiting.

Q: What are your differential diagnoses?

Gastrointestinal	Other
Gallstones / Cholangitis	MI
GORD	AAA
Gastroenteritis	
Peptic Ulcer Disease	
Pancreatitis	
Small Bowel Obstruction	

Q: After further questioning, your patient states he has had similar episodes in the past & has been advised to reduce his alcohol intake. Which of your differential diagnoses is now most likely?

Acute pancreatitis.

Q: What is your immediate management of this patient?

This requires **ALS** resuscitation (with appropriate **history** & **clinical examination**) & includes:

- **High Flow O$_2$**   (15L non re-breathing bag)
- **2 x Wide Bore Cannulae** (1 per antecubital fossa)
- **N/Saline or Hartmann's** (1L over 1 hour – then reassess haemodynamic status)
- **ECG Monitoring**
- **NGT**
- **Urinary Catheter**
- **Fluid Balance Chart**
- **Investigations**

Q: What relevant investigations would you consider?

Investigation	Interpretation
Observations	O_2 Saturations, BP, HR, Temperature & Urine Output.
ECG	Arrhythmias.
Bloods	FBC, WCC, U&E, LFT, CRP, Amylase, Ca^{2+}, LDH.
ABG	Blood Gases & pH.
CXR	Acute Lung Injury & Pneumoperitoneum.

Q: Below are the results of the ABG. What do they show?

pH	= 7.21
PaO_2	= 7.9 (on 21% O_2)
$PaCO_2$	= 5.0
HCO_3^-	= 16
Base Excess	= -10
Lactate	= 5

Metabolic acidosis & type 1 respiratory failure.

Q: How would you decide where this patient is best managed?

Patients will require ICU assessment for admission & management under the following conditions:
- Glasgow Criteria / Ranson's Score ≥3.
- CRP >210 in the 1st 72 hours of admission.
- Poor response to resuscitation.

Q: What additional radiological investigations will be necessary during admission?

Investigation	Explanation
USS	Exclude underlying gallstone disease as cause.
CT	Look for pancreatic necrosis & splenic artery thrombosis. Perform 2–3 days after admission.
MRI	Look for pancreatic pseudocyst. Perform 2–3 weeks after admission.

Case 3: You assess a 23 year old man, with a painful lump in his right groin. This has been discharging offensive smelling liquid over the last few weeks.

Q: What are the most common underlying causes of this clinical picture?

Drugs	Medical	Surgical
Steroids	DM	Abscess
Immunosuppressants	Hidradenitis Suppurativa	Wound Infection
IVDU	HIV	IBD

Q: What questions would you like to ask in your history?

Medical / Surgical History	Past Medical History
Change in Bowel Habit	DM
Weight Loss	HIV
PR Bleeding	IVDU
Oral / Anal Ulcers	Previous Abscesses
Drug History	Recent Leg Infections
Steroids / Immunosuppressants	Family History
	IBD

Q: He admits that his bowel habit has changed & he is losing weight. How would you like to investigate this patient?

Investigation	Explanation
Bloods	FBC, WCC, U&E & CRP.
Colonoscopy	In a young otherwise fit & well patient, IBD should be high on your list of differentials, given the history of bowel habit change, weight loss & groin abscess.
CT Abdomen	To assess abscess extent & involvement of surrounding structures e.g. bowel.

Q: Following your investigations, you discover he has patchy inflammation of his colon & an enterocutaneous fistula. How would you treat his fistula?

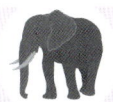

> Memory: 'SNAP' for acute management of enterocutaneous fistulae.

Acute	Interpretation
Sepsis	Prevention of Sepsis
Nutrition	Dietician Advice
Anatomy	CT Abdomen
Plan	Operate if Required
Long Term	**Interpretation**
Gastroenterology Referral	The British Society of Gastroenterology advises inpatient referral to a gastroenterologist with an IBD interest. Confirmation of diagnosis via thorough history & clinical examination, biochemical, endoscopic, radiological & histological investigations should be undertaken.
Endoscopy	Patients with mild to moderate disease should undergo colonoscopy & biopsy. Patients with severe disease should undergo flexible sigmoidoscopy. UC patients should have follow up colonoscopy every 8–10 years. CD patients should have follow up colonoscopy every 1–3 years.

Q: The patient is a little overwhelmed by all that is going on. He would like you to explain his primary diagnosis to his mother. What are some of the features you would explain?

Diagnosis	Explanation
Crohn's Disease	This is the most likely diagnosis due to the age of the patient, bowel habit change, presence of enterocutaneous fistula & patchy involvement of the colon (skip lesions / cobblestones). This condition is an inflammatory condition of the entire gastrointestinal tract & may be associated with other clinical manifestations e.g. abscess & enteric fistula.
Enterocutaneous Fistula	An abnormal communication between skin & bowel. Likely to be intimately related to his underlying CD & treatment should include that of the underlying cause (CD). Lifelong gastroenterology follow up with regular colonoscopy is appropriate. The patient may live a normal life despite this.

Case 4: You are the CT2 on-call & are asked to see a 70 year old male who has decompensated, after perforation of a known duodenal ulcer. His only other history is of AF, for which he is on warfarin.

Q: Outline your immediate management of this patient.

This requires **ALS** resuscitation (with appropriate **history** & **clinical examination**) & includes:

- **High Flow O$_2$** (15L non re-breathing bag)
- **2 x Wide Bore Cannulae** (1 per antecubital fossa)
- **Fluid Resuscitation**
- **Blood Tests** (including 2U cross match & clotting profile)
- **ECG Monitoring**
- **NGT**
- **Urinary Catheter**
- **Fluid balance chart**
- **CXR**
- **Theatre Preparation**

Q: Who else should be contacted with regards to this patient's further care?

Speciality	Explanation
ICU	Bed status & admission assessment.
Anaesthetics	Discuss plan for theatre.
Theatres	Book patient for operation.
Haematology	Reversal of INR e.g. FFP.
Senior	Discuss with your ST / Consultant.

Q: Following successful over-sewing of his ulcer & ICU admission, the patient is now back on the ward. When would you restart his warfarin & what measures would you keep in place until this is done?

When the patient requires no further surgery & it is felt clinically appropriate, warfarin may be restarted. This is likely to be approximately 1–2 weeks post theatre. Whilst the patient is being re-warfarinised, it is important to ensure appropriate anticoagulant cover for AF. Either (IV) heparin or a prophylactic dose of LMWH may be used for this purpose. The APTTR should be maintained around 2.5 in the case of (IV) heparin.

Q: How would you manage his anticoagulation?

- A conventional loading dose is 10mg (day 1), 10mg (day 2) & 5mg (day 3).
- Check INR daily until target (2–3) is reached & stable for 3 consecutive days.
- Liaise with community anticoagulation team to re-instate INR monitoring after discharge.
- Monitor anticoagulation 'cover' appropriately.
- Stop anticoagulation 'cover' when target INR is reached & stable.

Case 5: **The medical ST5 on call has asked you to come & give an urgent surgical opinion on a 75 year old man, whom they have admitted with a possible DVT. He has had 2 hours of left leg swelling & has developed some deep bruising. He has no significant medical history. Please study the clinical photograph below (Fig 11.2).**

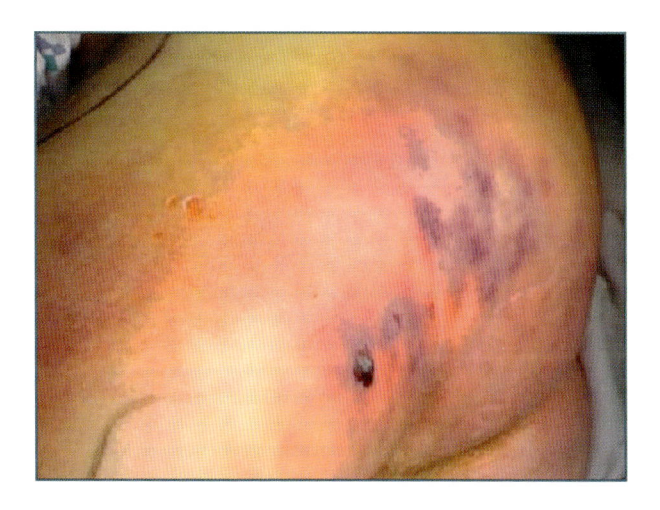

Q: What surgical emergency are you concerned about?

Necrotising fasciitis.

Q: How do you manage this condition?

This requires **ALS** resuscitation (with appropriate **history** & **examination**) & includes:
- **High Flow O$_2$** (15L non re-breathing bag)
- **2 x Wide Bore Cannulae** (1 per antecubital fossa)
- Fluid Resuscitation
- Blood Tests (including group & save)
- Blood Cultures
- Wound Swabs (MC+S)
- Broad Spectrum Antibiotics (until sensitivities known)
- Theatre Preparation
- Early Aggressive Debridement to Healthy Tissue

Q: What complications will you discuss with this patient, with regards to his consent form?

Immediate	Early	Late
Anaesthetic Risks e.g. CVA / MI	Further Debridement	Loss of Function
Bleeding & Transfusion	Reconstruction Requirement e.g. Skin Graft	Severe Scarring
Structural Damage	SIRS / MODS	Poor Cosmesis
Amputation	DVT & PE	
Death	Death	

Q: What organisms will microbiology be testing for?

Necrotising fasciitis may be monomicrobial or polymicrobial, hence organisms may be classified as follows:

Monomicrobial	Polymicrobial
Group A Haemolytic *Streptococcus*	*Pseudomonas*
Clostridium perfringens	*Staphylococcus*
	Bacteroides
	Coliforms
	Diphtheroids

Q: What is the mortality rate associated with this condition?

25–75% (depending on severity).

Case 6: You are in outpatients clinic & are faced by a 65 year old lady who has had some problems with dysphagia. She explains that she has also had some indigestion, but this has been treated by her GP.

Q: What aspects in her history are you particularly interested in?

Question	Explanation
Onset & Duration	When did these symptoms start? How long do they last for?
Course	Has dysphagia been progressive for solids then liquids?
Weight Loss	Has there been weight loss? How much & over what time period?
Smoking	How many pack years?
Alcohol	How many units per week?
Family Hx	GI cancers
Ideas, Concerns & Expectations	When taking any patient history, consider the patient's position. A good framework to use is **ICE** *(see book 2 communication skills & ethics chapter).*

Q: What specific investigations would you order for this lady & why?

Investigation	Explanation
FBC	Check for anaemia.
Haematinics	Further investigation of anaemia cause e.g. iron, B12 & folate deficiency.
LFT	There may be a history of alcohol or presence of liver metastases.
U&E	Dehydration, with raised urea : creatinine ratio, may be present.
CXR	There may be mediastinal lymphadenopathy or evidence of lung cancer.
OGD	Allows direct visualisation & biopsy of lesion.

Q: After returning to clinic, you are pleased to inform the patient that her investigations ruled out cancer & that the problem is related to a benign oesophageal stricture. What would you do next?

- **Reassurance:** This may be enough for patients with mild symptoms.
- **Stricture Dilation:** Particularly in patients with severe symptoms or weight loss.

Q: What complication would you be most concerned about if the patient decides to have a procedure to treat their stricture & how would you diagnose it?

Perforation of the oesophagus may occur. Features include surgical emphysema & pneumomediastinum which may be seen on a CXR.

Q: If the patient suffers this complication, what would your management be?

Successful management requires **early diagnosis**, **ALS** resuscitation (with appropriate **history & examination**) & includes:

- **High Flow O$_2$**   (15L non re-breathing bag)
- **2 x Wide Bore Cannulae**   (1 per antecubital fossa)
- **Fluid Resuscitation**
- **Broad Spectrum Antibiotics** (until sensitivities known)
- **Blood Tests**   (including 2U cross match & clotting profile)
- **NBM**
- **Urinary Catheter**
- **NG Tube**
- **Fluid Balance Chart**
- **Senior Review**   (consider definitive treatment as appropriate)

Q: What are the options for definitive management?

This depends on the site & size of the tear & patient co-morbidities. Options include:

- Conservative Treatment
- Drain
- Stent
- Primary Repair
- Resection

Case 7: Whilst on call, you admit an 82 year old lady with possible ischaemic bowel. She is acutely acidotic & unfortunately dies overnight. You are asked to complete her death certificate.

Q: What deaths must be referred to the coroner?

- Deaths <24 hours after admission.
- Doubt over cause of death.
- Sudden, unexplained or suspicious deaths.
- Suspected unnatural events contributing to cause of death.
- Clinical incident involved in cause of death.
- Deaths relating to accidents / operations.
- Deaths related to fractures / falls.
- Deaths due to drugs / overdose.
- Acute alcohol related death.
- Occupational / industrial diseases involved in cause of death.
- Deaths during police custody.

TRAUMA & ORTHOPAEDICS

Case 8: You are asked to see a 76 year old lady, on a medical ward. She is complaining of knee pain & swelling. On examination, she is afebrile & haemodynamically stable, both knees are swollen with an effusion on the right, there is no erythema or bony tenderness.

Q: What are your differential diagnoses?

- Septic Arthritis   (most important not to miss)
- Gout / Pseudogout
- Traumatic Haemarthrosis
- Rheumatoid Arthritis Flare-Up
- Osteoarthritis Arthritis Flare-Up

Q: What aspects of her history are you particularly interested in?

Question	Explanation
Onset & Duration	When did these symptoms start? How long do they last for?
Course	Do the symptoms come & go? Are the symptoms progressive?
Previous Episodes	Recurrence may be associated with a rheumatological condition.
Other Joints	Polyarthropathy may be associated with a rheumatological condition.
Trauma	Any recent history of trauma / falls may be associated with a fracture.
Anticoagulants	Aspirin / warfarin use may be associated with a large haemarthrosis, even after a simple fall.
Wounds	Open wounds / infected toenails may be associated with septic arthritis.
Systemic Symptoms	Pyrexia, nausea & vomiting etc. May be associated with septic arthritis.
Alcohol	Overconsumption may be associated with gout.
Ideas, Concerns & Expectations	When taking any patient history, consider the patient's position. A good framework to use is **ICE** *(see book 2 communication skills & ethics chapter)*.

Q: Which investigations would you order?

Investigation	Reasoning
Hb	Anaemia of chronic disease.
WCC	Increased in septic arthritis.
Urate	Raised in gout.
CRP	Acute phase reactant.
ESR	This may be increased in chronic disease & some rheumatological diseases.
Blood Cultures	Indication of systemic illness & enables you to treat with more specific antibiotics.
Imaging	AP & lateral radiographs of both knees will rule out fractures, assist diagnosis of e.g. OA & show any underlying bony destruction / changes*.
Joint Aspiration	This is diagnostic & should be sent for gram stain, MC+S & crystal analysis.

*Note: A diagnosis of septic arthritis cannot be excluded on the appearance of the radiograph alone. Bony destruction takes time to evolve & appear on the radiograph.

Q: The investigation results are now available.

    CRP   = 252
    WCC   = 14
    Joint Aspirate = no organisms seen
                   = monosodium urate crystals (positive)
                   = moderate numbers of leucocytes

Q: What is your diagnosis & treatment?

This patient has acute gout, affecting both knees. Treatment options may be classified as follows:

Conservative	Medical Treatment	Medical Prophylaxis
Reduce Alcohol	NSAID	Allopurinol
Reduce Purine Rich Foods	Colchicine	

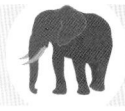

Memory: Colchicine whilst it's seen & Allopurinol once it's been!
(Medical Treatment)   (Medical Prophylaxis)

Q: Before writing on the drug chart, you carefully look through the patient's notes & see that she has been suffering with renal impairment. What is the significance of this?

NSAIDs should be avoided in patients with renal impairment, due to risk of analgesic nephropathy.

Case 9: **You are called by A&E for a 2nd opinion. The patient is a 35 year old woman who fell over yesterday & has right anatomical snuffbox tenderness. Here is one of her radiographs (Fig 11.3):**

Q: How would you manage this patient?

Anatomical snuffbox tenderness is associated with a scaphoid fracture, one of the most commonly missed traumatic diagnoses. Acute management is as follows:

- ATLS Resuscitation (if acute trauma)
- History
- Clinical Examination
- Appropriate Investigations:
  X-Ray
- Treatment:
  Analgesia
  > Scaphoid Cast (2 weeks)
  > Follow Up (2 weeks) & Further Radiographs

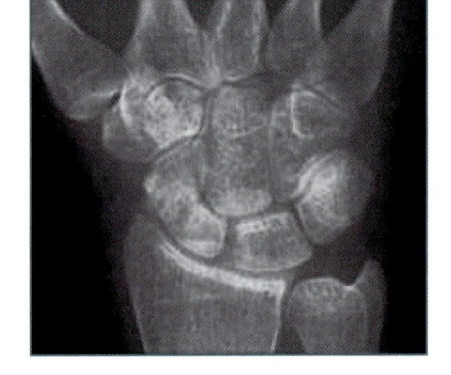

Q: What does this radiograph (Fig 11.4) show after 2 weeks?

Fractured waist of right scaphoid.

Q: What problem is faced with the management of this injury?

Avascular necrosis (AVN) of the proximal segment occurs as the blood supply to the scaphoid bone is from distal to proximal. The blood supply is from the palmar branch of the radial artery. The scaphoid bone spans both rows of the carpus, so if AVN ensues, there may be severe pain & limitation of mobility.

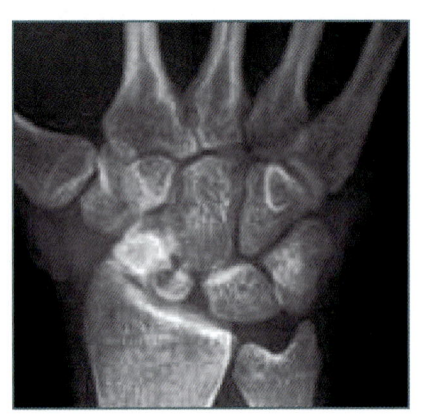

Q: What other bones are commonly affected by this problem when fractured?

The femoral head & talus.

Q: What are the repair options for this lady?

Repair Option	Explanation
Scaphoid Cast (6–12 weeks)	For undisplaced & simple fractures.
Open Reduction & Internal Fixation	For displaced or non-healing fractures e.g. K-wires / cannulated screws.
Bone Grafting	For severe displacement or non-union.

Case 10: **The following radiograph (Fig 11.5) is of an 85 year old woman who fell at home last night in her kitchen. She was found by her neighbour this morning.**

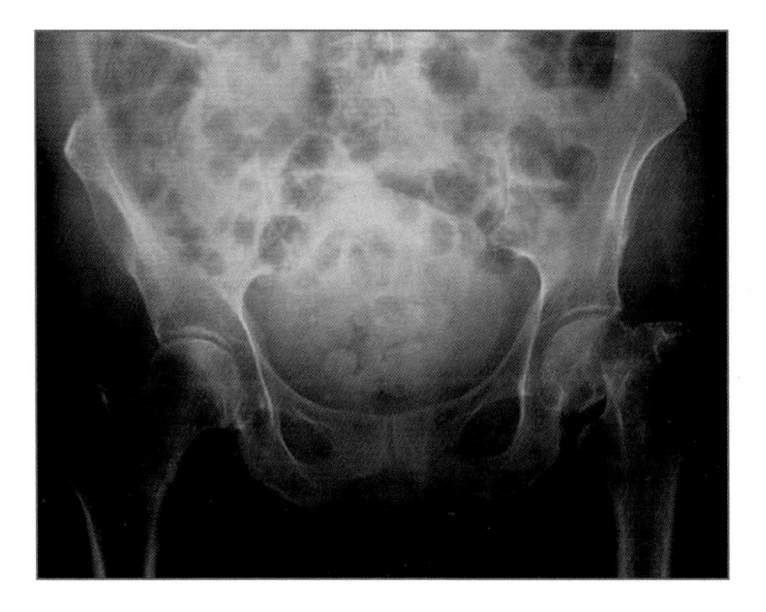

Q: What does this image show?

This is a radiograph of the pelvis. There is a displaced left sided intracapsular fracture.

Q: How are these fractures classified?

Garden's Classification. This classification guides repair of intracapsular fractures of the femoral neck. Grading is according to displacement & extent as follows (Fig 11.6):

Grade	Displacement	Extent	Repair
I	None	Incomplete	• Dynamic Hip Screw (Fig 11.7)
II	None	Complete	• Cannulated Hip Screw
III	Partial	Complete	• Hemiarthroplasty (Fig 11.7)
IV	Full	Complete	

Fig 11.6: Garden's Classification of femoral neck fractures.

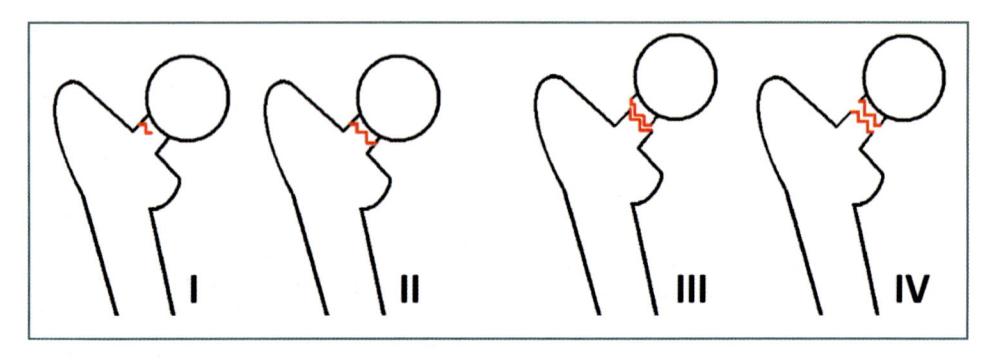

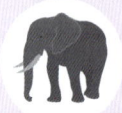

Memory: '1, 2, Do a Hip Screw   &   3, 4, Austin Moore'

Garden's Grade 1: DHS / cannulated hip screws may be used for repair.
Garden's Grade 2: Hemiarthroplasty (Austin Moore is a type of hemiarthroplasty).

Q: How should this fracture be fixed & why?

Hemiarthroplasty. There is a high risk of AVN of the femoral head. This occurs due to vessel trauma, with resulting haematoma that may expand, increasing pressure on the vasculature & reducing blood supply. Radiographic examples of hip repair / replacement are shown in Fig 11.7.

Fig 11.7: Right hip prostheses. Hemiarthroplasty (a), dynamic hip screw (b), total hip replacement (c).

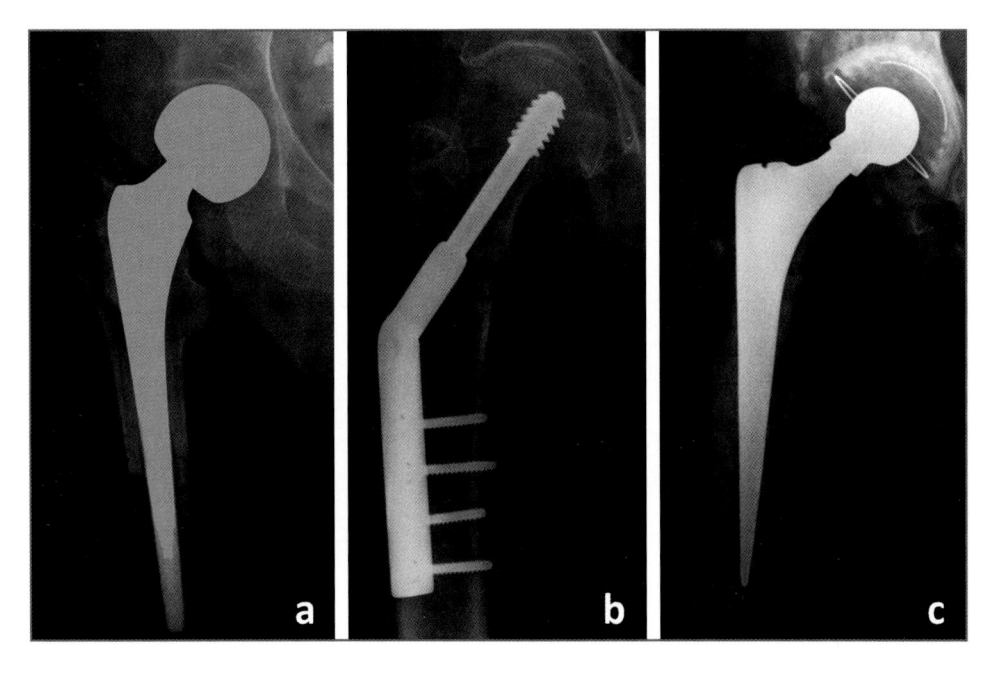

Q: What is the blood supply of the femoral head?

Intracapsular	Extracapsular
Retinacular Vessels	Profunda Femoris
Ligamentum Teres	
Medullary Vessels	

Q: What other investigations should be carried out & why?

Investigation	Reasoning
FBC	Is there anaemia? Is there underlying infection?
U&E	Dehydration is a common cause of falls. Are there electrolyte Imbalances that may be associated with arrhythmias?
CRP	Acute phase reactant.
Blood Glucose	Hypoglycaemia is a common cause of falls.
CK	The patient may have been lying on the floor for hours. Rhabdomyolysis may have ensued, with a risk of renal failure.
Cross Match	2U for hemiarthroplasty, otherwise group & save.
Urine Biochemistry	Myoglobinuria may be detected in association with rhabdomyolysis.
Urine Dipstick / MC+S	UTI is a common cause of falls.
CXR	Pneumonia is a common cause of falls. Are there rib fractures? For pre-anaesthetic purposes.
ECG	Is there a new arrhythmia?
Osteoporosis Screen	If underlying osteoporosis is present, treatment should be commenced in hospital. The GP should also be notified.

Q: What is the % mortality at 1 year following this?

25%

Case 11: You are in outpatient clinic & see a 65 year old man, complaining of pain in both knees. This has been going on for several years. His only other medical history is that of occasional psoriasis.

Q: When taking your history what particular questions would you ask about the pain?

These should be centred around the SOCRATES pain framework *(see book 2 history taking chapter)*.

Memory: **'SOCRATES'** for pain.

Site
Onset
Character
Radiation
Associations
Time
Exacerbating & Relieving Factors

Q: On examination, he walks without aids, has good range of movement, moderate bilateral crepitus on knee flexion bilaterally & slight medial joint line tenderness on the right. Ligaments are clinically intact. What simple investigations would you order for this gentleman?

Investigation	Reasoning
FBC, U&E & CRP	These will help to exclude infection, inflammation & should also be performed as a baseline.
Urate	Urate levels may help to exclude gout.
AP & True Lateral X-Rays	Check for bony changes of osteoarthritis *(see book 2 orthopaedics chapter)*.
Skyline X-Rays	Check for patellofemoral osteoarthritis.

Q: You conclude this man has osteoarthritis, what are your treatment options?

Conservative	Medical	Surgical
Diet & Exercise	Analgesic Ladder	Arthroscopic Debridement & Washout
Physiotherapy	Steroid Injection	Osteotomy (realign)
Occupational Therapy		Arthrodesis (fuse)
Aids e.g. Walking Stick		Arthroplasty (replace)

Q: Your patient admits that the only pain he has is when kneeling in the garden, but his friend had a knee replacement & it went really well. Because of this successful outcome, he tells you that he would like the same operation on his knee. How do you handle this?

- Elicit **I**deas, **C**oncerns & **E**xpectations (**ICE**) *(see book 2 communication skills & ethics chapter).*
- Explain he currently has minimal symptoms.
- Discuss trying conservative & medical options first.
- Explain that it is a major procedure with many complications.
- Address any questions.
- Give written advice on the operation.
- Arrange a follow up appointment.
- If the situation arises, always be receptive to the patient's right for a 2nd opinion.

Case 12: You are called to see an 85 year old lady who has slipped over in the bathroom at home. She trapped her leg as she fell & sustained the injury below (Fig 11.8).

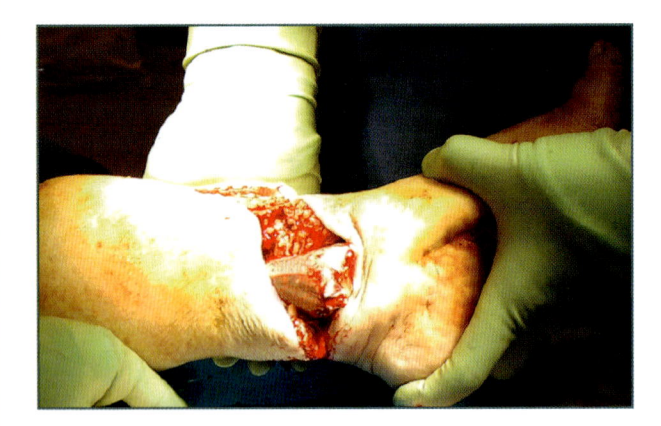

Q: How would you manage this patient?

This patient has an open fracture involving the left tibia. Management of such trauma may be thought of in terms of general fracture management principles & those relating to open fractures:

General Principles	Explanation
ATLS Resuscitation	All trauma requires this approach.
Analgesia	Effective analgesia is important.
Blood Tests	Full pre-operative work up e.g. FBC, U&E, CRP, clotting, group & save.
Imaging	AP & true lateral X-rays, including the knee & ankle joints.
Reduce	Fracture reduction should be immediate. A combination of Entonox™, (IV) diazepam & (IV) morphine may be required.
Hold	Backslab cast initially.
Rehabilitate	Remember that physiotherapy involvement is always important, once initial treatment / surgery has been completed.
Transfer	May require transfer to specialist centre for definitive management.
Open Fractures	Explanation
Photograph Wound	Allows inspection without continuous undressing/redressing of wound.
Irrigate Wound	Clean the wound
Cover Wound	Wash & dress wound with e.g. saline soaked gauze & impermeable film.
Prophylaxis	Tetanus & antibiotic prophylaxis.
Theatre Preparation	Mark & consent the patient. Alert theatres & the anaesthetist.
Theatre	• Liaison between Orthopaedics & Plastic Surgery. • Wound debridement. • Fracture fixation e.g. intramedullary nail / external fixation device. • Definitive wound cover may require flap or graft *(see bones & soft tissues chapter)*. This should be completed <72 hours & not exceeding 7 days.

UROLOGY

Case 13: You are referred a 15 year old boy by a GP who has a 2 hour history of a painful testicle.

Q: What are the differential diagnoses for an acutely painful testicle? (most important first)

- Testicular Torsion
- Epidymitis & Orchitis
- Hydatid of Morgagni Torsion
- Referred Pain e.g. Appendicitis / Renal Tract Colic
- Strangulated Inguinal Hernia
- UTI

Q: What investigations would you order to separate these differentials?

Investigation	Diagnosis
Temperature	Raised in epididymitis, orchitis & UTI.
WCC & CRP	Raised in epididymitis, orchitis & UTI. May be raised in appendicitis & renal colic.
Urinalysis	Positive in UTI, epididymitis, orchitis, orchitis & renal colic.
USS Renal Tract & Testis	Diagnostic for renal tract stones, testicular torsion, epididymitis, orchitis & Hydatid of Morgagni torsion. **Note: With suspected testicular torsion, it is inappropriate to wait for USS, as emergency surgical exploration is required.**

Q: If the above patient were 65 years old, would your differential list be changed at all?

- Renal Tract Colic (referred pain)
- Prostatitis
- Orchitis & Epididymitis
- UTI
- Torsion

Q: What further investigations would you require in this age group?

- PR Examination
- PSA

Case 14: You are called to A&E to see a 68 year old gentleman with frank haematuria.

Q: What would you ask in his history?

History	Questions
Onset & Duration	When did this start? How long have you had this for?
Course	Does it come & go? Is it progressive?
Previous Episodes	Have you had this before? What was the cause then?
Trauma	Have you fallen over or sustained other injuries? Associated with loin / urethral trauma.
Loin Pain ± Groin Radiation	Is there renal pain? This may represent underlying renal pathology. Is there crampy loin to groin pain? This may be due renal tract calculi.
Dysuria	Is there any pain when you urinate? Associated with UTI & prostatitis.
Prostatic Symptoms	Is there a good urinary stream normally? Is there hesitancy, frequency or post-micturition dribbling? These may be present in BPH or prostatic carcinoma.
Weight Loss	Has there been weight loss? How much & over what period of time? This may suggest underlying carcinoma.
Bone Pain	Is there bone pain? Metastases due to underlying carcinoma e.g. vertebral column.
Anticoagulants	Are you on aspirin / warfarin? Both are associated with increased bleeding.
Systemic Symptoms	Have you been feverish, nauseous or vomiting? Systemic symptoms may indicate underlying infection.
Smoking	Do you smoke? How many per day? RCC & TCC are more common in smokers.
Professional	Do you / have you ever worked with dyes? Analine dye exposure is associated with TCC.
Ideas, Concerns & Expectations	When taking any patient history, consider the patient's position. A good framework to use is **ICE** *(see book 2 communication skills & ethics chapter)*.

Q: How are you going to manage this man initially?

- **History**
- **Clinical Examination:** PR exam must be done after PSA to prevent an increase secondary to prostatic trauma.
- **Appropriate Investigations:**

Investigation	Explanation	
Blood Tests	FBC, U&E, LFT, CRP, Group & Save, PSA	
Urine Biochemistry	Stone Analysis	
Urine Microbiology	MC+S	
Imaging	KUB X-Ray:	90% of stones are visible.
		Is there a malignant opacity in the renal area?
	USS Renal Tract:	Stones visible.
		Bladder filing defects visible.
		Masses visible.
	Intravenous Urography (IVU):	Renal tract excretion visible.
		Filling defects visible.
	Flexible Cystoscopy:	Direct vision of bladder & urethra.
		Histological biopsy obtainable.
		Treatment possible e.g. TCC bladder.

- **IV Fluids**
- **3 Way Catheter & Irrigation:** If passing clots
- **Urine Output Monitoring**
- **Admit**

Q: What are your current differential diagnoses?

Benign	Malignant
BPH	RCC
Trauma	TCC
Renal / Ureteric Stone	Prostate Carcinoma

Case 15: At the start of your night shift you are asked to see a 5 year old boy who has been at a birthday party this afternoon. On going to the toilet before bed his mother noticed his urine appeared red, on questioning it has been this colour since he was kicked on the bouncy castle during the party.

Q: What clinical features would you look for to confirm renal trauma?

- Loin / Abdominal Tenderness
- Loin / Abdominal Bruising
- Loss of Loin Contour   (peri-nephric haematoma)
- Loin Mass   (haematoma)

Q: How would you manage this boy?

- **History**
- **Clinical Examination**
- **Ensure Haemodynamic Stability**
- **Appropriate Investigations:**

Investigation	Explanation
Observations	HR & BP. This is to ensure haemodynamic stability.
Blood Tests	FBC, Group & Save. This is to ensure adequate baseline Hb, check for infection & anticipate possible requirement for surgical intervention. Anaemia is an indicator of haematuria severity.
Urine Dipstick	Haematuria, proteinuria & infection.
Urine Microbiology	MC+S
Imaging	KUB X-Ray: Loss of psoas shadow. Loss of renal outline.
	USS Kidneys: Peri-nephric haematoma. Renal capsule damage.
	CT Abdomen: Less sensitive than USS. Good for other organ damage if suspected.

- **Admit The Patient For Observation & Investigation**

Q: What proportion of renal trauma can be managed conservatively?

80% of renal trauma cases may be managed conservatively e.g. grade I & II injuries. Of the remaining injuries, those with significant lacerations, vascular or collecting system injuries, will require surgical intervention. Patients who are in physiological shock will also require surgical intervention *(see operative surgery chapter)*.

Case 16: Study this radiological image (Fig 11.9) & answer the following questions:

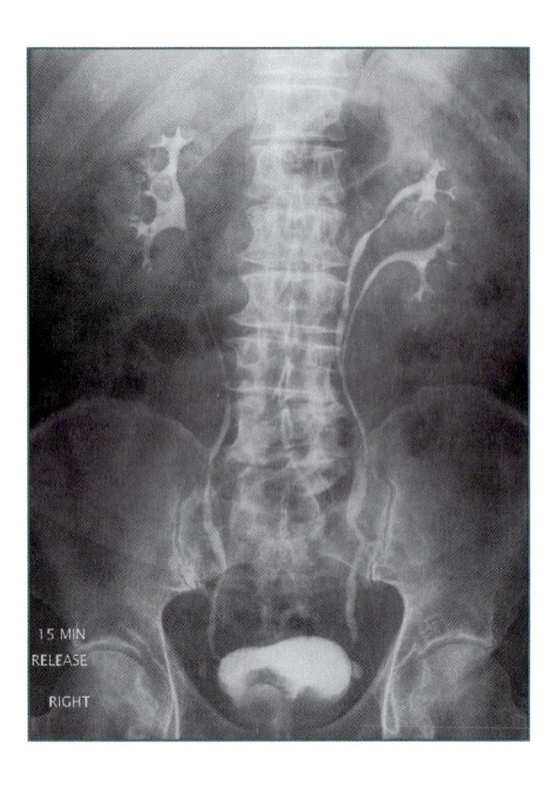

Q: What is this study?

(IV) Urogram / (IV) Pyelogram at 15 minutes.

Q: What anatomical anomaly does it show?

Duplex left ureter.

Q: What pathologies might you order this investigation for?

- Renal Tract Calculi
- BPH / Carcinoma
- Urinary Tract Outflow Obstruction
- Recurrent UTI

Q: What potential problems might a tablet control diabetic face with having a contrast study?

- Metformin may react with contrast, resulting in a potentially fatal lactic acidosis.
- Diabetic patients may have nephropathy that may be worsened by contrast (contrast induced nephropathy).

CARDIORESPIRATORY:

Case 17: You are examining a 65 year old man in pre-operative assessment. He has been booked for an anterior resection in 2 weeks. He has a metallic mitral valve following rheumatic fever as a child & is on lifelong warfarin.

Q: What advice will you give this gentleman regarding his warfarin.

Warfarin should be stopped 5–6 days pre-operatively (according to trust protocol). Pre-operative admission for heparin infusion should be arranged, or administration of LMWH (therapeutic dose) in the community.

Q: What instructions would you give your juniors with regards to managing his anticoagulation?

- Baseline coagulation profile e.g. INR, PrT, APTTR.
- 5000U IV bolus dose of heparin.
- 1000U in 1ml IV infusion of heparin.
- Check APTTR at 6 hours.
- Adjust either dose / rate of infusion according to trust protocol.
- Continue to check APTTR 6 hourly until target reached (usually 2.5).
- Continue to check APTTR 12 hourly until warfarin is re-instated & INR is therapeutic.
- Heparin infusion needs to be stopped 6 hours pre-, then started 12 hours post-operatively.

Q: Where would you like this patient cared for post-operatively & why?

Minimum of HDU for the following reasons:

- Elderly patient undergoing major operation.
- Potential for significant blood loss.
- Potential for significant electrolyte imbalances.
- Metallic heart valve counts as a significant co-morbidity.
- More likely to decompensate following theatre.
- Will need regular APTTR monitoring.

Q: Who else should be contacted with regards to this patient's admission?

Speciality	Explanation
Anaesthetics	Elective admission assessment.
	Discuss requirement for further investigations e.g. cardiac.
Cardiology	Assessment of cardiac function e.g. ECHO.
Microbiology	Antibiotic cover for infective endocarditis.

Case 18: You are the orthopaedic CT2 on-call & are asked to see an 85 year lady with a past medical history of 2 MIs & metastatic breast cancer. She sustained a pathological distal femoral fracture 3 days ago after a minor fall. She is currently post-operative by 12 hours & has developed chest pain & shortness of breath.

Q: What are your working differential diagnoses & why?

Diagnosis	Reasoning
Myocardial Infarction	Elderly patient with past history of 2 MIs.
	Major operation, increasing cardiac strain & chance of post-operative anaemia.
Left Ventricular Failure	Reduced functional reserve after previous MIs.
Pulmonary Embolism	Limited mobility due to long-bone fracture.
	Metastatic disease is a risk factor.
	Note that although post-operative, PE would be expected at 7–10 days.
Fat Embolus	Long bone fracture is a risk factor.
	Likely to have had an intramedullary nail repair which is a risk factor.

Q: What would your initial management of this lady be?

This requires **ALS** resuscitation (with appropriate **history** & **clinical examination**) & includes:

- **Sit Up Patient**
- **High Flow O$_2$** (15L non re-breathing bag)
- **2 x Wide Bore Cannulae** (1 per antecubital fossa)
- **Catheter**
- **Check Drug Chart & Check LMWH Prescribed**
- **Analgesia**

- **Appropriate Investigations:**

Investigation	Explanation
Observations	HR & BP. This is to ensure haemodynamic stability.
Blood Tests	FBC, U&E, CRP.
	Consider troponin T at 12 hours to exclude MI.
	D-dimer will help to exclude DVT & PE.
ABG	Exclude pH imbalance & assess respiratory failure.
ECG	Assess cardiac electrophysiology e.g. arrhythmia / MI.
	Check fo $S_I Q_{III} T_{III}$ pattern of PE.
CXR	Assess cardiac size & lung fields.

- **Treat Cause Acutely:**

Cause	Additional Acute Treatment
Myocardial Infarction	(SL) Aspirin (200mg) & Clopidogrel (200mg)
	(IV) Morphine (10mg) & Metoclopramide (10mg)
	(SL) GTN
Left Ventricular Failure	(IV) Furosemide
	(IV) Morphine (10mg) & Metoclopramide (10mg)
	(SL) GTN & GTN Infusion
Pulmonary Embolism	LMWH 175U/kg/24h
	(IV) Morphine (10mg) & Metoclopramide (10mg)
	Warfarin (start when diagnosis confirmed)
Fat Embolism	Suppportive
	Steroids (contraversial, but may have a small beneficial effect)

- **Medical Review / Referral**
- **Consider Anaesthetics Review for respiratory support & HDU / ICU Admission**

Q: What is your plan for the day team at handover?

- **Review Patient Immediately:** Establish Baseline State.
- **Review Patient Later:** Record Improvement / Deterioration.
- **Repeat / Review Investigations:** Blood Tests.
  ABG.
  ECG.
  Troponin T.
- **Organise Further Imaging:** Contact Radiology e.g. CTPA for PE.

Q: What are the features of fat embolism syndrome?

These are mostly dependent on the site of embolism & may be classified as follows:

Respiratory	Cutaneous	Cerebral	Other
Tachypnoea	Rash	Aphasia	Haematuria
Hypoxaemia		Confusion	Proteinuria
Hypocapnia		Hemiplegia	Right Heart Strain (ECG)
Inspiratory Crackles		Seizures	
Bilateral Fluffy Shadows (CXR)			

Case 19: This is the CXR of a 72 year old lady who has presented to A & E with an open fracture of her left radius & ulna after falling 10 feet from a ladder (Fig 11.10). She is sat comfortably in A&E & is not complaining of any chest symptoms.

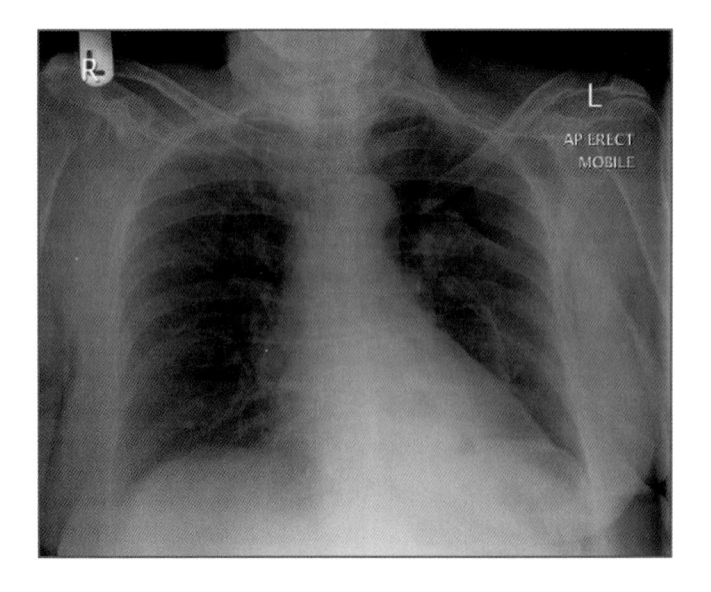

Q: What is the spot diagnosis?

Left fractured clavicle.

Case 20: What are your differential diagnoses for the abnormality on the CXR (Fig 11.11)? It belongs to an 86 year old gentleman, who has a long history of shortness of breath.

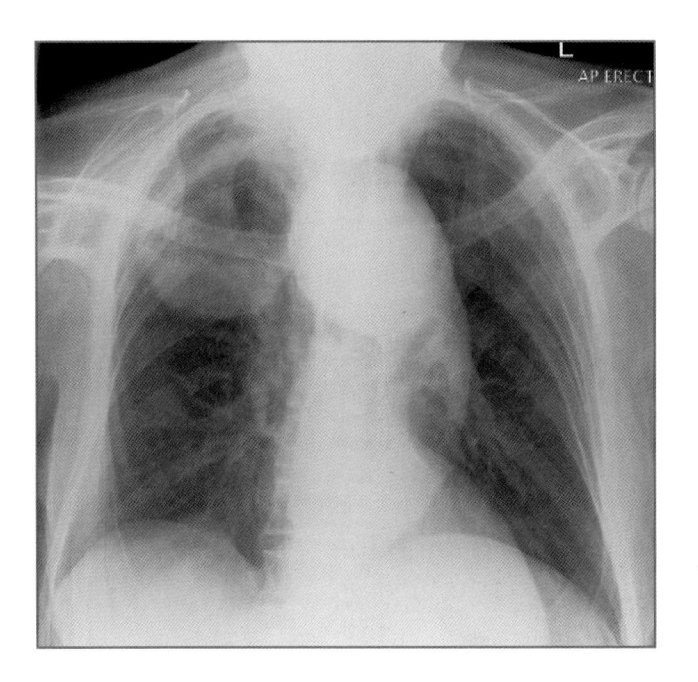

- Primary Lung Cancer
- Post Traumatic Lung Cyst
- Lung Abscess
- TB
- Granulmatosis
- Infected Bullae
- Aspergillosis

ABBREVIATIONS

+ve	Positive
-ve	Negative
1°	Primary
2°	Secondary
3°	Tertiary
2,3-DPG	2,3 Diphosphoglycerate
5-HIAA	5-Hydroxyindoleacetic Acid
A&E	Accident & Emergency
AAA	Abdominal Aortic Aneurysm
Ab	Antibody
ABC	Airway Breathing & Circulation
ABG	Arterial Blood Gas
ACE	Angiotensin-Converting Enzyme
ACh	Acetylcholine
ACL	Anterior Cruciate Ligament
ACTH	Adrenocorticotropic Hormone
ADP	Adenosine Diphosphate
ADPKD	Autosomal Dominant Polycystic Kidney Disease
AFB	Acid-Fast Bacilli
AG	Anion Gap
Ag	Antigen
AIDS	Acquired Immune Deficiency Syndrome
AKA	Above Knee Amputation
ALP	Alkaline phophatase
ALS	Advanced Life Support
ALT	Alanine Aminotransferase
AP	Anterior-Posterior
AgPC	Antigen Presenting Cell
APC	Adenomatosis Polyposis Coli
APTT	Activated Partial Thromboplastin Time
APTTR	Activated Partial Thromboplastin Time Ratio
APUD	Amine Precursor Uptake Decarboxylase
ARDS	Adult Respiratory Distress Syndrome
ARF	Acute Renal Failure
ASA	American Society of Anesthesiologists
ASIS	Anterior Superior Iliac Spine
AST	Aspartate Aminotransferase
ATLS	Advanced Trauma Life Support
ATN	Acute Tubular Necrosis
ATP	Adenosine Triphosphate
AVN	Avascular Necrosis

AXR	Abdominal Radiograph
BKA	Below Knee Amputation
BMI	Body Mass Index
BMR	Basal Metabolic Rate
BP	Blood Pressure
BPH	Benign Prostatic Hyperplasia
BTx	Blood Transfusion
BXO	Balanitis Xerotica Obliterans
c.f.u.	Colony Forming Units
Ca	Calcium
CA	Cancer Antigen
CABG	Coronary Artery Bypass Graft
CBD	Common Bile Duct
CBF	Cerebral Blood Flow
CCK	Cholecystokinin
CDK	Cyclin Dependent Kinase
CEA	Carcinoembryonic Antigen
CECT	Contrast Enhanced Computed Tomography
C_{IS}	Carcinoma in Situ
CKD	Chronic Kidney Disease
CML	Chronic Myeloid Leukaemia
CMV	Cytomegalovirus
COCP	Combined Oral Contraceptive Pill
COPD	Chronic Obstructive Pulmonary Disease
CPAP	Continuous Positive Airway Pressure
CPP	Cerebral Perfusion Pressure
CRF	Chronic Renal Failure
CRP	C-Reactive Protein
CRPS	Complex Regional Pain Syndrome
CSF	Cerebrospinal Fluid
CSL	Compound Sodium Lactate
CT	Computed Tomography
CVP	Central Venous Pressure
CVR	Cerebral Vascular Resistance
CXR	Chest Radiograph
DAI	Diffuse Axonal Injury
DCC	Deleted in Colon Cancer
DHS	Dynamic Hip Screw
DIC	Disseminated Intravascular Coagulation
DIEP	Deep Inferior Epigastric Perforator
DKA	Diabetic Ketoacidosis
DM	Diabetes Mellitus
DMARDS	Disease Modifying Antirheumatic Drugs
DNA	Deoxyribonucleic Acid
DVT	Deep Vein Thrombosis
EBV	Epstein-Barr Virus
ECG	Electrocardiogram
ECHO	Echocardiogram

EGF	Epidermal Growth Factor
EMG	Electromyogram
EPO	Erythropoietin
ERCP	Endoscopic Retrograde Cholangiopancreatography
ETOH	Alcohol / Ethanol
F	French Units
FAP	Familial Adenomatous Polyposis
FBC	Full Blood Count
FDP	Flexor Digitorum Profundus
FDS	Flexor Digitorum Superficialis
Fe	Iron
FFP	Fresh Frozen Plasma
F_iO_2	Fraction of Inspired Oxygen (i.e. concentration or percentage of oxygen in inspired gas)
FNAC	Fine Needle Aspiration Cytology
FOB	Faecal Occult Blood
FR	Free Radicals
FRC	Functional Residual Capacity
G6PD	Glucose-6-Phosphate Dehydrogenase
GA	General Anaesthetic
GAGS	Glycosaminoglycans
GB	Gallbladder
GFR	Glomerular Filtration Rate
GI	Gastrointestinal
GSD	Gallstone Disease
H^+	Hydrogen Ions
Hb	Haemoglobin
HBV / HCV	Hepatitis B Virus / Hepatitis C Virus
HCC	Hepatocellular Carcinoma
HCG	Human Chorionic Gonadotropin
HDU	High Dependency Unit
HHV	Human Herpesvirus
HIV	Human Immunodeficiency Virus
HLA	Human Leucocyte Antigen
HNA	Human Neutrophil Antigen
HOCM	Hypertrophic Obstructive Cardiomyopathy
HPV	Human Papilloma Virus
HR	Heart Rate
HRT	Hormone Replacement Therapy
HSV	Herpes Simplex Virus
HTLV	Human T-Cell Lymphotropic Virus
Htn	Hypertension
IBD	Inflammatory Bowel Disease
ICP	Intracranial Pressure
ICU	Intensive Care Unit
IFN	Interferon
Ig	Immunoglobulin
IGAP	Inferior Gluteal Artery Perforator
IGF	Insulin Like Growth Factor

IHD	Ischaemic Heart Disease
IL	Interleukin
IMV	Inferior Mesenteric Vein
INR	International Normalised Ratio
IPPV	Intermittent Positive Pressure Ventilation (=CMV)
ITP	Immune Thrombocytopenic Purpura
IV	Intravenous
IVC	Inferior Vena Cava
IVDU	Intravenous Drug User
IVU	Intravenous Urography
JVP	Jugular Venous Pressure
kPa	Kilopascal
LA	Local Anaesthetic
LBO	Large Bowel Obstruction
LDH	Lactate Dehydrogenase
LDL	Low Density Lipoprotein
LFT	Liver Function Tests
LIF	Left Iliac Fossa
LMN	Lower Motor Neurone
LMWH	Low Molecular Weight Heparin
LP	Lumbar Puncture
LRTI	Lower Respiratory Tract Infection
LSV	Long Saphenous Vein
LUQ	Left Upper Quadrant
MAC	Membrane Attack Complex
MAG3	Mercaptuacetyltriglycine
MAP	Mean Arterial Pressure
MEN	Multiple Endocrine Neoplasia
Mg	Magnesium
MI	Myocardial Infarction
ml	Millilitres
mmHg	Millimetres of Mercury
MODS	Multi Organ Dysfunction Syndrome
MOFS	Multi Organ Failure Syndrome
MRCP	Magnetic Resonance Cholangiopancreatography
MSU	Midstream Urine
MTPJ	Metatarsophalangeal Joint
N/Saline	Normal Saline
Na	Sodium
NaHCO$_3^-$	Sodium Bicarbonate
NGT	Nasogastric Tube
NO	Nitric Oxide
NSAID	Non-Steroidal Anti-Inflammatory Drugs
O$_2$	Oxygen
OA	Osteoarthritis
OCP	Oral Contraceptive Pill
OGD	Oesophagogastroduodenoscopy
OPSI	Overwhelming Post Splenic Infection

PA	Posterior-Anterior
PAC / PAFC	Pulmonary Artery (Flotation) Catheter
P$_a$CO$_2$	Partial Pressure of Arterial Carbon Dioxide
PAF	Platelet Activating Factor
P$_a$O$_2$	Partial Pressure of Arterial Oxygen
PCL	Posterior Cruciate Ligament
PCV	Packed Cell Volume (= Haematocrit)
PDGF	Platelet Derived Growth Factor
P$_{diast.}$	Diastolic Blood Pressure
PE	Pulmonary Embolism
PEA	Pulseless Electrical Activity
PEEP	Positive End Expiratory Pressure
PICC	Peripherally Inserted Central Catheter
PID	Pelvic Inflammatory Disease
POP	Plaster of Paris
PR	Per Rectum
PrT	Prothrombin Time
PSA	Prostate Specific Antigen
PSC	Primary Sclerosing Cholangitis
PSIS	Posterior Superior Iliac Spine
P$_{syst.}$	Systolic Blood Pressure
PT	Physiotherapy
PTH	Parathyroid Hormone
PTHRP	Parathyroid Hormone Related Peptide
PTSD	Post Traumatic Stress Disorder
RA	Rheumatoid Arthritis
Rb	Retinoblastoma
RBC	Red Blood Cell / Erythrocyte
RCC	Renal Cell Carcinoma
RCT	Randomised Control Trial
Rh	Rhesus
RIF	Right Iliac Fossa
ROM	Range of Motion
RR	Respiratory Rate
RRT	Renal Replacement Therapy
RSTL	Relaxed Skin Tension Lines
RSV	Respiratory Syncytial Virus
RTA	Road Traffic Accident
RUQ	Right Upper Quadrant
SBO	Small Bowel Obstruction
SCC	Squamous Cell Carcinoma
SFJ	Saphenofemoral Junction
SIMV	Synchronized Intermittent Mandatory Ventilation
SIRS	Systemic Inflammatory Response Syndrome
SL	Sublingual
SLE	Systemic Lupus Erythematosus
SLN	Sentinel Lymph Node
SLNB	Sentinel Lymph Node Biopsy

SMA	Superior Mesenteric Artery
SMV	Superior Mesenteric Vein
SNS	Sympathetic Nervous System
SOB	Short of Breath
SPJ	Saphenopopliteal Junction
SSG	Split Skin Graft
STI	Sexually Transmitted Infection
SV	Stroke Volume
SVC	Superior Vena Cava
SVR	Systemic Vascular Resistance
TB	Tubercle Bacillus / Tuberculosis
TBSA	Total Body Surface Area
TCC	Transitional Cell Carcinoma
TFT	Thyroid Function Tests
TGF	Transforming Growth Factor (sometimes referred to as Tumour Growth Factor)
TLC	Total Lung Capacity
TNF	Tumour Necrosis Factor
t-PA	Tissue Plasminogen Activator
TPN	Total Parenteral Nutrition
TRAM	Transverse Rectus Abdominis Myocutaneous
TRH	Thyrotropin Releasing Hormone
TSH	Thyroid Stimulating Hormone
TXA2	Thromboxane A2
U&E	Urea & Electrolytes (including creatinine)
UGT	Uridine-Diphospho-Glucuronosyltransferase
USS	Ultrasound Scan
UTI	Urinary Tract Infection
V / Q	Ventilation-Perfusion Ratio
VEGF	Vascular Endothelial Growth Factor
VIP	Vasoactive Intestinal Peptide
VTE	Venous Thromboembolism
vWF	von Willebrand Factor
WCC	White Cell Count
μl	Microlitres

INDEX

1,25-Dihydroxycholecalciferol 90, 115
1st Rib 5, 130, 131, 178, 390
2,3 Diphosphoglycerate (2,3-DPG) 110, 111
5-Hydroxyindoleacetic Acid (5-HIAA) 352
5% Dextrose 77
Abdominal Aorta 39, 142, 143
Abdominal Aortic Aneurysm (AAA) 26, 32, 85, 87, 203, 243, 315, 316, 317, 318, 412
Abdominal Aortic Aneurysm Repair 87, 203, 315, 316, 317, 318
Abdominal Radiograph (AXR) 12, 15, 16, 18, 21–5, 28, 376
Abdominal Radiograph OSCE Cases 21
Abdominoperineal Resection 270, 272
Abductor Hallucis 168
Abductor Pollicis Longus 153–4
ABO Blood Group 202–3, 206
Above Knee Amputation (AKA) 311
Abscess 32, 52, 65, 84, 87, 220, 226, 257, 277, 279, 282, 319, 334–6, 414–5, 441
Acetabulum 156, 301, 303
Achilles Tendon 48, 168, 309
Acidosis 56–8, 74, 77, 96, 114, 206, 413, 436
Acoustic Neuroma 49
Acral Lentiginous Melanoma 364
Actinic Keratosis 362
Action Potential 52, 90, 93–4, 100–1, 342
Acute Abdomen 11, 25
Acute Haemolytic Reaction 206
Acute Inflammation 218–9, 255, 334
Acute Lung Injury (ALI) 79–80
Acute Pancreatitis 82–4, 412
Acute Renal Failure (ARF) 63, 84
Acute Respiratory Distress Syndrome (ARDS) 63, 79–81, 84, 318
Addison's Disease 104
Adductor Brevis 155
Adductor Canal 162–3
Adductor Hiatus 162–3
Adductor Longus 155, 158–9, 162, 303
Adductor Magnus 155, 162, 303
Adductor Tubercle 155, 162
Adenoma 251, 346, 348–9, 368–9, 372, 376, 380–2
Adenoma-Carcinoma Sequence 382
Adrenaline 53–4, 105, 107, 256, 287, 322
Adrenergic Receptor 107, 353

Advanced Life Support (ALS) 12, 25, 39, 53, 83, 105–6, 113–4, 412, 416, 418, 420, 438
Advanced Trauma Life Support (ATLS) 34–5, 67, 106, 113–4, 279, 289, 307, 332, 424, 431
Air Flow 67, 392, 412, 416, 418, 420, 438
Alkalosis 56–8
Allen's Test 56
Allograft 216, 403
Alternative Pathway 212
Amelanocytic Melanoma 364
Amputations 309–12, 335, 337, 418
Amyloid 191–2
Anaemia 54, 75, 112–3, 192–8, 210, 239, 242, 334, 375, 382, 419, 423, 428, 435, 438
Anaesthetic 53–4, 392, 416, 418, 438–9
Analgesic Nephropathy 423
Anaphylaxis 72, 76, 105–6, 206, 210
Anaplastic Carcinoma 367
Anatomical Snuffbox 153, 424
Aneurysm 20, 31, 38–41, 56, 63, 240–4, 263, 315–9
Angiogram 40, 146, 157, 179
Angiosarcoma 373
Angiotensin 96–7, 105
Angiotensin Converting Enzyme (ACE) 98, 108
Angle of Louis 132–3
Ankle 48, 169, 184
Anrep Effect 97
Ansa Cervicalis 128, 178
Antecubital Fossa 128, 178, 412, 416, 418, 420, 438
Anterior & Posterior Triangles 128–9
Anterior Cardiac Vein 135
Anterior Cruciate Ligament (ACL) 44–5, 164
Anterior Resection 270–2, 384, 437
Anterior Rib 5
Anterior Superior Iliac Spine (ASIS) 159, 161–2, 280, 301–2
Anterior Tibial Artery 157, 166
Antero-Lateral Spinothalamic Tract 176
Anticoagulation 404, 417, 437
Antidiuretic Hormone (ADH) 96, 98, 116, 239
Antisepsis 393, 403
Anuria 70
Aorta 5, 30–3, 39–41, 103, 127, 132–4, 139, 142–3, 266, 271, 294, 316–8
Aortic Arch 96, 105, 127, 133, 137, 146, 178
Aortic Dissection 40–1, 244

Aortic Knuckle 5
Aortic Regurgitation 99
Aortic Stenosis 99
Aortic Valve 99, 132
Appendicectomy 275, 281–2
Appendicitis 26, 31–2, 280–2, 351, 432
Appendix 32, 266, 269, 280–2, 351
Appendix Mass 280, 282
Aqueduct of Sylvius 174
Arches of the Foot 147, 157, 169
Arterial Blood Gas (ABG) 56, 78, 83, 107, 114, 413, 439
Arterial Waveform 98–9
Ascending & Descending Spinal Pathways 176
Ascending Aorta 30, 41, 132, 134
Asepsis 393
Atheroma 240–3
Atlanto-Axial Joint 120
Atlas 120
Atrial Natriuretic Peptide (ANP) 96
Atrophy 95, 187, 283, 300, 320, 333, 350
Auditory Meatus 49, 125, 170–1, 251
Autograft 216
Autologous Blood Transfusion 203–4
Avascular Necrosis (AVN) 424, 427
Avoidance Bias 357
Avulsion 303, 314–5, 329
Axillary Artery 147
Axillary Nerve 171, 177
Axillary Node Clearance 258, 260
Axis 120, 329, 362, 371
Axonotmesis 92
Azygous Vein 133, 137–8
B12 Deficiency Anaemia 192–4, 419
Bacteraemia 86
Bare Area 140
Baroreceptor 95, 105–6
Basal Cell Carcinoma (BCC) 359–60
Base Excess 56–7, 413
Basilar Artery 63, 179
Basilic Vein 150
Battle's Sign 66
Beck's Triad 262
Below Knee Amputation (BKA) 309–10
Benign Oesophageal Stricture 419
Bias 357, 387
Biceps Brachii 148–9
Biceps Femoris 155, 165
Bicipital Aponeurosis 150
Bier's Block 52, 54, 395
Bile 47, 141, 185–6, 190, 273–6, 372–3
Bilirubin 185–6, 190–1
Bilirubin Metabolism 185–6, 190–1

Bipolar Diathermy   398–9
Bladder   31, 114, 143, 145, 189, 227–8, 235, 237–8, 266, 271, 288, 376–9, 434
Blastoma   237
Bleeding Varices   13
Blinding   387
Blood Groups   202–3
Blood Pressure (BP)   96–8, 104
Blood Pressure Regulation   96–8
Blood Products   43, 201, 204
Blood Transfusion   111, 194, 196, 203–4, 207
Blood Transfusion Reactions   206
Blood Transfusion Substitutes   207
Bohr Effect   111
Bone Structure   328
Bowditch Effect   97
Bowel Anastomoses   267
Bowel Resection   272
Bowen's Disease   362
Brachial Artery   56, 150, 151
Brachial Plexus   52, 129–30, 177, 307, 390
Brachial Plexus Block   52, 307
Brachialis   150
Brachiocephalic Trunk   134, 146
Brachioradialis   150–1
Bradykinin   85, 211, 239
Brainstem Death   88
Breast Cancer   258–61, 370–1, 438
Breast Reconstruction   261, 371
Breslow Thickness   365
Broca's Area   173
Burn   58–61, 80, 85, 87, 95, 112, 198, 410–11
Burns Assessment   410–11
Burr Hole   319–22
Caecal Volvulus   22
Calcification   17, 20, 31, 241, 343, 348
Calcitonin   90–1, 234, 346, 353, 367
Calcium   4, 83, 90–1, 94, 183, 189, 328, 341, 346, 349
Calcium Homeostasis   90
Calculus   26, 72, 188, 189, 226, 288
Calor   218
Calot's Triangle   274–5
Cancellous Bone   328
Capitate   152
Carcinogen   235, 378, 400
Carcinogenesis   234–5
Carcinoid Syndrome   351–2
Carcinoid Tumour   351–2
Carcinoma   72, 144, 233–5, 237–9, 268, 356–84, 433
Cardiac Action Potential   90, 101
Cardiac Cycle   98–9
Cardiac Output (CO)   72, 96–7, 102–4, 111
Cardiac Pericardiocentesis   262–3
Cardiac Tamponade   105, 262
Cardiogenic Shock   105–7

Cardiopulmonary Bypass   63, 114
Carotid Canal   170
Carotid Sheath   128–9, 178
Carpal Tunnel   54, 151–2, 300–1
Carpal Tunnel Decompression   300
Carpal Tunnel Syndrome   300–1
Cartilage   137, 164, 331, 338, 343
Caudate Lobe   140–1, 274
Celiac Trunk   143
Cell Cycle   232–3
Cell Saver   203–4
Central Sulcus   172
Central Venous Access   252
Central Venous Pressure (CVP)   61, 73, 252–4
Cephalic Vein   150
Cerebellum   66, 172–6, 180
Cerebral Autoregulation   64
Cerebral Hemisphere   172–3, 180
Cerebral Perfusion Pressure (CPP)   67, 321
Cerebrospinal Fluid (CSF)   43, 46, 50, 64–7, 171, 174, 322–4
Chemoreceptor   96, 105
Chest Drains   6, 9–10, 264–5
Chest Pain   40, 438
Chest Radiograph (CXR)   5–14, 79–80, 249, 254, 265, 350, 370, 376, 383, 413–9, 428, 439–41
Chest Radiograph OSCE Cases   7–14,
Cholangiocarcinoma   235, 373
Cholecystectomy   274–5
Chorda Tympani   123–5
Chronic Inflammation   191, 218–9, 378
Chronic Renal Failure (CRF)   71–5, 348
Circle of Willis   179–80, 243
Circumcision   295–7
Circumflex Artery   134, 147
Clark's Level   366
Classic Pathway   212–3
Clinical Evidence   387
Clinical Trials   386
Clinoid Process   170
Cloquet's Node   160
Clot   222, 240
Clotting Cascade   90, 183, 199–200, 222, 229, 240
Coffee Bean   21–2
Collateral Ligament   45, 164
Collecting Duct   116
Colloid   207, 353
Colon   17, 22, 25, 28, 143, 267–77, 290–1, 380–1, 384, 415
Colorectal Adenoma   381
Colorectal Carcinoma   380–4
Commensal Bacteria   230
Comminuted   35, 329
Common Carotid Artery   127, 129, 134, 146, 178
Common Hepatic Duct   140, 273–4

Common Iliac Artery   142
Compact Bone   328, 331
Compartment Syndrome   305–6, 333, 389, 397
Compartments of the Lower Leg   166–7
Complement Cascade   75, 183, 212–5, 229
Computed Tomography (CT)   12, 15, 23–6, 29–32
Computed Tomography OSCE Cases   33–40
Condylar Head   122
Continuous Positive Airways Pressure (CPAP)   81
Contrast Enhanced Computed Tomography (CECT)   39
Contrast Study   436
Cooperative Binding   111
Coracoacromial Ligament   148
Coracobrachialis   149
Coronary Artery   63, 134, 263
Coronoid Process   122
Corpus Callosum   173, 187
Corpus Cavernosum   144
Corpus Spongiosum   144–5
Corrected Calcium   83, 183
Cortical Bone   29, 43, 328
Corticospinal Tracts   176
Costodiaphragmatic Recess   138, 290
Coupling   342, 399
Cranial Nerves   66, 88, 174–5
Craniotomy   319–20
Cremasteric Vein   145
Cribriform Plate   170–1
Cricothyroidotomy   254–6
Crista Galli   170
Crohn's Disease (CD)   19, 68, 189, 193, 210, 269, 281, 415
Cross Match   203, 217, 279, 316, 416, 420, 428
Cruciate Ligament   45, 164
Cryoprecipitate   204–5
Crystalloid   76–7, 207
Cushing's Disease / Syndrome   188, 239, 320, 349–51
Cyst   20, 23, 220–1, 277, 281, 319, 368, 441
Cytokine   199, 215
Cytokinesis   232
Dartos Pouch   292
De Quervain's Tenosynovitis   153
Deep Cervical Fascia   129, 178, 249
Deep Ring   161, 283
Deep Vein Thrombosis (DVT)   87, 226, 240, 270–2, 276, 303, 315, 333, 388, 391, 396, 417, 418, 439
Delayed Haemolytic Febrile Transfusion Reaction   204, 206
Delayed Haemolytic Reaction   204, 206
Deltoid   149, 169

Depolarisation   93–5, 100–1
Dermoid Cyst   20, 220
Descending Aorta   5, 30, 40–1, 133, 139
Descending Genicular Artery   163
Descending Loop of Henle   116
Dextrose-Saline   59, 77
Diaphragm   18, 138–9, 265
Diaphragm Muscle   138
Diaphragm Tendon   138
Diathermy   258, 270, 391, 397–9
Digastric   125, 129
Discectomy   46
Disinfection   393
Disseminated Intravascular Coagulation (DIC)   201
Distal Convoluted Tubule   116
Diuretics   58, 67, 87, 116, 184, 198
Dolor   218
Doppler   103
Dorsal & Plantar Venous Arches   157
Dorsal Columns   176
Dorsalis Pedis   56, 157
Dorsum of the Hand   153
Double Blinding   387
Drains   17, 250, 264–5, 391, 402
Dressings   295, 303, 335, 403–4
Ductal Carcinoma   370
Duodenal Ulcer   416
Duodenum   141, 143, 190, 266, 269, 272–3, 276, 290, 323
Duplex Left Ureter   436
Duplication Cyst   23–4
Dupuytren's Fasciectomy   54
Dye Dilution Method   103
Dynamic Hip Screw (DHS)   426
Dysequilibrium Syndrome   75
Dysphagia   95, 320, 419
Dysplasia   233, 381
Echocardiogram (ECHO)   103, 316, 438
Ectopic Gallstone   25
Ejection Fraction   62, 98
Elastic Cartilage   343
Electrocardiogram (ECG)   7, 13, 53, 98, 114, 254, 316, 412–3, 416, 428, 439–40
Embolus   31, 58, 72, 80, 85, 240, 242, 438
End Diastolic Volume   98, 102, 262
Endocrine Tumour   374–5
Endotoxin   104, 228–9
Enterocutaneous Fistula   415
Epididymis   144, 292
Epidural Anaesthesia   54, 309, 311
Epigastric Pain   82, 374, 412
Erb's Palsy   177
Ethmoid   170
Excision Margins   361–5
Excitation-Contraction Coupling   342
Exotoxin   104, 228–9

Expiratory Reserve Volume (ERV)   108
Extensor Carpi Radialis Brevis   153–4
Extensor Carpi Radialis Longus   153–4
Extensor Carpi Ulnaris   154
Extensor Digiti Minimi   153–4
Extensor Digitorum Communis (EDC)   152–4
Extensor Digitorum Longus   166–7
Extensor Hallucis Longus   167–8
Extensor Indicis   152–4
Extensor Pollicis Brevis (EPB)   153–4
Extensor Pollicis Longus (EPL)   152–3
Extensor Retinaculum   153
External Carotid Artery & Branches   124, 128, 178
External Fixation   332, 431
External Oblique   145, 161–2, 281, 283, 291, 293–4
Extradural Haemorrhage   35–7
Extraluminal Gas   17–18, 32
Extrapyramidal System   176
Extrinsic Pathway   200
Exudate   10, 207, 221, 223, 404
Facet Joint   121
Facial Nerve (VII)   123–6, 171, 251–2, 320
Faecal Occult Blood (FOB)   357
Falciform Ligament   18, 140
False Aneurysm   318
Familial Adenomatous Polyposis (FAP)   381–2
Fasciotomy   306
Fat Embolism   303, 333, 439–40
Fe2+ Deficiency Anaemia   193
Femoral Angiogram   157
Femoral Artery   56, 158–63, 243, 253, 312, 315
Femoral Canal   160
Femoral Condyle   164
Femoral Embolectomy   312–3
Femoral Head   155–6, 301, 424–5, 427
Femoral Hernia Repair   284–5
Femoral Neck Fracture   426
Femoral Nerve   158, 302
Femoral Sheath   160
Femoral Triangle   158–9, 162, 253
Femoral Vein   157–60, 163, 253, 315
Femur   154–5, 162, 302–3, 311, 425–8
Fibrinolytic System   200–1
Fibrocartilage   164, 343
Fibroelastic Cartilage   343
Fibula   169
Fick Principle   103
Field Change   378
Final Common Pathway   200, 212, 213

Fine Touch   176
Fistula   25, 220, 252, 257, 272, 279, 287, 318, 405, 415
Flap   259, 261, 272, 310, 312, 338
Flexor Carpi Radialis (FCR)   152
Flexor Carpi Ulnaris (FCU)   150
Flexor Digitorum Brevis   168
Flexor Digitorum Longus   167
Flexor Digitorum Profundus (FDP)   152
Flexor Digitorum Superficialis (FDS)   152
Flexor Hallucis Longus   167–8
Flexor Retinaculum   152
Flexor Pollicis Longus (FPL)   152
Fluids   75–7, 207, 264
Focal Nodular Hyperplasia   372
Folate Deficiency   192, 194, 419
Follicular Carcinoma   367
Foot   48, 157, 169
Foramen Lacerum   170–1
Foramen Magnum   170–1
Foramen of Luschka   174
Foramen of Magendie   174
Foramen Ovale   170–1
Foramen Rotundum   170
Foramen Spinosum   170–1
Forced Vital Capacity (FVC)   108–9
Fovea Capitis   155
Fracture Healing   328, 331–2
Fracture Patterns   330
Fractured Clavicle   440
Fractured Neck of Femur   155, 425
Fractures   34, 156, 328–35, 348, 425–6, 428, 431
Frank-Starling Curve   102
Fresh Frozen Plasma (FFP)   76, 204–5, 416
Frontal Bone   170–1, 198, 322
Frontal Lobe   172–3, 180
Full Thickness Skin Graft   339
Functio Laesa   218
Function Anatomy of the Liver   140–1
Functional Residual capacity (FRC)   108–9, 389
Gallbladder   188, 190, 273–5, 323
Gallstone   190–1, 273–5, 412–3
Gallstone Disease (GSD)   190–1, 273–5, 412–3
Gallstone Ileus   25, 191
Gap 1 Phase   232
Gap 2 Phase   232
Garden's Classification   156, 426
Garden's Grade   426
Gastric Bubble   5
Gastrinoma   375
Gastrocnemius   155, 165–7
Gastrostomy   69
General Anaesthetic (GA)   52, 54, 332
Geniculate Ganglion   125

Genitofemoral Nerve (L2)   145
Genu   173
Glans Penis   144
Glenohumeral Joint   149
Glioblastoma Multiforme   50, 237
Glomerulus   116
Glossopharyngeal Nerve (IX)   123, 171
Glucagonoma   374–5
Gluteal Tuberosity   155
Gluteus Maximus   155, 302
Gluteus Medius   155–6, 301–2
Gluteus Minimus   155
Gonadal Vein   142
Gout   184–5, 422–4, 429
Grading   34, 358, 426
Graft   39, 63, 216, 316–8, 338–9
Graft Versus Host Disease   204, 206
Granuloma   72, 219
Great Saphenous Vein   157
Greater Auricular Nerve   128
Greater Trochanter   155–6, 301–2
Greenstick Fracture   329
Groove for Vertebral Artery   120
Group & Save   203, 418, 428, 431, 434, 435
Guyon's Canal   152
Gynaecomastia   346–7
Gyrus   172
Haemangioma   188, 372, 380
Haematoma   33, 35, 37, 40, 53, 55, 56, 62, 65, 171, 224, 243, 244, 250, 252, 283, 289, 298, 301, 306, 312, 315, 319, 320, 331, 397, 435
Haematuria   15, 26, 189, 288, 289, 376, 433–4
Haemodiafiltration   74, 87
Haemodialysis   74, 87, 114
Haemofiltration   74, 87
Haemolytic Anaemia   194, 196, 210
Haemorrhoidectomy   285–7
Haemorrhoids   285–7
Haemostasis   199, 250, 251, 256, 259, 261, 270, 271, 278–9, 291–5, 299, 395, 396, 403
Hamartoma   188, 380
Hamate   152
Hartmann's Procedure   268, 434
Hartmann's Solution   77
Hasselbach's Triangle   162
Haustra   17–18, 21, 22
Head Injury   58, 64–7, 79, 87, 321
Heart   6, 96–9, 102, 134–5, 262
Heart Rate (HR)   62, 96, 106
Heart Sound   99, 262
Heavy Chain   214
Helium Dilution Method   109
Hemiarthroplasty   26, 301, 426–8
Hemicolectomy   73, 269, 384
Hemi–Diaphragm   5, 18
Henry's Law   110, 111
Hepatic Artery   140, 141, 273

Hepatic Function   185
Hepatitis B Virus (HBV)   204, 231, 235, 373
Hepatitis C Virus (HCV)   204, 235, 373
Hepatoblastoma   373
Hepatocellular Carcinoma (HCC)   373
Hereditary Non-Polyposis Colorectal Carcinoma (HNPCC)   381–2
Hickman Line   69
High Dose Dexamethasone Suppression Test   350
Hinge Region   214
Hip Joint   154–6, 301–2
Histamine   85, 211, 352
Hook of Hamate   152
Horizontal Fissure   137
Hounsfield Scale   29
Howell-Jolly Body   196
Human Immunodeficiency Virus (HIV)   87, 204, 214, 224, 226, 334, 361, 414
Hyaline Cartilage   331, 343
Hydrocoele Repair   299
Hydrostatic Pressure   208–9
Hydroxyapatite   90, 328
Hypercalcaemia   91, 189, 239, 348–9, 377
Hyperchromatism   236
Hyperparathyroidism   91, 346–9
Hyperplasia   95, 187–8, 198, 216, 241, 348, 372
Hyperpolarisation   93, 100
Hypersensitivity   104, 206, 210–11, 215
Hypersensitivity Reaction   104, 206, 210–11, 215
Hyperthyroidism   347, 353–4
Hypertrophic Scar   339–40
Hypertrophy   188, 339–40
Hyperuricaemia   184–5
Hypocalcaemia   84, 91, 206, 250, 348, 374
Hypoglossal Canal   171
Hypoglossal Nerve (XII)   123, 171
Hypoparathyroidism   91, 250
Hypothermia   63, 88, 112–4, 195, 196
Hypothyroidism   88, 192–3, 250, 300
Hypovolaemic Shock   96, 106, 333
Hypoxaemia   78, 79, 84, 112, 440
Hypoxic Ventilatory Drive   82
Ilioinguinal Nerve   145, 283, 295
Iliopsoas   155, 158, 159
Immunisation   231
Immunity   214–5, 231
Immunodeficiency   214
Immunoglobulin   191, 214, 231
Infarction   62, 236, 241–4, 263, 269, 438, 439
Inferior Alveolar Nerve   122
Inferior Colliculus   173

Inferior Epigastric Artery   162
Inferior Mediastinum   133
Inferior Mesenteric Artery   142, 143, 268, 271, 316
Inferior Vena Cava (IVC)   139–43
Inflammation   32, 41, 65, 85, 218–9
Inflammatory Bowel Disease (IBD)   19
Infraorbital Foramen   171
Infraspinatus   149
Ingrown Toenail   303
Inguinal Canal   145, 161–2, 284
Inguinal Hernia Repair   283
Inguinal Ligament   158–62, 283, 284, 285, 312
Inguinal Lymph Nodes   144, 294
Inhalational Injury   60
Initiator   234
Innervation of the Tongue   123
Inotrope   107
Inotropic Effect   102
Inspiratory Reserve Volume (IRV)   108
Insulinoma   374, 375
Intensive Care Unit (ICU)   87–8
Intercondylar Fossa   155
Intermittent Positive Pressure Ventilation (IPPV)   81
Internal Auditory Meatus   49, 125, 170, 171
Internal Fixation   332, 425
Internal Jugular Vein (IJV)   7, 124, 129, 171, 178, 179, 253
Internal Laryngeal Nerve   127
Internal Oblique   145, 161, 162, 281, 291, 293
Interosseous Membrane   166, 381
Interosseous Vessels   156
Intervertebral Disc   46, 343
Intestinal Neoplasms   380
Intestinal Polyps   380
Intestinal Stenosis of Garre   285
Intracapsular Fracture   156, 425, 426
Intracranial Pressure (ICP)   64, 65, 81, 321–2
Intraluminal Gas   17, 18
Intraperitoneal Air   12
Intravenous Urography (IVU)   434, 436
Intrinsic Pathway   200
Involucrum   334
Ischaemia   22, 28, 58, 63, 67, 83, 85, 187, 195, 241–2, 250, 269, 272, 283, 306, 309, 317, 318, 397
Isograft   216
Jackson's Burn Model   58
Jaundice   69, 84, 185–6, 191, 195, 273, 373, 374, 382
Jejunostomy   69
Jenkins' Rule   266
Jugular Foramen   170, 171
Juxtaglomerular   97

Keloid Scar   339
Kessler Suture   308
Ketone   55
Kidney   16, 23, 30–4, 55, 90, 115–6, 140, 142, 186, 189, 290–2, 377, 435
Kidney Bean   22
Kidney Ureter Bladder (KUB)   189
Klumpke's Palsy   177
Knee Joint   163–4, 311
L4–5 Intervertebral Space   322, 324
Lacrimal Bone   170
Lactic Acid   31, 55, 114, 436
Lacunar Ligament   160
Lag Bias   357
Lamellar Bone   328, 331
Lamina   120
Laminar Air Flow   392
Laminectomy   46
Language Comprehension   173
Laparoscopic   284, 290
Laparoscopic Appendicectomy   282
Laparoscopic Cholecystectomy   274–6
Laparoscopic Splenectomy   278
Laparoscopy   276
Laparotomy   39, 266–72, 281, 291, 316
Large Bowel Obstruction (LBO)   272, 318, 351, 382
Lateral Cerebral Hemisphere   172–3, 180
Lateral Condyle   155
Lateral Epicondyle   150, 155
Lateral Mass   120
Lateral Sulcus   172
Lateral Ventricle   35, 36, 38, 50, 174
Latissimus Dorsi   149, 258, 261, 265, 291
Lead Bias   357
Lectin Pathway   212
Leeches   404
Left Atrium   61, 132
Left Hilum   5, 6
Left Varicocoele   377
Left Ventricle   5, 134, 243
Left Ventricular Failure   437–9
Lentigo Maligna Melanoma   364
Lesser Trochanter   155
Leukoplakia   362
Leukotrienes   229
Level of Evidence   387
Lichtenstein's Repair   283
Ligamentem Arteriosum   127
Ligaments of the Foot   169
Ligamentum Teres   140, 141, 155, 156, 427
Ligamentum Venosum   140
Light Amplification by Stimulated Emission of Radiation (LASER)   394
Light Chain   214
Linea Aspera   155

Linea Semilunaris   162
Liver   132, 140–1, 183, 185–6, 192, 199, 273, 274, 372–3
Liver Cancer   372–3
Lobular Carcinoma   370
Local Anaesthetic (LA)   52–3
Lockwood Approach   284
Long Saphenous Nerve   163
Long Thoracic Nerve of Bell   177, 259, 265
Low Dose Dexamethasone Suppression Test   350
Lower Leg Compartments   166–7
Lower Limb Vessels   157
Lumbar Puncture   322–4
Lund & Browder Chart   59, 410–11
Lung   79–80, 108, 136–7, 264–5, 441
Lung Function   108–9
Lymphoedema   207, 209, 259, 260
Lymphoma   214, 235, 237–9, 367
Macrocytic   192–4
Macrophages   80, 185, 215, 219, 220, 221, 222, 241
Macula Densa   97
Maggots   404
Magnetic Resonance Cholangiopancreatogram (MRCP)   47, 273
Magnetic Resonance Imaging (MRI)   41–50, 281, 350, 352, 368, 413
Magnetic Resonance Imaging OSCE Cases   44–50
Main Bronchus   13, 137
Malignancy   214, 233, 236–8, 240, 309, 368, 373, 374, 405
Malignant Melanoma   363–7
Malignant Tumours   237
Mamillary Body   175
Mandible   122, 124–6, 128, 129
Mandibular Foramen   122
Mandibular Nerve (V3)   122–3, 171
Manubrium   128, 132, 323
Marginal Mandibular Nerve   122
Masseter   124, 251
Mastectomy   258–61, 371
Maxilla   170
McEvedy Approach   285
Mean Arterial Pressure (MAP)   62, 65, 99
Mechanical Ventilation   81
Medial Cerebral Hemisphere   173
Medial Condyle   155, 390
Medial Cutaneous Nerve of the Arm   177
Medial Epicondyle   150, 155, 390
Medial Malleolus   157, 168, 169
Medial Plantar Nerve   168
Median Cubital Vein   150
Median Nerve   150, 151, 152, 177, 300, 301
Mediastinum   13, 32, 96, 132–3, 237

Medulla   96, 116, 125, 171, 175, 176, 289, 324
Medullary Carcinoma   192, 346, 367
Membrane Attack Complex (MAC)   212, 213
Menisci   164, 343
Meniscus   10, 122, 164
Mental Foramen   122
Mental Nerve   122
Mesencephalon   175
Metabolic Acidosis   56–8, 206, 413
Metabolic Alkalosis   56–8
Metaplasia   233
Microcytic   192, 193, 197
Midstream Urine (MSU)   114, 228
Mitosis Phase   232
Modified Glasgow Criteria   83
Moh's Micrographic Surgery   360, 361, 363
Monopolar Diathermy   398–9
Monro-Kellie Doctrine   64
Motor Cortex   172
Multi-Hit Hypothesis   86, 382
Multiorgan Dysfunction Syndrome (MODS)   69, 86–7, 418
Multiorgan Failure Syndrome (MOFS)   87
Multiple Endocrine Neoplasia (MEN)   346, 367, 375
Multiple Hit Hypothesis   86, 382
Muscle   90, 94–5, 149–50, 155, 166–7, 341–2
Muscle Relaxant   94–5
Musculocutaneous Nerve   177
Myasthenia Gravis   58, 79, 95–6
Myocardial Infarction   263, 438–9
Nasogastric Tube (NGT)   6, 7, 412, 416
Necrotising Fasciitis   85, 309, 417–8
Negative Pressure Therapy (VACTM)   338, 405
Neoplasia   232–3, 319
Nephrectomy   289–92, 378, 380
Nephroblastoma   237, 376, 379
Nephron Function   115
Nerve Action Potential   93
Nerve Injuries   92
Nerve to Vastus Medialis   163
Neurohumoral Response   104–5
Neuromuscular Junction   94–5
Neuropraxia   92
Neurotmesis   92
Neurovascular Bundles   139, 307, 311
Nodes of Ranvier   94
Nodular Basal Cell Carcinoma   360
Nodular Melanoma   364
Non-Haemolytic Febrile Transfusion Reaction   206
Non-Invasive Stabilisation   332
Normal Saline   77, 207
Normocytic   192
Nosocomial Infection   230

Nutrition 68–70, 230, 267, 332, 415
Oblique Fissure 137
Occipital Condyle 170
Occipital Lobe 172, 173
OctreoScanTM 352
Odontoid Process 120
Oedema 14, 50, 68, 207–9
Oesophagus 15, 127–9, 132, 133, 139, 143, 187, 233, 237, 238, 256, 257, 368, 419, 420
Oliguria 70, 73, 106
Omental Bursa 141
Omohyoid 128, 129
Oncological Principles 356–8
Oncotic Pressure 183, 208
Open Fracture 431, 440
Optic Canal 170, 171
Optic Nerve 171, 173, 187
Orbital Fissure 171
Orchidectomy 292, 294–5
Osteoarthritis 337, 422, 429–30
Osteomyelitis 195, 219, 220, 306, 333–7, 405
Over Diagnosis Bias 357
Oxygen Dissociation Curve 110–11
Oxygen Therapy 81–2
Oxygen Transport 110–12
Pacemaker Potential 100
Painful Testicle 432
Pampiniform Plexus 145
Pancreas 20, 82–4, 143, 188, 190, 237, 238, 374–5
Pancreatic Carcinoma 374–5
Pancreatitis 15, 20, 63, 80, 82–4, 85, 87, 91, 191, 273, 374, 412
Panda / Raccoon Eyes 66
Papillary Adenocarcinoma 367
Papillary Cystadenoma 369
Para-Aortic Lymph Nodes 144, 294, 379
Paraneoplastic Syndromes 91, 238–9, 377, 382
Parathyroid Glands 128, 129, 250, 348
Parathyroid Hormone (PTH) 90, 348
Parietal Lobe 172, 173
Parietal Pleura 135, 137
Parkland Formula 59
Parotid Duct 124, 251, 252
Parotid Gland 124–6, 128, 251, 368–9
Parotidectomy 251–2, 369
Patella 157, 164
Patellar Ligament 164
Patient Positioning 389–90
Patient Safety for Theatre 391
Pectineal Line 155, 160
Pectineus 155, 159, 160
Pectoral Nerve 177, 259
Pectoralis Major 149, 258, 265
Pectoralis Minor 147, 149, 260
Pedicle 120, 287, 289, 291, 399

Penis 53, 144–5, 237
Pericardiocentesis 262–3
Pericardium 133, 135, 138
Perioperative Care 386–91
Peripheral Nerve 92
Peripherally Inserted Central Catheter (PICC) 69
Peritoneal Dialysis 74, 75, 87
Peroneal Artery 157, 166
Peroneal Vein 166
Peroneus Longus 166, 167
pH 52, 55–8, 74, 108, 110, 397, 413, 439
Phrenic Nerve 130, 139
Physeal Cartilage 343
Physiological Shock 104–5, 435
Piriformis 155, 156, 302
Plantar Aponeurosis 168
Plantaris 155, 165, 167
Plasma Proteins 55, 90, 183, 199
Plastibell Technique 296
Platelets 199, 201, 204, 205, 222, 240, 277
Pleomorphic Adenoma 369
Pleomorphism 233, 236
Pleura 8, 135, 137
Pleural Effusion 6, 10, 14, 20, 32, 79, 84, 226, 264
Pneumobilia 24–5
Pneumomediastinum 13, 276, 420
Pneumonia 79, 85, 95, 113, 182, 224–6, 230, 231, 257, 272, 280, 333, 428
Pneumothorax 8, 9, 226, 264–5, 440
Polycythaemia 198, 239, 377
Polyps 380–1
Pons 125, 173, 175
Popliteal Artery 157, 165
Popliteal Fossa 156, 165
Popliteus 166, 167
Porta Hepatis 32, 140
Positive End Expiratory Pressure (PEEP) 80, 81
Post-Central Gyrus 172
Posterior Cruciate Ligament (PCL) 45, 164
Posterior Interventricular Artery 134, 135
Posterior Rib 5
Posterior Tibial Artery 157, 166, 167, 168
Posterior Tibial Nerve 166
Posterior Tibial Vein 157, 166, 168
Posterior Triangle 128
PostTourniquet Syndrome 397
Pre-Central Gyrus 172
Pre-Operative Assessment 437
Pressure Sores 390
Pressure Support Ventilation (PSV) 81
Primary Pneumothorax 9
Pringle's Manoeuvre 141
Processus Vaginalis 145

Promoter 234
Pronator Teres 150
Properitoneal Fat Plane 16, 18
Proprioception 176
Prostaglandins 85, 211, 229
Proximal Convoluted Tubule 116
Pseudocyst 84, 220, 413
Psoas 16, 20, 23, 290, 435
Psoas Shadow 16, 20, 435
Pterion 171
Pubic Tubercle 157, 159, 161, 283, 285, 315
Pulmonary Artery 5, 6, 30, 40, 61–2, 80, 132, 137
Pulmonary Artery Catheter (PAC) 6, 61–2
Pulmonary Embolism (PE) 79, 105, 333, 438, 439
Pulmonary Oedema 14, 58, 68, 79, 105
Pulmonary Trunk 99, 134
Pulmonary Vein 137
Pus 220–1
Pyelogram 436
Quadrate Lobe 140
Radial Artery 56, 152, 424
Radial Nerve 150, 177, 397
Radiograph Densities 4
Radiography 4–28
Randomisation 386
Raynaud's Disease 54
Raynaud's Syndrome 396
Reconstructive Ladder 338
Rectal Tumours 270
Rectum 21–2, 143, 270–2, 380, 384
Recurrent Laryngeal Nerve 127, 129, 250, 256–7, 348
Red Blood Cell (RBC) 198
Referral to Coroner 421
Refractory Period 93, 101
Renal Artery 72, 142, 289, 291
Renal Calculi / Renal Stones 26–7, 91, 184, 189
Renal Cell Carcinoma (RCC) 376–8
Renal Failure 15, 63, 70–3, 84, 184, 192, 206, 209, 227, 318, 428
Renal Function 115–6
Renal Replacement Therapy (RRT) 74–5
Renal Trauma 289–90, 435
Renal Tumour 376
Renal Vein 142, 377
Renin-Angiotensin-Aldosterone System 96, 97, 105
Repolarisation 93, 100–1
Residual Volume (RV) 108–9
Respiratory Acidosis 56–7
Respiratory Alkalosis 56–8
Respiratory Failure 57, 78–9, 81, 95, 413, 439
Resting Membrane Potential 93, 100–1

Syndrome (SIRS) 75, 84–7, 418
Systemic Vascular Resistance (SVR) 62, 96, 104–6
T1 & T2 Weighted Sequences 42–3
Target Cell 196–7, 212
Taste 123, 125
Temperature 58, 84, 103, 110–12, 205
Temperomandibular Joint 122
Temporal Lobe 172
Tendo Calcaneus 168
Tendon Repair 52, 307–8
Tensillon Test 96
Teratoma 220, 234, 237
Teres Major 149
Teres Minor 149
Testicular Artery 142, 145
Testicular Torsion 292, 294, 432
Testicular Vein 145, 377
Testis 144, 283, 292–4, 299, 351, 432
Thalamus 174, 237, 353
Thalassaemia 192, 194, 196–7, 277
Theatre Design 392
Thermoregulation 112, 224
Thoracic Duct 133, 139, 253
Thoracic Outlet Syndrome 131
Thoracodorsal Nerve 177, 259
Threshold Potential 93, 100
Thromboembolic Deterrent Stockings (TEDS) 209, 315, 388
Thromboprophylaxis 388
Thrombus 240–2
Thymus 95, 239
Thyroid Artery 127, 250, 348
Thyroid Cancer 367
Thyroid Function Tests (TFT) 96, 113, 249, 354, 368
Thyroid Gland 127, 249–50, 348, 353
Thyroid Hormones 353
Thyroid Isthmus 127, 256
Thyroid Lobe 127
Thyroid Vein 127, 249
Thyroidectomy 249–50, 354
Tibia 166, 169, 306, 309, 430–1
Tibial Nerve 165–8
Tibialis Anterior 166–8
Tibialis Posterior 166–8
Tibioperoneal Trunk 157
Tidal Volume (TV) 108
Tissue Expansion 338
TNM Staging System 358
Tongue 123, 125
Tophi 184, 185

Total Hip Replacement 427
Total Lung Capacity (TLC) 108, 109, 389
Total Parenteral Nutrition (TPN) 69, 70, 77, 252
Tourniquets 300–1, 304, 307, 395–7
Trabecular Bone 328, 331
Trachea 5, 6, 30, 127, 129, 132–3, 250, 255–7, 343
Tracheostomy 7, 254–7
Transfusion Related Acute Lung Injury 206
Transitional Cell Carcinoma (TCC) 376, 378–9, 433–4
Transplant Rejection 210, 217
Transplantation 216–17
Transudate 10, 207
Transversalis Fascia 145, 161, 162, 284, 285
Transverse Process 20, 120–1, 137
Transversus Abdominis 161–2, 290
Trapezium 152–3
Trapezoid 152
Triangles of the Neck 128–9
Triple Assessment 370
Trousseau's Sign 91, 374
True Aneurysm 243
Tubercle 120, 130, 152, 155, 157, 159, 161–2, 283, 285, 315
Tumor 218
Tumour Markers 233–4
Tunica Adventitia 244
Tunica Intima 241, 244
Tunica Media 244
Tunica Vaginalis 144, 292–3, 299
Type I Hypersensitivity 104, 210, 215
Ulcerative Colitis (UC) 28, 380–1, 415
Ulnar Artery 152
Ulnar Nerve 152, 301
Ultrasound (USS) 23, 26, 83, 103, 249, 253–4, 260, 273, 281–2, 288, 315, 368, 370, 376, 383, 413, 432–5
Universal Donor 202
Universal Recipient 202
Upper Limb Vessels 146–7
Upper Lobe Collapse 13
Urate 184, 189, 423, 429
Urate Crystals 423
Ureter 20, 27, 31, 72, 142–3, 226–7, 237, 268, 272, 290–1, 318, 379, 434, 436

Urethra 72, 144–5, 189, 226–30, 272, 297, 376, 378–9, 433–4
Urinary Calculi 188–9
Urinary Tract Infection (UTI) 85, 226–8, 272, 288, 428, 432–3, 436
Urogram 436
Vaccination 225, 231, 280, 373
Vagus Nerve (X) 123, 171
Valvulae Conniventes 17–18
Varicose Vein 315
Varicose Vein Surgery 315
Vas Deferens 145, 294, 297
Vasectomy 247, 297–8
Vasopressor 107
Vastus Intermedius 155
Vastus Lateralis 155
Vastus Medialis 155, 162–3
Vaughan-Williams Classification 101
Venous Thromboembolism (VTE) 388
Ventilation 56, 67, 80–2, 87–8, 224, 230, 256,
Ventricle 5, 35, 36, 50, 61, 103, 132, 134, 173–4, 243
Ventricular Action Potential 100
Vertebra 30, 121
Vibration 176
VIPoma 375
Virchow's Triad 240
Visceral Pleura 8, 137
Von Willebrand Factor 199, 205, 222
Wallace's Rule of Nines 59
Wallerian Degeneration 92
Warfarin 38, 416, 422, 433, 437, 439
Warthin's Tumour 369
Wernicke's Area 173
Whipple's Procedure 375
Wide Local Excision 259
Wilms' Tumour 376, 379–80
Windowing 29
Winslow's Foramen 141
Wound Healing 68, 222–3, 339
Wound Infection 224, 276, 283, 304, 318, 320, 333, 336, 414
Woven Bone 328, 331
Xenograft 216, 403
X-ray 4–11, 29, 302, 424–5, 436, 440–1
Zadek's Procedure 303–4
Zygoma 124–6, 170–2, 251
α-Fetoprotein 373

Resting Phase 232
Restriction Point 232
Retinacular Vessels 156, 427
Retromandibular Vein 124
Retroperitoneum 143, 266
Rhesus System 202–3
Rib 5, 6, 30, 34, 119, 130–1, 137, 277, 290, 291, 323, 390, 428
Right Atrium 5, 61, 63, 134, 135
Right Hemicolectomy 73, 269–70, 384
Right Hilum 5, 6
Right Pulmonary Artery 5, 30, 132, 137
Right Ventricle 61, 103, 132, 134
Rigler's Sign 18, 25
Robson's Staging 377
Rodent Ulcer 359
Roos' Test 131
Rostrum 173
Rotator Cuff 148–9
Rubor 218
Rule of Thirds 75–7
Sacroiliac Joint 16, 19
Salivary Gland Neoplasms 368–9
Saltatory Conduction 94
Salter-Harris Classification 330–1
Saphenofemoral Junction (SFJ) 157, 314–5
Sarcoma 235, 237, 309, 373, 380
Sarcomere 342
Sartorius 158, 162, 302
Scalene Tubercle 130
Scaphoid 152–3, 424–5
Scaphoid Fracture 424
Scars 339–40
Schwann Cell 92, 94
Sciatic Nerve 156, 167, 302, 311
Sclerotherapy 13, 286, 314
Screening 29, 204, 315, 355–7, 381
Screening Programmes 356–7
Scrotal Approach 292, 294
Scrotum 144, 292–9
Sebaceous Cyst 221
Secondary Brain Injury 64, 67
Secondary Pneumothorax 9
Selection Bias 357
Sella Turcica 170
Semimembranosus 165
Semitendinosus 165
Sensitivity 357
Sensory Cortex 172
Sentinel Lymph Node (SLN) 260, 367, 371
Sentinel Lymph Node Biopsy (SLNB) 260, 367, 371
Sepsis 56, 58, 62, 68–9, 72, 75, 80, 85–7, 105, 107, 112, 415
Septic Arthritis 226, 304, 306, 335–7, 422–3
Septic Shock 86, 107, 229
Septic Syndrome 86

Septicaemia 86, 87, 194, 226, 228, 335
Sequestration Crisis 195
Sequestrum 334
Severe Sepsis 86
Shock 58, 77, 86, 96, 104–7, 201
Shortness of Breath 8, 10, 14, 438, 441
Sickle Cell Anaemia 54, 192, 195–6, 334
Sigmoid Sinus 170
Sigmoid Volvulus 21, 268
Silhouette Sign 11
Simon's Classification 347
Single Blinding 387
Sinus 96, 105, 135, 141, 170, 179, 220, 329
Skeletal Muscle 242, 341–2
Skin Cancer 359–67
Skin Graft 216, 338–9, 418
Skull 35, 64, 66, 129, 170–1, 319–20
Skull Foramina 171
Small Bowel Obstruction (SBO) 285, 412
Small Saphenous Vein 157, 167
Smooth Muscle 90, 211, 241, 285, 341
Snuffbox Tenderness 153, 424
SOCRATES 429
Soleus 166–7
Specificity 357
Speech Production 173
Spermatic Cord 144–5, 283, 294, 297–8
Sphenoid 170–1, 351
Spinal Accessory Nerve 128
Spinal Anaesthesia 52, 54, 306
Spinocerebellar Tracts 176
Spinothalamic Tract 176
Spinous Process 5, 6, 120
Spirometry 103, 108–9
Splachnic Nerves 139
Spleen 16, 33–4, 192, 266, 276–80, 323
Splenectomy 34, 275–80
Splenic Injury 33–4
Splenium 173
Split Thickness Skin Graft 338
Squamous Cell Carcinoma (SCC) 361–2
Staghorn Calculus 26, 27, 189
Staging 29, 358
Stanford Classification 41
Stapedius 125
Starling Curve 102
Starling's Law of the Capillaries 183, 208–9
Starling's Law of the Heart 102, 106, 111
Sterilisation 393
Sternocleidomastoid 124, 128–9, 178, 251, 253, 256

Sternohyoid 128
Sternum 132, 137, 258, 343
Stroke Volume (SV) 62, 96, 98, 102, 262
Stylohyoid 125, 251
Stylomastoid Foramen 125–6, 171
Subarachnoid Haemorrhage 38, 65
Subclavian Artery 127, 134, 146–7, 253
Subclavian Steal Syndrome 146
Subdural Haemorrhage 36–7
Submandibular Gland 127–8, 368
Subscapular Nerve 177
Subscapularis 148–9
Substitute Blood Products 206–7
Superficial Femoral Artery 162–3, 312, 315
Superficial Petrosal Nerve 125, 171
Superficial Ring 161, 283
Superficial Spreading Melanoma 364–5
Superficial Temporal Artery 124
Superior Colliculus 173
Superior Epigastric Vessels 139
Superior Mediastinum 133
Superior Mesenteric Artery 143, 323
Superior Orbital Fissure 171
Superior Vena Cava (SVC) 61, 133, 134, 137
Supinator 150
Supraorbital Foramen 171
Suprapubic Catheterisation 288
Suprascapular Nerve 177
Supraspinatus 148–9
Surface Anatomy 124, 128, 135–7, 156–9, 161–2
Surgical Airways 254–7
Surgical Emphysema 13, 257, 265, 420
Surgical Site Infection 223
Surgical Technology 392–405
Sustentaculum Tali 168–9
Suture Characteristics 400
Suture Materials 400–1
Suture Needles 401
Suture Sizes 401
Sympathetic Chain 129, 133
Sympathetic Trunks 139
Synchronised Intermittent Mandatory Ventilation (SIMV) 81
Synovial Joint 120, 122, 149, 164
Synthesis Phase 232
Systematic Interpretation of Computed Tomography Scans 31–2
Systematic Interpretation of Magnetic Resonance Imaging Scans 42–3
Systematic Interpretation of the Abdominal Radiograph 15–20
Systematic Interpretation of the Chest Radiograph 5–6
Systemic Inflammatory Response